Textbook of
Community Health Nursing-II

For BSc Nursing Students

(As per the Syllabus of INC for BSc Nursing)

Nursing Knowledge Tree
An Initiative by CBS Nursing Division

Textbook of
Community Health Nursing-II

For BSc Nursing Students
(As per the Syllabus of INC for BSc Nursing)

Nursing Knowledge Tree
An Initiative by CBS Nursing Division

Shyamala D Manivannan RN, RM, MSc(N), PhD(N)

Professor and Director (Faculty of Nursing)
Dr M G R Educational and Research Institute Deemed University
Chennai, Tamil Nadu, India

Foreword
Indarjit Walia

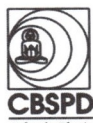

CBSPD
Dedicated to Education

CBS Publishers & Distributors Pvt Ltd

• New Delhi • Bengaluru • Chennai • Kochi • Kolkata • Lucknow • Mumbai
• Hyderabad • Jharkhand • Nagpur • Patna • Pune • Uttarakhand

Textbook of
Community Health Nursing-II
For BSc Nursing Students
(As per the Syllabus of INC for BSc Nursing)

ISBN: 978-93-86827-22-7

Copyright © Publishers

Reprint: 2025

First Edition: 2018

Published by Satish Kumar Jain and produced by Varun Jain for

CBS Publishers & Distributors Pvt Ltd
4819/XI Prahlad Street, 24 Ansari Road, Daryaganj, New Delhi 110 002, India.
Ph: +91-11-23289259, 23266861, 23266867   Website: www.cbspd.com
Fax: 011-23243014
e-mail: delhi@cbspd.com; cbspubs@airtelmail.in.

Corporate Office: 204 FIE, Industrial Area, Patparganj, Delhi 110 092
Ph: +91-11-4934 4934   Fax: 4934 4935
e-mail: feedback@cbspd.com; bhupesharora@cbspd.com

Branches

- **Bengaluru:** Seema House 2975, 17th Cross, K.R. Road, Banasankari 2nd Stage, Bengaluru 560 070, Karnataka
  Ph: +91-80-26771678/79   Fax: +91-80-26771680   e-mail: bangalore@cbspd.com
- **Chennai:** 7, Subbaraya Street, Shenoy Nagar, Chennai 600 030, Tamil Nadu
  Ph: +91-44-26680620, 26681266   Fax: +91-44-42032115   e-mail: chennai@cbspd.com
- **Kochi:** 68/1534, 35, 36-Power House Road, Opp. KSEB, Cochin-682018, Kochi, Kerala
  Ph: +91-484-4059061-65   Fax: +91-484-4059065   e-mail: kochi@cbspd.com
- **Kolkata:** Hind Ceramics Compound, 1st Floor, 147, Nilganj Road, Belghoria, Kolkata-700056, West Bengal
  Ph: +033-2563-3055/56   e-mail: kolkata@cbspd.com
- **Lucknow:** Basement, Khushnuma Complex, 7-Meerabai Marg, (Behind Jawahar Bhawan), Lucknow-226001 Uttar Pradesh
  Ph: +0522-4000032   e-mail: tiwari.lucknow@cbspd.com
- **Mumbai:** PWD Shed, Gala No. 25/26, Ramchandra Bhatt Marg, Next to J.J. Hospital Gate No. 2, Opp. Union Bank of India, Noor Baug, Mumbai-400009
  Ph: +91-22-66661880/89   Fax: +91-22-24902342   e-mail: mumbai@cbspd.com

Representatives

- **Hyderabad**   +91-9885175004
- **Patna**   +91-9334159340
- **Jharkhand**   +91-9811541605
- **Pune**   +91-9623451994
- **Nagpur**   +91-9421945513
- **Uttarakhand**   +91-9716462459

Printed at : Goyal Offset Works Pvt. Ltd. Haryana

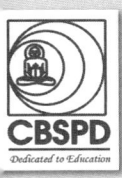

CBS Nursing Knowledge Tree

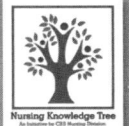

Extends its Tribute to

Florence Nightingale

> *For glorifying the role of women as nurses,*
> *For holding the title of " The Lady with the Lamp,"*
> *For working tirelessly for humanity—*
> *Florence Nightingale will always be*
> *remembered for her*
> *selfless and memorable services to the*
> *human race.*

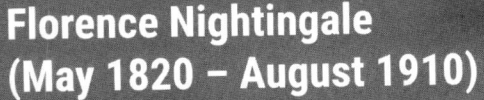

Florence Nightingale
(May 1820 – August 1910)

This book is dedicated to
my beloved husband Mr A Manivannan,
my family members
&
all nursing students...

Foreword

Community Health Nursing is certainly a very important subject of Nursing Curriculum. Therefore, it becomes essential for the students to have a panoramic view and a basic understanding of all the important concepts in the subject. I want to congratulate Dr Shyamala D Manivannan, Professor and Director (Faculty of Nursing), Dr MGR Educational and Research Institute Deemed University, Chennai, for presenting such a well-written compendium on the subject.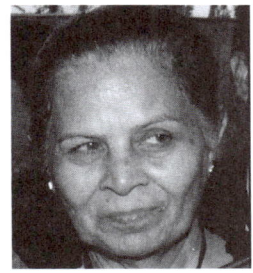

I personally liked the presentation of the book. The bulleted points interspersed between the texts would help in enhancing the readability of the book. Relevant figures and tables at various places will complement the learning experience of the students. This is so far the most updated textbook on community health nursing with profound emphasis on practical orientation most vitally needed in nursing. Each chapter has ended with summary that will give the students a gist of the complete chapter. The most frequently asked questions in Assess Yourself section at the end of each chapter will help the students in assessing their knowledge and learning.

I am sure this book will prove to be a boon for the students and will help in making them aware of their important roles and responsibilities in implementing primary health care.

Indarjit Walia
PhD (Community Medicine), MSc (CHN)
Former Principal, PGI NINE
Chandigarh, India

Preface

Previous work in collaboration with the prestigious CBS publishers, "Textbook of Community Health Nursing-I" for the second year BSc Nursing students gave a podium to contribute once again to my beloved nursing fraternity and students. First of all, I would like to thank all Principals of nursing colleges, friends and students for showing admirable interest in my previous textbook. Once again it gives me immense pleasure to meet you all with "Textbook of Community Health Nursing-II" exclusively written for 4th year BSc Nursing students strictly based on the INC syllabus.

Aim and Ambition

The intended aim is to bring out a friendly, informative, updated and simplified community health nursing textbook for 4th year BSc nursing students as per the INC syllabus. Over and above, students should be able to find all the essential contents in the single book to achieve the learner-centered objectives of community health nursing syllabus.

Organization

The content of the book is organized under seven units. To avoid boredom and enhance the interest and understanding of the students, various measures have been adopted throughout the book: meaningful flow charts, diagrams that speak concepts, meticulous tables, highlights of current message and boxes with key points would definitely keep the interest of the students at the most acceptable levels. Every unit ends with "Summary" followed by "Assess Yourself" that is very useful for evaluating self and a drawing plan to prepare further for theory and practical examinations in community health nursing.

Unit 1

In this unit, significant concepts and scope are explained. The historical events in the development of community health and community health nursing in the context of the entire world and India are presented. The historical development of community health and community health nursing is presented with the pictures of pioneers in this field. This would help the students to remember them better and would promote the interest in learning the history.

Unit 2

This unit talks about the health planning, policies and health problems. NITI Aayog that has replaced planning commission of India is well explained. All the five-year plans have been briefly explained with its general and health-related goals.

Unit 3

The planning and delivery of community health services at various levels with organization and staffing for both urban and rural areas are explained well as per the current norms.

Unit 4

This unit talks about the various approaches used in providing care in the community: Some of the basic nursing theories and models used in the community health nursing practice have been explained adequately. In addition, the other measures like epidemiological approach, evidence-based practice and empowering people to care for themselves has expanded the horizon of caring practices in the community. The concept and principles of primary health along with the roles and responsibilities of community health nurses in various areas like family health services, maternal and child health, IEC activities and the management and information system have been discussed in depth.

All the related phenomena like health workers functioning at village level, their training and supervision and treatment for minor ailments are discussed using simple language. The designed content would give more room for the vertical and horizontal integration of learning.

Unit 5

Although provision of care is the core concept of community health nurses, the recent trend stresses on equipping the people with necessary knowledge and skills to promote health, prevent diseases and seek treatment for the diseases. This unit would help the learners to empower the community in caring practices for self, family and community.

Unit 6

Since the time of independence of our county, "National Health Programs" have been designed for a parallel journey along with the five year plans to shoulder the share in controlling/combating specific diseases that pull down the health and socioeconomic status of the country. Various programs have been implemented time to time to meet the public health challenges and these programs have undergone many changes in structure, administration, sponsors, staffing, etc. One of the examples is present RCH that includes the components of many programs, which were started earlier for mothers and children. After learning this unit, students will be able to gain knowledge on different milestones of various national health programs and their current state. It is worthy to state here that the roles and responsibilities of community health nurses in national health programs is attended by giving significant importance.

Unit 7

National and international health agencies have been well described including structure, purpose and functions. Following this, the most important voluntary health organizations have been explained.

I hope that this book will be of great help to the fourth year nursing students in learning and achieving the objectives of community health nursing-II. Most of the times students have stated that they could not find relevant content that matches to 4th year community health nursing syllabus; this student-friendly book will definitely do the justice in fulfilling the desires and expectations of the students.

Shyamala D Manivannan

Acknowledgments

"God You Stand first, and your child here….."

First, I submit my heartfelt thanks to God for giving me necessary wisdom, health and energy to accomplish this project. I have read, learnt, served, reflected, taught and walked through the path of many learning facilities and sought to learn repeatedly through series of discussions and debates. Continuous commitment to learning perpetuates a teacher to meet the needs of the students taught.

I thank all my teachers, who played an important role in shaping me as today's author. I am thankful to all my colleagues and friends for supporting me in my intellectual journey.

I am indebted to my students whose feedback and appreciation took the most important place in my journey of teaching.

I thank my husband, Capt. A. Manivannan, who always stood as a moral support and encouragement for finishing this project. I also thank my entire family for their support.

I would like to convey my special thanks to madam Dr Indarjit Walia and the other experts who served as reviewers.

I would like to thank **Mr Satish Kumar Jain** (Chairman) and **Mr Varun Jain** (Managing Director), M/s CBS Publishers and Distributors Pvt Ltd for providing me the platform in bringing out the book. I have no words to describe the role, efforts, inputs and initiatives undertaken by **Mr Bhupesh Aarora**, Sr. Vice President – Publishing and Marketing (Health Sciences Division) for helping and motivating me.

I sincerely thank the entire CBS team for bringing out the book with utmost care and attractive presentation. I would like to thank Ms Nitasha Arora (Assistant General Manager Publishing – Medical and Nursing), Ms Daljeet Kaur (Assistant Publishing Manager) and Dr Anju Dhir (Product Manager and Medical Development Editor) for their publishing support. I would also extend our thanks to Mr Shivendu Bhushan Pandey (Sr. Manager and Team Lead), Mr Ashutosh Pathak (Sr. Proofreader cum Team Coordinator) and all the production team members for devoting laborious hours in designing and typesetting the book.

Reviewers

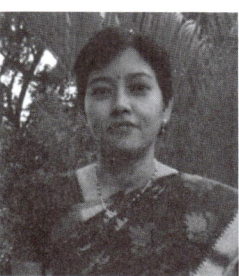

Dr Anita Yuvraj Nawale
MSc, PhD (CHN)
Assistant Professor
BVDU, Bharati Vidyapeeth College
of Nursing,
Pune, Maharashtra, India

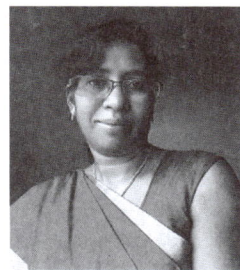

Prof (Mrs) Bernice Margaret
Principal
NDRK College of Nursing
Hassan, Karnataka, India

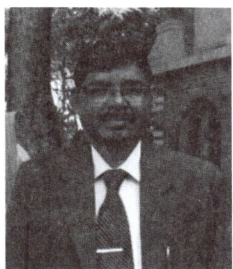

Prof David A Kola
Principal
SDM College of Nursing
Manjushri Nagar, Sattur, Dharwad
Karnataka, India

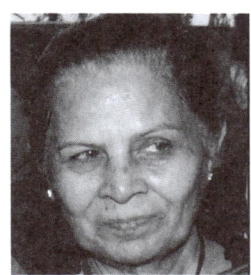

Dr Indarjit Walia
MSc (CHN), PhD (Community Medicine)
Former Principal
PGI NINE, Chandigarh, India

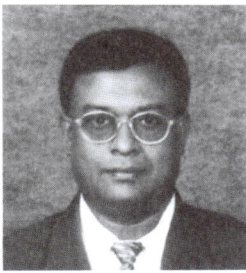

Dr Jeyaseelan M Devadason
PhD
Dean
Annai JKK Sampoorani
Ammal College of Nursing
Komarapalayam, Tamil Nadu, India

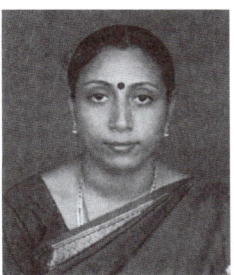

Prof (Mrs) Lakshmi Sivaramakrishnan
PhD
Principal
Chettinad College of Nursing
Chettinad Academy of Research
and Education
Chennai, India

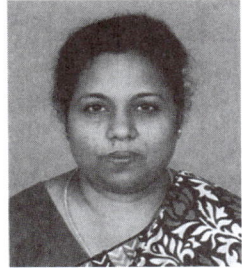

Lt Col Dr Rosy KO
Principal
Nehru College of Nursing
Ottapalam, Palakkad
Kerala, India

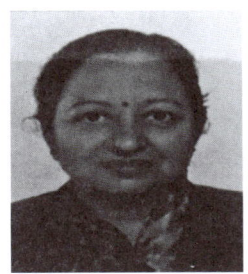

Dr Sushma Saini
Lecturer
National Institute of Nursing
Education
PGIMER, Chandigarh, India

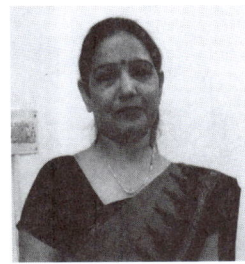

Dr Samta Soni
Lecturer
Government College of Nursing
Jaipur, Rajasthan, India

Publisher's Desk

Dear Reader,

Nursing Education has a rich history, often characterized by traditional teaching techniques that have evolved over time. Primarily, teaching took place within classroom settings. Lectures, textbooks, and clinical rotations were the core teaching tools; and students majorly relied on textbooks by local or foreign publishers for quality education. However, today, technology has completely transformed the field of nursing education, making it an integral part of the curriculum. It has evolved to include a range of technological tools that enhance the learning experience and better prepare students for clinical practice.

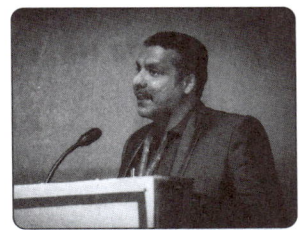

As publishers, we've been contributing to the field of Medical Science, Nursing and Allied Sciences and earned the trust of many. By supporting **Indian authors**, coupled with **nursing webinars and conferences**, we have paved an easier path for aspiring nurses, empowering them to excel in national and state level exams. With this, we're not only enhancing the quality of patient care but also enabling future nurses to adapt to new challenges and innovations in the rapidly evolving world of healthcare. Following the ideology of **Bringing learning to people instead of people going for learning**, so far, we've been doing our part by:

- Developing quality content by qualified and well-versed authors
- Building a strong community of faculty and students
- Introducing a smart approach with Digital/Hybrid Books, and
- Offering simulation Nursing Procedures, etc.

Innovative teaching methodologies, such as modern-age Phygital Books, have sparked the interest of the Next-Gen students in pursuing advanced education. The enhancement of educational standards through **Omnipresent Knowledge Sharing Platforms** has further facilitated learning, bridging the gap between doctors and nurses.

At Nursing Next Live, a sister concern of CBS Publishers & Distributors, we have long recognized the immense potential within the nursing field. Our journey in innovating nursing education has allowed us to make substantial and meaningful contributions. With the vision of strengthening learning at every stage, we have introduced several plans that cater to the specific needs of the students, including but not limited to **Plan UG** for undergraduates, **Plan MSc** for postgraduate aspirants, **Plan FDP** for upskilling faculties, **SDL** for integrated learning and **Plan NP** for bridging the gap between theoretical & practical learning. Additionally, we have successfully completed seven series of our **Target High** Book in a very short period, setting a milestone in the education industry. We have been able to achieve all this just with the sole vision of laying the foundation of diversified knowledge for all. With the rise of a new generation of educated, tech-savvy individuals, we anticipate even more remarkable advancements in the coming years.

We take immense pride in our achievements and eagerly look forward to the future, brimming with new opportunities for innovation, growth and collaborations with experienced minds such as yourself who can contribute to our mission as Authors, Reviewers and/or Faculties. Together, let's foster a generation of nurses who are confident, competent, and prepared to succeed in a technology-driven healthcare system.

Mr Bhupesh Aarora
(Sr Vice President – Publishing & Marketing)
bhupeshaarora@cbspd.com| +91 95553 53330

Special Features of the Book

Unit Outline will summarize what the students will learn after studying the chapter.

Unit Outline

- Important Definitions
- Scope of Community Health Nursing
- Roles of Community Health Nurses
- Work sites of Community Health Nurse
- Community Health Nurses and their Education in India
- Principles of Community Health Nursing
- History of Development of Community Health—Globally
- Development of Community Health Nursing—Globally
- Development of Public Health Nursing: Significant Events Worldwide
- Challenges of 21st Century for Community Health Nursing
- Community Health in British India
- Development of Community Health Nursing in India—Preindependence
- Development of Community Health Nursing—PostIndependence
- Twenty-first Century and Challenges for Community Health Nursing

Learning Objectives

At the end of this unit the learners will be able to:

- Define health, public health, community, community health, community health nursing, public health nursing and population health
- Describe the scope of community health nursing
- State the various roles of community health nurses
- List down the principles of community health nursing practice
- Describe briefly on the historical development of community health in the world
- Describe briefly on the historical development of community health nursing in the world
- Describe briefly on the development of community health in India during pre and post-independence
- Describe briefly on the development of community health nursing in India during pre and post-independence

Given in the starting of the chapter, these enlist what the students will learn after reading the chapter.

Important terms used in the chapter are highlighted.

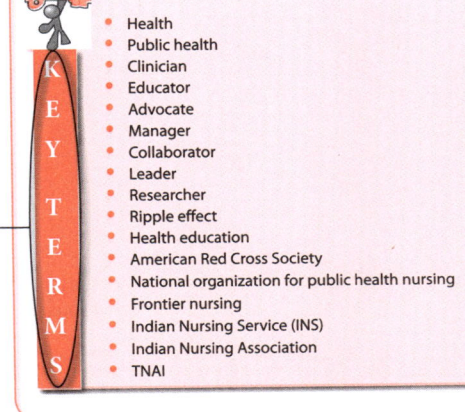

KEY TERMS

- Health
- Public health
- Clinician
- Educator
- Advocate
- Manager
- Collaborator
- Leader
- Researcher
- Ripple effect
- Health education
- American Red Cross Society
- National organization for public health nursing
- Frontier nursing
- Indian Nursing Service (INS)
- Indian Nursing Association
- TNAI

Numerous boxes summarizing important information have been included wherever necessary.

Box 1: The occupational health team

The professionals involved in the occupational health team includes, some or all of the following:
- Occupational health nurses
- Occupational health physicians
- Industrial hygienists
- Safety engineers
- Work organization specialists
- Psychologists
- Counselors
- Physiotherapists.
- Ergonomists
- Health economists
- Academic researchers and others.

Table 15: Patterns of delivery of medical services

Direct pattern	Indirect Pattern
In areas having 1,000 or above service dispensaries established with medical and paramedical personnel On an average a doctor attends 80 outpatients/day and makes one home visit	A panel of medical practitioners recognized to provide services
In areas with less than 750 employees part time dispensaries are established If employees scattered in a long distance mobile dispensaries established	Registered medical practitioners under this system designated as, "Insurance Medical practitioners" This system is known as "Panel system"

Numerous Tables summarizing important information have been included wherever necessary for quick recall.

Numerous Figures and Flowcharts are used to make learning easy for students.

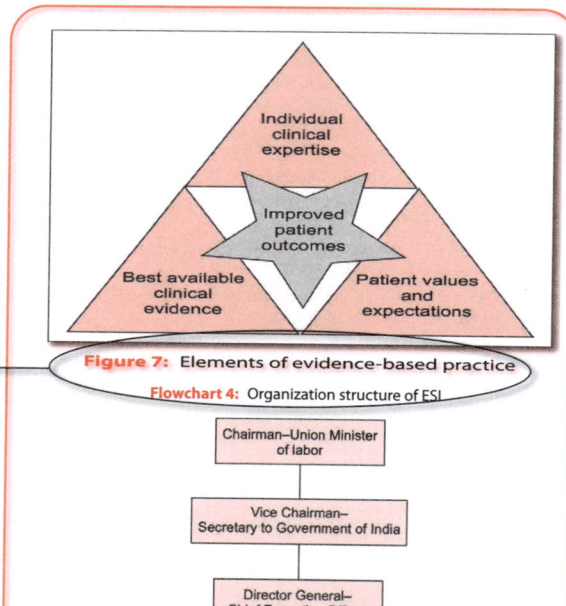

Figure 7: Elements of evidence-based practice

Flowchart 4: Organization structure of ESI

Summary

Health is a state of complete physical, mental and social well-being and not merely the absence of disease or infirmity. The IOM defines public health as "organized community efforts aimed at the prevention of disease and promotion of health." "Community" implies people acting together in some way as a group, and the whole meaning more than the sum of its parts. According to ANA (1999), public health nursing is a population-focused community nursing practice with the goal of prevention of disease and disability by creating the conditions where people can be healthy. Community health nurses are on the front lines of health care and prevention of diseases and promotion of health. The term population health, which is similar to community health, has emerged in recent years.

Community health nurses play various roles like clinician, educator, advocate, manager, collaborator, leader, and researcher. Community health nurses' work in various settings like home, school, industry, clinics, community health centers, maternity homes and primary health centers and as educators in nursing schools and colleges and in training centers.

After much contradiction, Shattuck's report was considered as one of the most farsighted and influential documents in the history of the decline of Roman dynasty pulled down the developments in community health organization. There was no provision for clean water, waste disposal and sanitation. People threw the garbage on the street and no health behavior seen in people. Practice of nurses joining military orders during the time of Crusades started between 1091 and 1291.

In 1601, the Church of England introduced, "Elizabethan poor law" and made it compulsory. This made people care for poor, blind, orphans and lame. Initially the neighbors in local communities cared people with physical and mental illnesses. Later this became official in England by adoption of "1601- poor law". Toward mid-nineteenth century there was tremendous advancement in public health. This period was referred to **the great sanitary awakening.**"(Winslow, 1923). **Chadwick** proposed to build a drainage network to remove sewage and waste. **Lemuel Shattuck,** a Massachusetts bookseller and statistician published a survey *Report of the Massachusetts Sanitary Commission* in 1850. The Greeks showed interest in community sanitation.
American public health system: Edward Jenner of Berkeley had saved many lives with his discovery of **"Smallpox Vaccination. William Farr** (1839) stressed the importance of "vital statistics" for studying health problems. In **1854, Snow** discovered that the cholera epidemics occurred due to polluted water. **John Snow** was given the title of **"father**

of modern epidemiology." In **1877 Louis Pasteur,** a French chemist, proved that anthrax is caused by bacteria.

During 20th century, people started look beyond the traditional concept of protecting people from polluted environment and communicable diseases. People started to understand the relationship between bacteria and communicable diseases. In the early 20th century, home visits offered by public health nurses in New York and Baltimore. School health clinics were established in Boston (1894), New York (1903) and in Rhode Island (1906) to support and promote the health of school going children.

Elders of the families who had lived in experiences on handling health-related issues provided consultation to their own family members and guided them.

In the **middle ages,** family members only took care of the sick and ill. From the 1500s through the 1700s, the renaissance in **Europe** stimulated the rise of scientific thought and social consciousness.The Sisters (or Daughters) of Charity or "Grey Sisters," was founded in 1617 in **France,** with the aim of providing care to the sick poor. People were afraid to go to hospitals and addressed hospitals as, "death houses". In **Holland,** women appointed by churches to care for the poor called as deaconess-groups. **Florence Nightingale,** daughter of Wealthy English family, committed to prevent illness and death. Florence took a lead role with a team of nurses and assisted soldiers during the **Crimean War** (1854–1856).

In 1859 William Rathbone, a Quaker merchant and philanthropist of England hired **Mary Robinson,** a nurse (who later named as the **first district nurse**) to take care of people in one of the poorest parish districts in Liverpool. Nightingale started the first school of nursing, and Rathbone hired several graduates as district nurses. Two years later, with Nightingale's assistance, he established a nursing school in Liverpool. In 1813, the **Ladies' Benevolent Society of Charleston,** South Carolina, started to provide organized home care services to the sick. In 1912, Wald assisted to found the **National Organization for Public Health Nursing.** Mary Breckinridge the founder of "Frontier nursing" traveled on horseback, and assessed the health situations and needs of the mountain people. In 1939, she helped to establish the Frontier Graduate School of Midwifery, one of the first midwifery programs in the country.

Many unexpected changes may occur in this 21st century all over the world in the field of health/nursing /community health nursing. There are chances for serious transformation that may dominate the environment along with the changes in other areas like culture, beliefs, practice, technology and economy.

Summary has been included at the end of every chapter. This will act as revision for the students to focus on the important concepts discussed in the chapter.

Assess Yourself

I. Multiple Choice Questions (Choose the Correct Answers)

1. **Which of these following theories focuses on pure air, water and ventilation?**
   a. Betty Neuman's theory
   b. Florence Nightingale's theory
   c. Callista Roy's theory
   d. Orem's theory
2. **Which of these following theories categorizes nursing care based on dependency?**
   a. Environmental theory
   b. Roy's adaptation theory
   c. Neuman's theory
   d. Orem's self care deficit theory
3. **Which of these following theories states that man responds to internal and external stimuli?**
   a. Environmental theory
   b. Roy's adaptation theory
   c. Neuman's theory
   d. Orem's self-care deficit theory
4. **Which of these following states that "every person has unique personal characteristics and experiences that affect subsequent actions"?**
   a. Health promotion model
   b. Health belief model
   c. Orem's model
   d. Adaptation model
5. **Which of these following is *not* an element of primary health care?**
   a. Provision of maternal and child health care
   b. Provision of immunization
   c. Provision of essential drugs
   d. Provision of employment
6. **Primary prevention activities of a community health nurse includes all *except*:**
   a. Encouraging elderly people to install and use safety devices
   b. Teaching young adults healthy lifestyle behaviors
   c. Larva control measures for prevention of malaria
   d. Teaching a postsurgery patient to walk with crutches at home
7. **Minimizing disability and restoring or preserving function equals:**
   a. Primary prevention
   b. Secondary prevention
   c. Tertiary prevention
   d. Early detection
8. **ASHA covers the population of**
   a. 1000
   b. 2000
   c. 3000
   d. 4000
9. **In rural areas what is the supervisor to Anganwadi worker (AWW) ratio?**
   a. 1:20
   b. 1:25
   c. 1:30
   d. 1:35
10. **Which of the following weeks before which antenatal mothers should be registered?**
    a. 10
    b. 12
    c. 14
    d. 16

II. Write Short Answers:

1. Mention four qualities of community health nurse.
2. Write purpose of standing order.
3. Define occupational health.
4. Define epidemiology.
5. Write four importance of maintaining records and reports.
6. List down four functions of female health worker.
7. List down four functions of male health worker.
8. List down four functions of "Male health assistant/Male supervisor".
9. List down four functions of "Female health assistant/ Female supervisor".
10. Write four uses of management information system.
11. Principles of home visit.
12. List down four principles of primary health care.
13. Write any two qualities of community health nurse.

III. Write Short Notes on:

1. Epidemiological approach
2. Home visit
3. Components of school health program
4. Role of community health nurse at maternal and child health center.
5. Roles and responsibilities of community health nurse in school health services.
6. Treatment of minor ailments
7. Maintenance of records and reports
8. Problem solving approach
9. Concepts of primary health care
10. Evidence based approach
11. Empowering people to care for themselves.

IV. Write Essays on:

1. List various health committees of India. Describe Bhore and Mudaliar committee.
2. Explain in detail about home visit. Write the job description of community health nurse.
3. Define occupational health. Discuss in detail the role of occupational health nurse.
4. Define occupational health services. Explain in detail about occupational hazards and role of community health nurse in its prevention.
5. Explain in detail about the various approaches used by community health nurses in caring practice.

Important questions and MCQs of the chapters are enlisted to help students assess their learning.

ANSWERS

| I | 1. | b | 2. | d | 3. | b | 4. | a | 5. | d | 6. | d | 7. | c | 8. | a |
| | 9. | a | 10. | b | | | | | | | | | | | | |

Syllabus

COMMUNITY HEALTH NURSING–II

Placement: *Fourth Year*

Time (Theory) : *90 hours*
(Practical) : *135 hours*

Course Description : This course is designed for students to practice community health nursing for the individual, family and groups at both urban and rural settings by using concept and principles of health and community health nursing.

Unit	Time (Hrs)	Learning Objectives	Contents	Teaching Learning Activities	Assessment Methods
I.	4	Define concepts, scope, principles and historical development of community health and community health Nursing	**Introduction** • Definition, concept & scope of Community Health and Community Health Nursing • Historical development of ▪ Community health ▪ Community health Nursing – Preindependence – Postindependence	Lecture discussion	• Essay type • Short answers
II.	6	Describe health plans, policies, various health committees and health problems in India	**Health Planning and Policies and Problems** • National health planning in India Five-Year Plans • Various committees and commissions on health and family welfare ▪ Central council for health and family welfare (CCH and FW) ▪ National health policies (1983, 2002) ▪ National population policy • Health problems in India	• Lecture discussion • Panel discussion	• Essay type • Short answers
III.	15	• Describe the system of delivery of community health services in rural and urban areas • List the functions of various levels and their staffing pattern • Explain the components of health services • Describe alternative systems of health promotion and health maintenance. • Describe the chain of referral system	**Delivery of Community Health Services** • Planning, budgeting and material management of SCs, PHC and, CHC • **Rural:** Organization, staffing and functions of rural health services provided by government at: ▪ Village ▪ Subcenter ▪ Primary health center ▪ Community health center/subdivisional ▪ Hospitals ▪ District ▪ State ▪ Center	• Lecture discussion • Visits to various health delivery systems • Supervised field practice • Panel discussion	• Essay type • Short answers

Contd…

Unit	Time (Hrs)	Learning Objectives	Contents	Teaching Learning Activities	Assessment Methods

			• **Urban:** Organization, staffing and functions of urban health services provided by government at:
			  ▪ Slums
			  ▪ Dispensaries
			  ▪ Maternal and child health centers
			  ▪ Special Clinics
			  ▪ Hospitals
			  ▪ Corporation/Municipality/Board
			• Components of health services
			  ▪ Environmental sanitation
			  ▪ Health education
			  ▪ Vital statistics
			  ▪ M.C.H.-antenatal, natal, postnatal, MTP Act, Female Foeticide Act, Child Adoption Act
			  ▪ Family Welfare
			  ▪ National health programs
			  ▪ School health services
			  ▪ Occupational health
			  ▪ Defence services
			  ▪ Institutional services
			• Systems of medicine and health care
			  ▪ Allopathy
			  ▪ Indian System of Medicine and Homeopathy
			  ▪ Alternative health care systems like yoga. Meditation, social and spiritual healing etc
			• Referral system		

IV.	25	• Describe Community Health Nursing approaches and concepts
		• Describe the roles and responsibilities of community health nursing personnel
			Community Health Nursing Approaches, Concepts and Roles and Responsibilities of Nursing Personnel
			• Approaches
			  ▪ Nursing theories and Nursing process
			  ▪ Epidemiological approach
			  ▪ Problem solving approach
			  ▪ Evidence-based approach
			  ▪ Empowering people to care for themselves
			• Concepts of Primary Health Care:
			  ▪ Equitable distribution
			  ▪ Community participation
			  ▪ Focus on prevention
			  ▪ Use of appropriate technology
			  ▪ Multisectoral approach
			• Roles and responsibilities of community health nursing personnel in
			  ▪ Family health services
			  ▪ Information Education Communication (IEC)
				• Lecture discussion
				• Demonstration
				• Practice session
				• Supervised field practice
				• Participation in camps
				• Group project
					• Essay type
					• Short answers

Contd…

Unit	Time (Hrs)	Learning Objectives	Contents	Teaching Learning Activities	Assessment Methods
			▪ Management Information System (MIS): Maintenance of Record & reports ▪ Training and supervision of various categories of health works ▪ National Health Programs ▪ Environmental sanitation ▪ Maternal and child health and family welfare ▪ Treatment of minor ailments ▪ School health services ▪ Occupational health ▪ Organization of clinics, camps: Types, preparation, planning, conduct and evaluation ▪ Waste management in the center, clinics etc. • Home visit: Concept, Principles, Process, Techniques: Bag technique home visit • Qualities of community health nurse • Job description of community health nursing personnel		
V.	15	• Describe and appreciate the activities of community health nurse in assisting individuals and groups to promote and maintain their health	**Assisting Individuals and Groups to Promote and Maintain their Health** • Empowerment for self-care of individuals, families and groups in- • **Assessment of self and family** ▪ Monitoring growth and development – Mile stones – Weight measurement – Social development ▪ Temperature and blood pressure monitoring ▪ Menstrual cycle ▪ Breast self-examination and testicles ▪ Warning signs of various disease ▪ Tests: Urine for sugar and albumin. Blood sugar • **Seek health services for** ▪ Routine checkup ▪ Immunization ▪ Counseling ▪ Treatment ▪ Follow • **Maintenance of health records for self and family** • **Continue medical care and follow-up in community for various diseases and disabilities** • **Carryout therapeutic procedures as prescribed/required for self and family**	• Lecture discussion • Demonstration • Practice session • Supervised filed practice • Individual/group/ family/community health education	• Essay type • Short answers

Contd…

Unit	Time (Hrs)	Learning Objectives	Contents	Teaching Learning Activities	Assessment Methods

			• **Waste Management**
			Collection and disposable of waste at home and community
			• **Sensitize and handle social issues affecting health and development for self and family**
			  ▪ Women empowerment
			  ▪ Women and child abuse
			  ▪ Abuse of elders
			  ▪ Female foeticide
			  ▪ Commercial sex workers
			  ▪ Food adulteration
			  ▪ Substance abuse
			• **Utilize community resources for self and family**
			• Trauma services
			• Old age homes
			• Orphanage
			• Homes for physically and mentally challenged individuals
			• Homes for destitute		

VI.	20	• Describe national health and family welfare programs and role of a nurse • Describe the various health schemes in India	**National Health and Family Welfare Programs and the Role of a Nurse** • National ARI program • Revised National Tuberculosis • National Anti-Malaria • National Filaria control program • National Guinea worm eradication program • National Leprosy eradication program • National AIDS control program • STD control program • National program for control of blindness • Iodine deficiency disorder program • Expanded program on immunization • National Family Welfare Program-RCH Program historical development, organization, administration, research, constraints • National water supply and sanitation program • Minimum Need program • National Diabetics control program • Polio Eradication: Pulse Polio Program • National Cancer Control Program • Yaws Eradication Program • National Nutritional Anemai Prophylaxis program • 20 point program • ICDS program	• Lecture discussion • Participation in national health programs • Field visits	• Essay type • Short answers

Contd...

Unit	Time (Hrs)	Learning Objectives	Contents	Teaching Learning Activities	Assessment Methods
			• Mid-day meal applied nutritional program • National mental health program ▪ Health schemes – ESI – CGHS – Health insurance		
VII.	5	Explain the roles and functions of various national and international health agencies	**Health Agencies** **International**—WHO, UNFPA, UNDP, World Bank, FAO, UNICEF, DANIDA, European commission (EC), Red Cross, USAID, UNESCO, Colombo Plan, ILO, CARE etc. National—Indian Red Cross, Indian Council for Child Welfare, Family Planning Association of India (FPAI,) Tuberculosis Association of India, Hindu Kusht Nivaran Sangh, Central Social Welfare Board, All India Women's Conference, Blind Association of India etc.	• Lecture discussion • Field visits	• Essay type • Short answers

Contents

Unit 4	Community Health Nursing Approaches, Concepts and Roles and Responsibilities of Nursing Personnel	103

Unit 7 | Health Agencies ... 270

Recent Updates 2022

AYUSHMAN BHARAT (AB)

Prime Minister Narendra Modi announced the launch of **Ayushman Bharat National Health Protection Scheme (AB-NHPS)** in 2018. It is considered as the biggest government-sponsored health scheme in the world and was launched on 23 September 2018 by the Prime Minister Mr Narendra Modi in Ranchi, the capital of Jharkhand. It became operational on 25 September which marks the birth anniversary of Pandit Deendayal Upadhyaya.

SALIENT FEATURES OF AYUSHMAN BHARAT

- Ayushman Bharat, a national health protection mission, will have a defined benefit cover of Rs. 5 lakh per family per year.
- Benefits of the scheme are portable across the country and a beneficiary covered under the scheme will be allowed to take cashless benefits from any public/private empaneled hospitals across the country.
- Ayushman Bharat National Health Protection Mission will be an entitlement-based scheme with entitlement decided on the basis of deprivation criteria in the Socio-Economic and Caste Census (SECC) database.
- The beneficiaries can avail benefits in both public and empaneled private facilities.
- To control costs, the payments for treatment will be done on package rate (to be defined by the government in advance) basis.
- One of the core principles of Ayushman Bharat National Health Protection Mission is co-operative federalism and flexibility to states.
- For giving policy directions and fostering coordination between Center and States, it is proposed to set up Ayushman Bharat National Health Protection Mission Council (AB-NHPMC) at apex level chaired by Union Health and Family Welfare Minister.
- States would need to have State Health Agency (SHA) to implement the scheme.
- To ensure that the funds reach SHA on time, the transfer of funds from Central Government through Ayushman Bharat - National Health Protection Mission to State Health Agencies may be done through an escrow account directly.
- In partnership with NITI (National Institution for Transforming India) Aayog, a robust, modular, scalable and interoperable IT platform will be made operational which will entail a paperless and cashless transaction.

COMPONENTS OF AYUSHMAN BHARAT

Ayushman Bharat National Health Protection Scheme (AB-NHPS) has been launched with two major components to achieve universal health coverage. The two components are:

1. Comprehensive Primary Health Care (CPHC) through Health and Wellness Centers (HWCs)
2. Pradhan Mantri Jan Arogya Yojana (PMJAY)

Comprehensive Primary Health Care (CPHC) through Health and Wellness Centers (HWC)

The National Health Mission (NHM), country's key program for strengthening the health care delivery system specifically focusing on primary and secondary health care, visualizes "attainment of universal access to equitable, affordable and quality health care which is accountable and responsive to the needs of people." National Health Mission (NHM) invested time and money to strengthen Reproductive and Child Health (RCH) services and control the burden of some communicable diseases such as Tuberculosis, HIV/AIDS and vector-borne diseases. However, this was unable to meet the challenges of range of services delivered at the primary care level; growing disease burden and mounting costs of care because of chronic diseases have been a constant problem.

The National Health Policy (2017) of India recommended strengthening the delivery of Primary Health Care, by converting health subcenters and primary health centers as **Health and Wellness Centers** to provide **Comprehensive Primary Health Care.** Two-thirds of the health budget is committed to strengthening primary health care. Following this in 2018 India proposed for 1,50,000 Health and Wellness Centers (HWCs) from transforming the existing Sub Health Centers and Primary Health Centers to deliver Comprehensive Primary Health Care.

Comprehensive primary health care focuses on:

- Universal Access
- Affordability
- Quality
- Equity

Key Principles of Comprehensive Primary Health Care (CPHC)

1. Transform existing Sub Health Centers and Primary Health Centers to Health and Wellness Centers to ensure universal access to an expanded range of Comprehensive Primary Health Care services.

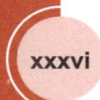

2. Ensure a people-centered, holistic, equity sensitive response to people's health needs through a process of population empanelment, regular home and community interactions and people's participation.

3. Enable delivery of high quality care that spans health risks and disease conditions through a commensurate expansion in availability of medicines and diagnostics, use of standard treatment and referral protocols and advanced technologies including IT systems.

4. Instill the culture of a team-based approach to delivery of quality health care encompassing: preventive, promotive, curative, rehabilitative and palliative care.

5. Ensure continuity of care with a two-way referral system and follow up support.

6. Emphasize health promotion (through school education and individual-centric awareness) and promote public health action through active engagement and capacity building of community platforms and individual volunteers.

7. Implement appropriate mechanisms for flexible financing, including performance-based incentives and responsive resource allocations.

8. Enable the integration of Yoga and AYUSH as appropriate to people's needs.

9. Facilitate the use of appropriate technology for improving access to health care advice and treatment initiation, enable reporting and recording, eventually progressing to electronic records for individuals and families.

10. Institutionalize participation of civil society for social accountability.

11. Partner with not-for-profit agencies and private sector for gap filling in a range of primary health care functions.

12. Facilitate systematic learning and sharing to enable feedback and improvements, and identify innovations for scale up.

13. Develop strong measurement systems to build accountability for improved performance on measures that matter to people.

As per information provided by the States/UTs on HWC portal, the state wise details of operationalized HWC as on 04.02.2019 are as under (Table 1):

Table 1: State wise details of operationalized HWC

State/UT	Operational HWCs status on portal 04/02
Andaman and Nicobar Islands	30
Andhra Pradesh	1,361
Arunachal Pradesh	54

State/UT	Operational HWCs status on portal 04/02
Assam	301
Bihar	211
Chandigarh	10
Chhattisgarh	199
Dadra and Nagar Haveli	27
Daman and Diu	24
Goa	14
Gujarat	347
Haryana	133
Himachal Pradesh	2
Jammu and Kashmir	36
Jharkhand	333
Karnataka	548
Kerala	350
Madhya Pradesh	97
Maharashtra	248
Manipur	29
Meghalaya	1
Mizoram	1
Nagaland	5
Odisha	486
Puducherry	2
Punjab	373
Rajasthan	451
Sikkim	5
Tamil Nadu	1318
Telangana	445
Tripura	71
Uttar Pradesh	467
Uttarakhand	51
West Bengal	0
Total	**8,030**

Staffing of HWC at the Sub Health Center Level

Middle Level Health Provider (MLHP) leads the team consisting of multi-Purpose workers (male and female) and ASHAs. Together they will deliver an expanded range of services. A Primary Health Center (PHC) linked to a cluster of HWCs serves as the first point of referral. The Medical Officer at the PHC is responsible for ensuring CPHC services in all the HWCs linked to it. Key Elements of Health and Wellness Center (HWC) are shown in Figure 1.

Contd...

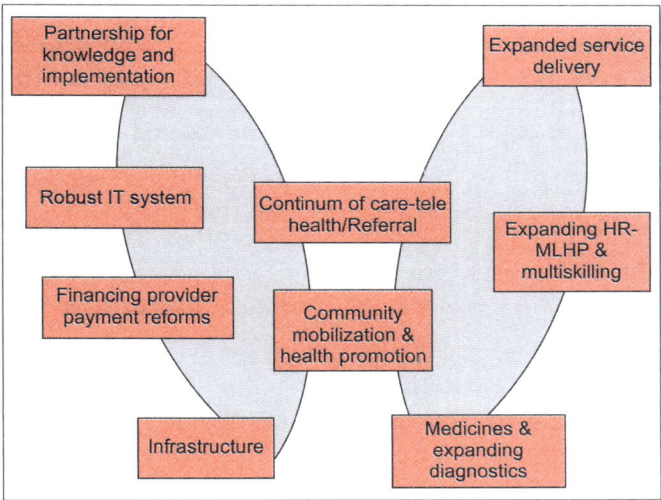

Figure 1: Key elements of health and wellness center (HWC)

Abbreviations: HR, Human Resource; IT, Information Technology; MLHP, Mid-level Health Care Provider

Expanded Range of Services Provided in HWCs

- Care in pregnancy and childbirth
- Neonatal and infant health care services
- Childhood and adolescent health care services
- Family planning, contraceptive services and other reproductive health care services
- Management of communicable diseases including National Health Programs
- Management of common communicable diseases and outpatient care for acute simple illnesses and minor ailments
- Screening, prevention, control and management of non-communicable diseases
- Care for common ophthalmic and ears, nose and throat (ENT) problems
- Basic oral health care
- Elderly and palliative health care services
- Emergency medical services
- Screening and basic management of mental health ailments

Structural Frame and Workflow in HWC

Primary health care team is responsible to deliver the expanded range of services.

At the Upgraded Sub Health Center (SHC)

Staffing: A team of at least three service providers including Mid-level provider-1, Multi-Purpose Workers (MPW)-3 (two female and one male)

A team of ASHAs at the norm of one per 1000.

At the Strengthened Primary Health Center (PHC)

Primary Health Center (PHC) staffing as per Indian Public Health Standards (IPHS): Primary health centers provide 24/7 in-patient care but this is not happening in all the states due to various reasons. An additional nurse included in staffing where cervical cancer screening is a routine work.

In the urban areas, the team would consist of the MPW-F (for 10,000 population) and the ASHAs (one per 2500 population).

Data Base at HWC: Database created for all families and individuals in the area served by an HWC. This ensures that every individual empaneled to an HWC. Health cards issued to enable continuum of care to the families and individuals. The family health folders kept in HWC or nearby PHC as either hard copy or digital.

Advantages of HWC

- Improved population coverage
- Reduced out of pocket expenditure
- Risk factor mitigation
- Decongestion of secondary and tertiary health facilities
- Improved population health outcomes
- Increased responsiveness

Organization of Services

Services are delivered at three levels: (i) Family/Household and community levels (ii) Health and Wellness Centers (iii) Referral facilities/Sites

Mid-Level Health Provider (MLHP)

An important change made in the primary health team at the SHC-HWC is the addition of Mid-level Health Provider (MLHP) who would be a Community Health Officer (CHO).

Qualification Required for MLHP

Bachelor of Science (BSc) in Community Health or a Nurse [General Nursing and Midwifery (GNM) or BSc] or an Ayurveda practitioner, trained and certified through Indira Gandhi National Open University (IGNOU)/other State Public Health/Medical Universities for a set of competencies in delivering public health and primary health care services.

Purposes of Introducing MLHP

- To enhance the capacity of the Health and Wellness Center to provide the expanded range of services

- To improve clinical management, care coordination and ensure continuity of care
- To improve public health activities and the measurement of health outcomes of the population served by the HWC.

Selection of Mid-Level Health Providers for the Health and Wellness Centers

- State level advertisement that clearly indicates district wise positions and preference for selection of local candidates.
- States can reserve a proportion of seats for women candidates.
- State to supervise and assist every district for initial screening of applicants based on the qualifications.
- A written examination and interview.

Role of Mid-Level Health Provider

- Ensures that all households are covered through maintaining a database.
- Provides clinical care and standard treatment guidelines for the range of services expected of the HWC.
- Coordinates care/case management for chronic illnesses based on the diagnosis and treatment plan and dispenses drugs as per standing orders.
- Focuses on screening activities and initiates the treatment based on appropriate Standard Treatment Guidelines (STGs) or on the basis of plans made by medical officer/specialists.
- Coordinates and leads local response to diseases outbreaks, emergencies and disaster situations.
- Supports the team of MPWs and ASHAs that include supervision, monitoring and administrative functions of the HWC.
- Supports and supervises the collection of population-based data by frontline workers and works with the team to develop a local action plan with measurable targets.
- Plays key role to promote behavior change for improved health outcomes.
- Addresses the issues of social and environmental determinants of health with extension workers of other departments (e.g. gender based violence, education, etc.)

Pradhan Mantri Jan Arogya Yojana (PMJAY)

The Pradhan Mantri Jan Arogya Yojana (PMJAY) provides financial protection for secondary and tertiary care to about 40% of India's households. The success and affordability of this scheme considerably lie in the efficient delivery of **Comprehensive Primary Health Care (CPHC) through Health and Wellness Centers (HWCs).**

It offers insurance cover of ₹5 lakh per family. About 50 crore citizens of poor and economically backward segment avail the benefit of this program. The scheme used the data from the Socio-Economic Caste Census (SECC) 2011 to identify the beneficiaries.

Aim

To provide health insurance coverage for more than 10 crore poor families who live in urban and rural areas of India.

The scheme also aims at addressing the shortcomings of Rashtriya Swasthya Bima Yojana (RSBY). The scheme includes the beneficiaries of the RSBY scheme in all the states where it is active.

Eligibility Criteria for Rural Beneficiaries

- Families living in only one room with kachcha walls and kachcha roof
- Families with no adult members aged between 16 and 59
- Female-headed family with no adult male member in the 16-59 age group
- Families having at least one disabled member and no able-bodied adult member
- SC/ST households
- Landless households deriving a major part of their income from manual casual labor
- Destitutes and those surviving on alms
- Manual scavenger families
- Tribal groups
- Legally-released bonded laborers

Eligibility Criteria for Urban Beneficiaries

The following 11 occupational categories of workers are included in the list by the government:

- Ragpicker
- Beggar
- Domestic worker
- Street vendor/cobbler/hawker/other service providers working on the streets
- Construction worker/plumber/mason/labor/painter/welder/security guard/coolie and other head-load workers
- Sweeper/sanitation worker/gardener
- Home-based worker/artisan/handicrafts worker/tailor
- Transport worker/driver/conductor/helper to drivers and conductors/cart-puller/rickshaw puller

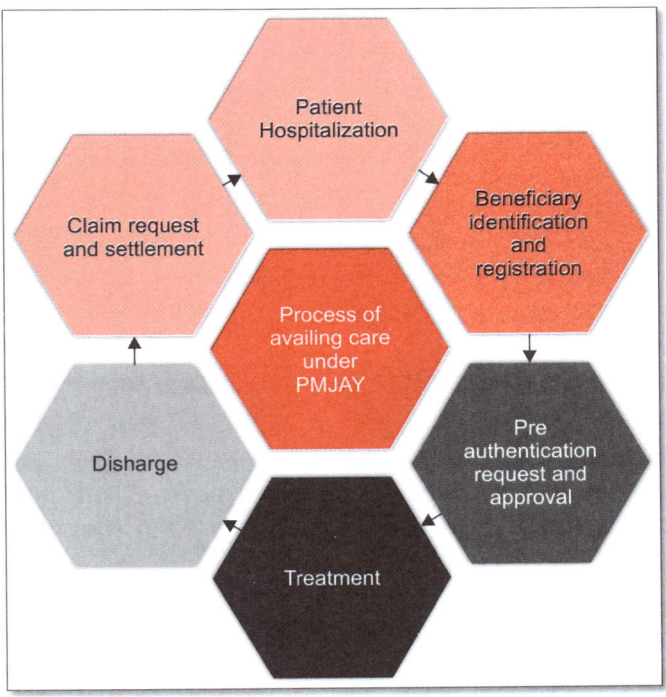

Figure 2: Ayushman Bharat-PMJAY

o Shop worker/assistant/peon in small establishment/helper/delivery assistant/attendant/waiter

o Electrician/mechanic/assembler/repair worker

o Washerman/chowkidar

Nature of the Scheme

o Focuses on poor and economically backward people of urban and rural areas.

o No premium required from the beneficiaries for the insurance cover.

o Cashless and paperless transaction for beneficiaries.

o Medical expenses for secondary and most tertiary care procedures covered.

o A defined transport allowance per hospitalization paid to the beneficiary.

o The beneficiaries can avail services from both public and empaneled private facilities.

o To contain cost the government sets the predetermined treatment packages.

o Empaneled hospitals have recruited 'Ayushman Mitras', who coordinate with beneficiaries and assist patients. Empaneled hospitals identify eligible patients and assist in documentation.

o QR codes of beneficiaries are verified for authentication.

o Individual bank account is necessary to avail the benefits.

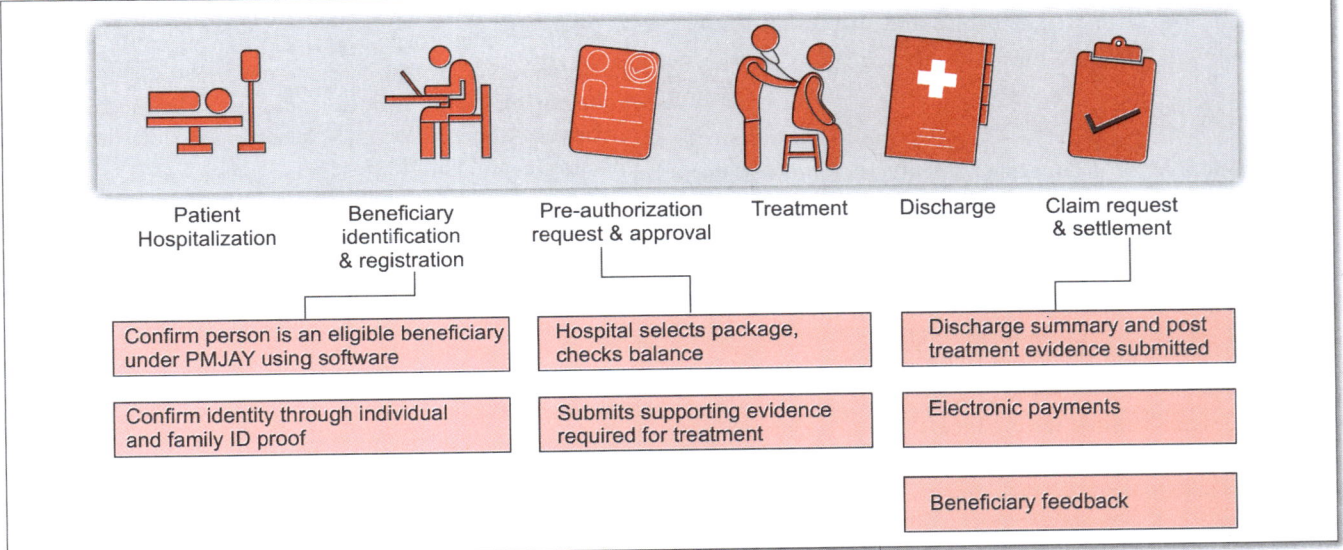

Figure 3: Process of getting care under PMJAY

HEALTH PROMOTION AND BEHAVIORAL CHANGE COMMUNICATION SKILLS

Health promotion and information delivery at the community level is the vital element of the expanded range of services under Comprehensive Primary Health Care.

According to National Health Policy 2017, all states should plan to focus on seven areas identified as priority to improve the environment for health:

o The Swachh Bharat Abhiyan (SBA)

o Balanced, healthy diets and regular exercises

- Addressing tobacco, alcohol and substance abuse
- Yatri Suraksha–preventing deaths due to rail and road traffic accidents
- Nirbhaya Nari–action against gender violence
- Reduced stress and improved safety in the workplace
- Reducing indoor and outdoor air pollution

This becomes states' responsibility to draw strategies and institutional mechanisms to develop a social movement for health in the form of Jan Andolan named **Swasth Nagrik Abhiyan.** This social movement is expected in all the seven priority areas.

HEALTH PROMOTION STRATEGIES FOR BEHAVIORAL CHANGE

Primary Prevention for General Population

Some examples for **primary prevention among general population**:

- Providing mass education to general population on lifestyle modifications such as healthy diet, regular exercise to prevent cardiovascular diseases and diabetes.
- Initiate education on sanitation and clean surroundings to prevent the spread of communicable diseases malaria, gastroenteritis, etc.
- Nutrition counselling to adolescents and women to prevent low birth weight babies and to promote early initiation of breastfeeding.

Population at Risk

This is for population groups that are **high risk** for developing a disease/disorder.

Example: Strategies for population at risk of HIV/AIDS: Promote healthy behaviors delivering health educative messages:

(A) (i) Decrease the number of sexual partners
   (ii) Safe sexual intercourse
   (iii) Counselling and testing for HIV
   (iv) Adherence to biomedical strategies—avoid sharing of needles and syringes, and decrease substance use, etc.
(B) Promote regular screening for non-communicable diseases.

For Individuals with Symptoms

This is for individuals and population groups with signs of a disease condition.

Example: Early identification of diseases through home visits, prompt referral and follow up of cases like high-risk pregnancies, high-risk new born, malnourished children, and passive surveillance for malaria, etc.

Ensuring Wellness and Health Promotion through Yoga

- Identify yoga instructors at the local level (ASHA, NGO, Physical instructor from village, etc.).
- Schedule of classes for community yoga training at the HWCs.
- Provision of incentive/honorarium for these yoga teachers/per session basis annually.
- Dissemination of the schedule.

Coordination of Health Promotion Activities

Mid-level Healthcare Providers (MLHP) will provide individual and family-based health promotion in HWCs and community. The MLHP will coordinate the health promotion activities via frontline workers, Village Health Sanitation and Nutrition Committees (VHSNCs), MAS (Mahila Arogya Samitis) SHGs (Self-Help Groups), NGOs and patient support groups. The MLHP will ensure that it reaches all segments of population.

Inter-Sectoral Convergence for Health Promotion

Convergence initiatives are in position to address the spread of outbreaks of communicable diseases, such as dengue, chikungunya, malaria for sanitation drives, vector control, controlling water coagulation, through cleaning of drains, etc. Intersectoral convergence is necessary for **community mobilization**. This would build on the accountability initiatives under National Health Mission leading to universality and equity.

FAMILY PLANNING 2020

The population of India as per 2011 census is 121 crore (1.21 billion). It is second (next to China) most populous country in the world. India accounts for 2.4% of the world's surface area and supports more than 17.5% of the world's population. India's population has increased about 18.1 crore (181 million) between 2001 and 2011.

The decadal population growth rate of India has declined from 21.54% in 1991-2001 to 17.64% in 2001-2011. This (2001-2011) decade has actually added lesser population compared to the previous decades with the exception of 1911-1921.

India's crude birth rate is 21.6 as per SRS 2012. The CBR is showing a consistent decline each year recording total decline of 16% from the year 2000 to 2012. India is in latter half of the third stage of demographic transition whereby the death rate has declined substantially and the birth rate is also declining. India's TFR according to SRS 2012 was 2.4.

Family Planning 2020 (FP 2020) is a global partnership that supports the rights of women and girls to decide on whether, when, and how many children they want to have.

LONDON SUMMIT ON FAMILY PLANNING

India launched child survival and development in February, 2013 and the comprehensive Reproductive, Maternal, Newborn, Child and Adolescent Health (RMNCH+A) strategy in May, 2013. Gaining a huge momentum in improvement of maternal and child health outcomes, family planning became the first pillar of the operational strategy RMNCH+A.

The 'Plus' in the strategy denotes the inclusion of adolescence as an important 'life stage' that forms the basis for a healthy life. This strategy also connects maternal and child health to reproductive health components, like family planning and community. Besides, this approach focuses on health system strengthening, reducing out of pocket expenditure and providing services in underserved areas.

FAMILY PLANNING (FP 2020) COMMITMENTS OF INDIA

- Overarching FP2020 goals to increase the modern contraceptive usage from 53.1% (2017-Track 20 estimate) to 54.3% by 2020 and ensure that 74% of the demand for modern contraceptives is satisfied by 2020.
- Expanding range and reach of contraceptive options by 2020: (i) The rolling-out of injectable contraceptives, Progesterone only Pills (POPs) and Ormeloxifene (nonhormonal weekly pill: Centchroman – Indian brand) in the public health system; (ii) Exploring introduction of new LARCs (Long Acting Reversible Contraceptives).
- Delivering quality assured services to the hardest-to-reach in rural and urban areas—providing a full-service package at all levels in all 146 Mission Parivar Vikas (MPV)
- Strengthening supply chain and commodity tracking in all states of India.
- Increased awareness and demand through 360-degree communications campaign rolled out across all states of India.
- Expanded role for the private sector for ensuring family planning services.
- Enabling young people to access sexual and reproductive health information and services.
- Civil society commitments for creating awareness on family planning commodities and services and mobilizing community for increasing uptake of services through civil society organizations, plus providing services.

The initial strategy and design of the FP2020 Partnership was built upon a theory of change that reflected the 2012 environment and is no longer fit for the purpose. Specifically, new strategy has to be based on three assumptions which were not given weightage in FP2020s:

1. More donor and domestic money for FP would be forthcoming;
2. A coordinated partnership would enhance accountability for progress; and
3. Harmonizing and aligning FP efforts would achieve greater efficiencies.

CLIMATE CHANGE AND ITS IMPACT ON HEALTH

Climate is the average daily weather for an extended period of time at a certain location.

"Climate" is a very common term used by all of us. What is the climate there now? How do you like this climate? Such kinds of questions are part of people's conversation. Actually climate talks about the regularly observed weather condition of a specific area.

The key factors of climate change are:

- Climate change affects the social and environmental determinants of health such as clean air, safe drinking water, sufficient food and secure shelter.
- Between 2030 and 2050, climate change is expected to cause approximately 2,50,000 additional deaths per year, from malnutrition, malaria, diarrhea and heat stress.
- The direct damage costs to health (i.e. excluding costs in health-determining sectors such as agriculture and water and sanitation), is estimated to be between USD 2-4 billion/year by 2030.
- Areas with weak health infrastructure, mostly in developing countries, will be the least able to cope without assistance to prepare and respond.
- Reducing emissions of greenhouse gases through better transport, food and energy-use choices can result in improved health, particularly through reduced air pollution.

Climate change affects every nook and corner of our lives. This has been shown in Figure 4.

Climate is the product of combination of meteorological factors. They are:

- Atmospheric pressure
- Air temperature
- Humidity
- Precipitation
- Speed and direction of wind
- Movement of clouds

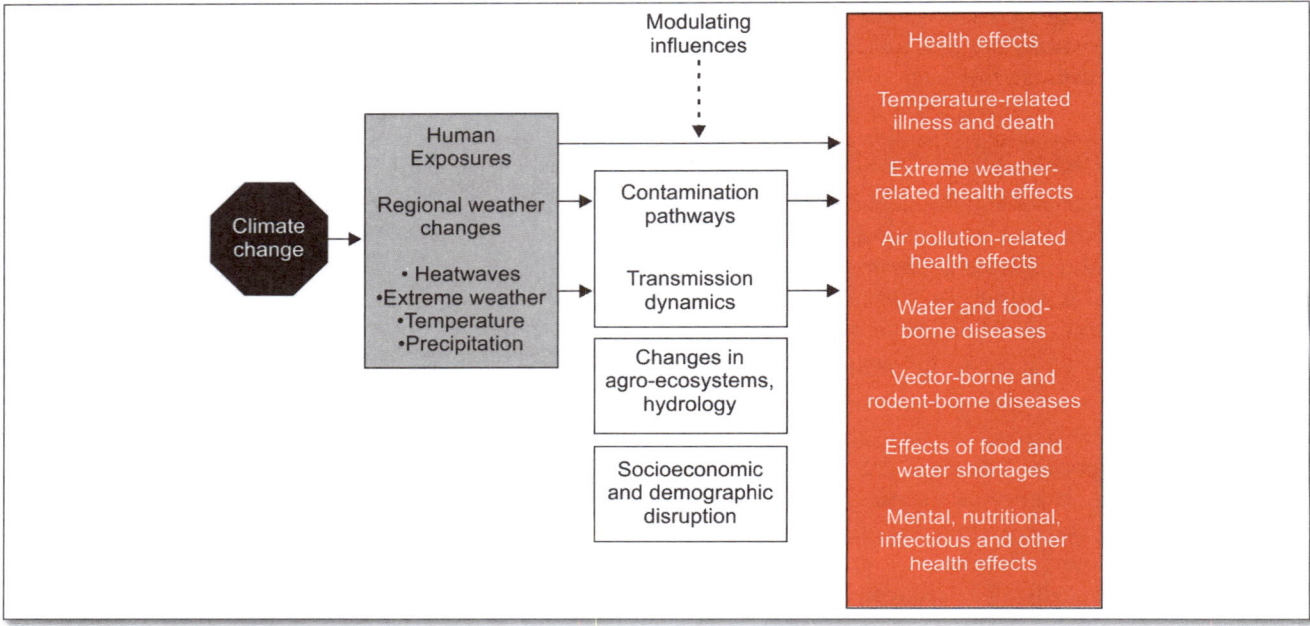

Figure 4: Pathways by which climate change affects human health (Modified)

ATMOSPHERIC PRESSURE

Atmospheric pressure and altitude are inversely proportional to each other. As the altitude increases the atmospheric pressure falls. So the high altitudes will have low atmospheric pressure. A special instrument called barometer is used to measure atmospheric pressure.

AIR TEMPERATURE

Latitude of the place, altitude, direction of wind and proximity to sea are the factors that influence the air temperature.

Thermometers Used to Measure Air Temperature

There are many kinds of thermometers which are used to measure air temperature. They are as follows:

- Dry bulb thermometer
- Wet bulb thermometer
- Maximum thermometer
- Minimum thermometer
- Globe thermometer
- Wet globe thermometer
- Silvered thermometer
- Kata thermometer

HUMIDITY

Humidity refers to the constant presence of moisture in the atmosphere. It is measured in either relative terms (relative humidity) or absolute terms (dewpoint temperature). Dry and wet bulb thermometer and Sling psychometer are used to measure the humidity.

PRECIPITATION

Precipitation is the term that encompasses all forms of water, like snow, hail, dew, frost and rain. Rain gauges are used for measuring rain fall. Symon's rain gauge is used in India for measuring the rain fall.

SPEED AND DIRECTION OF WIND

The velocity or the rate of speed of the wind decides the consequences of the wind. An instrument named anemometer is used for measuring the speed of the wind.

Wind directions are mainly grouped into North, South, East and West with 8-16 directions. A special instrument named wind vane is used for observing the direction of the wind.

MOVEMENT OF CLOUDS

The movement of the cloud is one of the phenomena used for making meteorological assessments. Meteorological satellites are used to observe the form, amount, direction, and height of the clouds.

ENERGY BALANCE OF THE EARTH

Earth is a planet that always maintains the flow of energy. Earth gets warmed by absorbing the solar energy. Earth does not accept sun energy when it reaches a particular threshold. Here sun's energy is allowed into space. Earth starts cooling at this point to get into the process-cycle. This is how earth maintains energy balance.

FACTORS THAT INFLUENCE EARTH'S ENERGY BALANCE

- There are natural and human factors which contribute to changes in earth's energy balance.
- Changes in the greenhouse effect, which affects the amount of heat retained by earth's atmosphere.
- Greenhouse effect influences the retention of heat by earth's atmosphere.
- Any changes or differences in the sun's energy reaching earth.
- Any changes found in the reflectivity of atmosphere.
- Many activities of man, like burning of woods, land alteration for living, and increased urbanization increase the levels of greenhouse gases in atmosphere.

GREENHOUSE EFFECT

Water vapor (H_2O), ozone (O_3) carbon dioxide (CO_2), and methane (CH_4) are the gases found in the earth's atmosphere capable of absorbing outgoing infrared energy from earth to space. These greenhouse gases function like a blanket by retaining the heat and increasing the earth's temperature and warming up the earth excessively. This act is called the "greenhouse effect".

Global warming is a change in earth's climate likely to become permanent with a gradual increase in the average temperature of the earth's atmosphere and its oceans.

HOW GREENHOUSE GASES AFFECT GLOBAL WARMING

There are three factors that affect the degree to which any greenhouse gas will influence global warming. They are as follows:

1. Its abundance in the atmosphere
2. How long it stays in the atmosphere
3. Its global-warming potential

CLIMATE CHANGE AND ITS IMPACT ON HEALTH

- Climate change may have crucial impact on health by disturbing the basic needs of human beings, like air, drinking water, food and housing.

Table 2: Climate, sicknesses and preventive measures

Climate component	Health problem	Prevention
Atmospheric pressure- High altitude Low altitude	Mountain sickness Pulmonary edema Increase in -respiration, hemoglobin concentration and cardiac output	Carry proper breathing equipment
Exposure to heat	Heat stroke, hyperpyrexia, heat exhaustion, heat cramps, heat syncope	Proper clothing, protective work place, Intake of water, protective devices
Effects of cold stress- Wet cold condition conditions Dry cold conditions	Trench foot Frost bite	Intake of hot fluids Proper clothing

- It is expected that climate change of earth may add approximately 25,000 deaths per year due to various causes like malnutrition, diarrhea, etc.
- Climate change also adds the costs to individual and country by causing damage to health.

HEAT WAVES AND ITS IMPACT ON HEALTH

Heat exposure can cause wide range of physiological impacts and this may even lead to death and disability.

As forecasted, global temperature is increasing and the frequency and intensity of heatwaves are crossing their usual patterns due to changes in climate.

Although the rising global ambient temperatures affect all populations, some are at higher levels of risk. They are: the elderly, infants and children, pregnant women, outdoor and manual workers, athletes, and the poor. Gender can play an important role in determining heat exposure.

PREVENTIVE MEASURES TO PROTECT FROM HEAT WAVES

- Stay in coolest room in the home or under the shade
- Ideal room temperature is <32°C during the day and 24°C during the night
- Keep all windows open during the night and the early morning
- Turn off unwanted lights
- Avoid going outside during the hottest time of the day

- Avoid strenuous physical activity if you can and select morning time between 4 a.m. and 7:00 a.m.
- Stay under the shade
- Do not leave children or animals in parked vehicles
- Take cool baths
- Wear light, loose-fitting clothes of natural materials
- Wear a hat or cap and sunglasses
- Use light bed linen and sheets
- Drink more fluids, avoid alcohol and caffeine and sugar
- Eat small meals and eat more often
- Avoid high protein foods

Table 3: Heat waves and its impact

Direct impact of heat waves on health	Indirect impact of heat waves on health
- **Heat illness:** Dehydration, heat cramps and heat stroke - **Accelerated death from:** Respiratory disease, cardiovascular and other chronic diseases - **Hospitalization:** Respiratory disease, diabetes, renal disease, Stroke, mental health disturbances	- **Impact on health services:** Increased hospital calls, strokes, Increased admissions - **Increased risk of accidents:** Drowning, work related accidents, injuries and poisoning - Increased transmission of foodborne and waterborne diseases - **Potential fistruption of infrastructure:** Power, water, transport and productivity

FOODBORNE ILLNESSES

Foodborne illnesses are specifically man made that occur knowingly or unknowingly.

Foodborne illnesses are serious health issues. An incident of foodborne illness will be treated as an outbreak when two or more cases of a similar illness occur as a result of eating the same food.

A foodborne outbreak indicates that something went wrong in the food safety system and that has to be rectified. The food safety system includes:

- Production
- Processing
- Packing
- Distribution/Transportation
- Storage
- Preparation

Foodborne illnesses occur as the result of ingestion of foods contaminated with microorganisms or chemicals. It is quite possible that the foodborne infection can occur at any point between manufacturers to consumers. Contamination can be favored from various environmental sources including but not limited to pollution of water, soil or air. Natural and manufactured chemicals found in food products also may cause sickness.

There are many foodborne diseases. They can be caused by bacteria, viruses, or parasites.

Foodborne illnesses are classified as:

- Foodborne intoxication
- Foodborne infections

Foodborne intoxication is caused by ingesting food containing toxins released by bacterial growth in the food item. Here, live bacteria need not have to be ingested.

Foodborne infection results from consuming foods containing live bacteria which grow and stabilize themselves in the intestinal tract of man.

Dealing with Suspected Foodborne Illness

- Initially we need to preserve the food sample under suspicion. Suspected food should be wrapped in a cover marked as "DANGER" and placed in freezer. All items used for packing like containers or cans or cartons should be kept under care. A record of food type, the date and other identities of the package must be kept. The most essential is noting of the time the food was consumed, and when the onset of symptoms occurred. Save any similar unsealed products.
- Seek medical aid. Vulnerable group like children, pregnant women and elderly should get immediate medical aid.
- Local health department has to be informed if suspect food was served to many people (for example, big get together or marriage or any large gathering) from a hotel or any other common food service facility, or a commercial product.

Diseases that occur due to food toxicants and their food sources are shown in Figure 5.

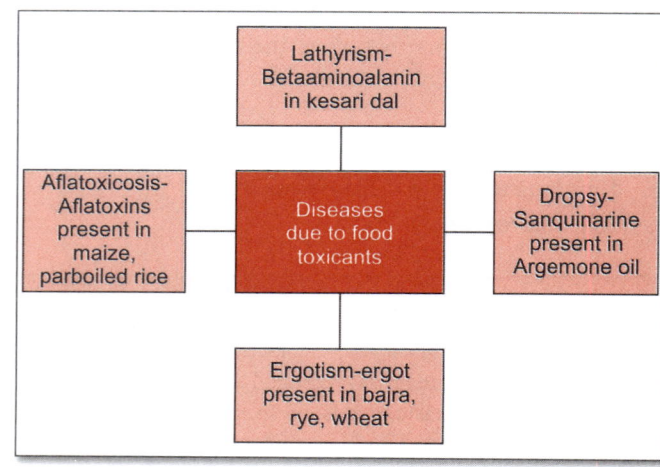

Figure 5: Diseases that occur due to food toxicants

FOOD POISONING

Food poisoning is an acute sickness that appears with gastroenteritis caused by the ingestion of food or drink contaminated with bacteria, their toxins or inorganic chemical substances and poisons resulting from plants or animals.

Literature states that the following are the commonly found causes of food poisoning and this accounts for approximately 90 percent of the of food poisoning cases every year. The course of disease followed has been shown in Figure 6.

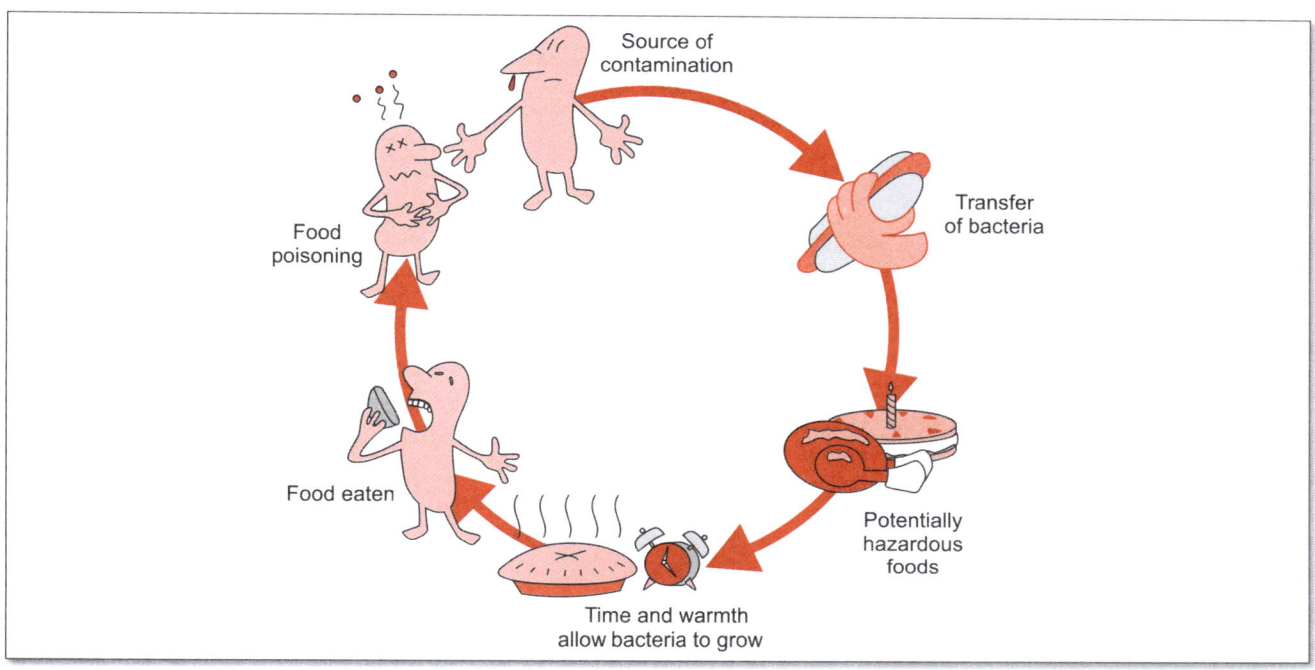

Figure 6: Course of disease

Types

Bacterial and nonbacterial are types of food poisoning.

Bacterial: This is caused by consumption of food contaminated with live bacteria or their toxins

Nonbacterial: This is caused by chemicals like arsenic, certain sea foods, fertilizers, pesticides, etc.

The following bacteria are usually found in raw foods. Some of them are diseased here:

- **Salmonella**
- **Staphylococcus aureus**
- **Clostridium perfringens**
- **Campylobacter**
- **Listeria monocytogenes**
- **Vibrio parahemolyticus**
- **Bacillus cereus**
- **Enteropathogenic Escherichia coli**

Salmonella Food Poisoning

Salmonella Food Poisoning is the most common, caused by Salmonella. Disease spread through contaminated animal foods like milk and milk products.

Causes

- Increased communal feeding

- Higher incidence of salmonellosis in animals
- Increased international trade in food
- Expanded use of household detergents
- Wide distribution of prepared food.

Symptoms

- Chills, fever, nausea, vomiting
- Acute enteritis and colitis
- Profuse watery diarrhea

Staphylococcal Food Poisoning

Staphylococcal Food Poisoning is caused by enterotoxins of certain strains of Staphylococcus aureus. Staphylococcus aureus is predominantly found on skin, nose and throat of man and animals.

Symptoms

Common symptoms of staphylococcal food poisoning are: vomiting, diarrhea with or without blood and mucus, and abdominal cramps. Fever is unusual and the disease is not a life-taking phenomenon but still requires immediate medical attention.

Botulism

It is a serious illness, occurs rarely and is fatal. An exotoxin of *Clostridium botulinum* causes botulism. The organism, *Clostridium botulinum* is found in soil, dust, and in the intestinal tract of infected animals. It makes its entry into food as spores.

Some of the main sources of infection are home preserved foods, canned foods, smoked or pickled fish, and other low acid foods.

Symptoms

The symptoms of the disease include dysphagia, blurring of vision, muscle weakness, quadriplegia and could even result in death due to cardiac or respiratory failure.

Bacillus cereus Food Poisoning

B. cereus is found in dust, soil and spices. *B. cereus* can comfortably grow when under cooked food is stored at mismatched temperature. It is capable of surviving as a heat resistant spore in temperature produced during cooking.

Later it would produce more number of cells if the storage temperature is not a correct one. To avoid the growth of *B. cereus* food must be served hot or cooled rapidly.

Enteropathogenic Escherichia coli

Enteropathogenic *E. coli* is the most frequent cause of diarrhea in unhygienic conditions and common in underdeveloped and developing countries. There are four subgroups of enteropathogenic *E. coli*:

1. Enterotoxigenic
2. Enteroinvasive
3. Hemorrhagic
4. Enteropathogenic

The major source of the bacteria is the feces of infected humans and animal reservoirs. Feces and untreated water are the most likely sources for contamination of food.

CONTROL OF FOODBORNE PATHOGENS

Use adequate holding times, and temperatures while cooking. Avoid recontamination of cooked meat. Do not appoint food handlers who have infection and screen them periodically.

Personal hygiene of food handlers should be monitored continuously.

PREVENTION OF FOOD POISONING

○ To prevent recontamination of cooked foods, hand washing should be done before and after handling raw foods

○ Refrigerate foods below 40°F

○ Serve hot foods immediately or keep them heated above 140°F

○ It is safe to store food in small portions for fast cooling. It is not advised to refrigerate big volumes of hot foods since they can raise the temperature of foods that were already cooled.

○ Remember the danger zone is between 40° F and 140° F.

○ Heat canned foods thoroughly before tasting.

○ If suspicion arises on any food discard it immediately.

HYGIENE OF FOOD HANDLERS

The "WHO five keys to safer food" (Figure 7) help us provide educational programs to train food handlers and the consumers. These are significant practices in preventing foodborne illnesses.

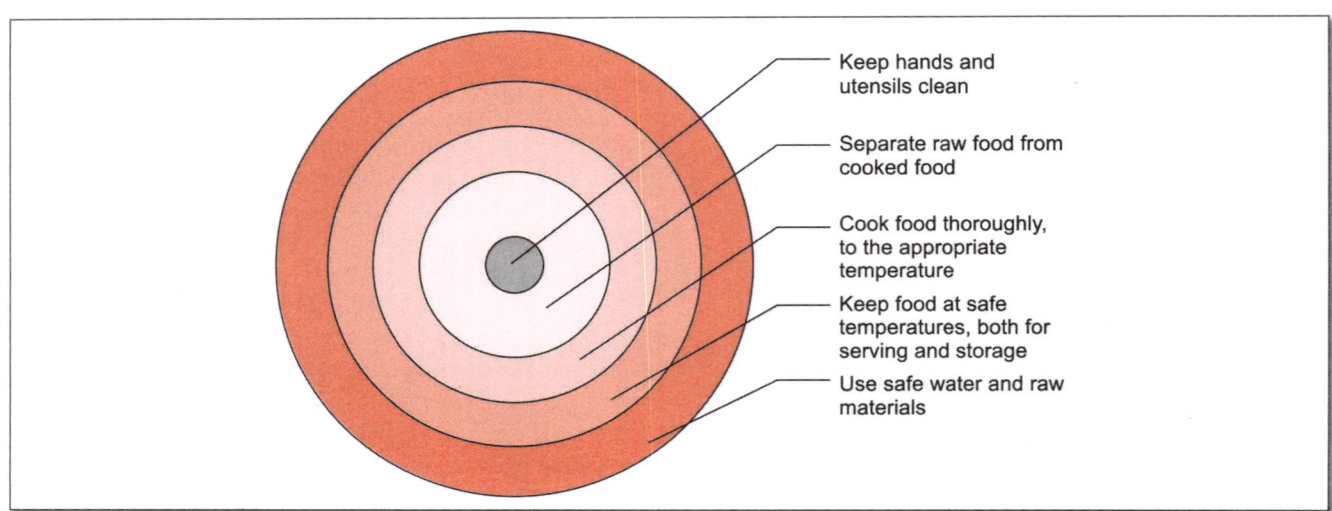

Keep hands and utensils clean

Separate raw food from cooked food

Cook food thoroughly, to the appropriate temperature

Keep food at safe temperatures, both for serving and storage

Use safe water and raw materials

Figure 7: WHO five keys to safer food

General Guidelines for Food Handlers' Health Maintenance

- Provide complete medical examination to food handlers to find out any infections.
- Look for medical fitness before employing food handlers.
- Do not appoint if there is any history of communicable diseases like typhoid fever, diphtheria, chronic dysentery, tuberculosis, etc.
- Continuous monitoring on their health.
- Notify all health problems of food handlers.
- Food handlers should be taught on the prime important factors, like hand washing, trimming finger nails and keeping clothes and hair clean.
- Avoid activities such as coughing, sneezing, licking fingers, nose picking, smoking, etc. while preparing and serving food. They must use clean kitchen napkins.

Hygiene of the Eating Places

- Eating place should be clean and aesthetic.
- It must be located away from the sources of contamination.
- It must be well ventilated and illuminated well.
- There should be provisions for adequate and continuous safe water.
- The raw and cooked food should be kept separately.
- The eating place should be a highly protected area, free from rats, cockroaches, flies and other parasites.
- Raw food should be stored in air-tight containers.
- All measures should be in place to avoid flies and other insects; proper disposal of garbage must be practiced.

The Goal of Home Food Storage

- Maintain the quality and safety of food.
- Adopt proper storage to enhance the shelf life of food by particularly taking care of proper temperature and humidity.
- Storage should not decrease the quality of food significantly.

SAFE CHILDBIRTH CHECKLIST

Childbirth is a multifaceted process, and it requires the availability of trained personnel and necessary facilities to make the "birth journey" as a safe one. According to World Health Organization (WHO) 289,000 women died in the year 2013 because of pregnancy and childbirth; and 2.8 million neonatal deaths occurred in the same year. To highlight the fact majority of these deaths reported were from poor resource settings had no necessary support.

The WHO designed a "Safe Childbirth Checklist" to improve the quality of care provided to women before, during and after the process of birth. The WHO Safe Childbirth Checklist is intended for use at four pause points during facility-based births:

PAUSE POINT 1: ON ADMISSION (AT THE TIME OF ADMISSION)

- Detect for any complications the mother already carries.
- Confirm whether she needs to be referred to another facility.
- Prepare mother and her companion for labor and delivery and educate them about danger signs for which she should call for help.

PAUSE POINT 2: JUST BEFORE PUSHING (OR BEFORE CESAREAN)

- Check the mother just before pushing (or before Cesarean) to detect and treat complications that may occur during labor.
- Prepare for routine events and probable crisis situations that may occur after birth.

PAUSE POINT 3: SOON AFTER BIRTH (WITHIN ONE HOUR)

- Check the mother and newborn soon after birth (within 1 hour) to detect and treat complications that can occur after delivery.
- To educate the mother (and her companion) about danger signs for which she should call for help.

PAUSE POINT 4: BEFORE DISCHARGE

- Check the mother and newborn before discharge to be sure that the mother and newborn are healthy before discharge.
- To ensure follow-up has been arranged, family planning discussed and offered to the mother (and her companion).
- To ensure that education provided on danger signs to look out for, both in the mother and her baby and readiness for immediate skilled care, if needed.

NATIONAL AIR QUALITY MONITORING PROGRAMME (NAMP)

The government is executing a nationwide programme of ambient air quality monitoring known as NAMP.

OBJECTIVES OF NAMP

- To determine the status and trends of ambient air quality
- To ascertain whether the prescribed ambient air quality standards are violated
- To identify non-attainment cities
- To obtain the knowledge and understanding necessary for developing preventive and corrective measures
- To understand the natural cleansing process undergoing in the environment through pollution dilution, dispersion, wind-based movement, dry deposition, precipitation, and chemical transformation of the pollutants generated.

NAMP monitors four air pollutants regularly:

1. SO_2
2. NO_2
3. Suspended particulate matter (PM10)
4. Fine particulate matter (PM2.5)

The monitoring activity runs for 24 hours/twice a week that equals 104 observations/year. The monitoring is being carried out with the help of the Central Pollution Control Board (CPCB), State Pollution Control Board (SPCB), Pollution Control Committees (PCC), National Environmental Engineering Research Institute (NEERI).

NATIONAL AIR QUALITY INDEX (NAQI)

The AQI was launched by the Prime Minister in April 2015 starting with 14 cities and now extended to 71 cities in 17 states. The AQI functions like an effective tool to communicate air quality status to people using simple terms. It transforms complex air quality data of various pollutants into a single number (index value), nomenclature and color.

There are six AQI categories, namely, Good, Satisfactory, Moderately Polluted, Poor, Very Poor, and Severe. Each of these categories is decided based on the ambient concentration values of air pollutants and their likely health impacts known as "health breakpoints." The AQ sub-index and health breakpoints are evolved for eight pollutants (PM10, PM2.5, NO_2, SO_2, CO, O_3, NH_3, and Lead [Pb]) for which short-term (up to 24 hours) National Ambient Air Quality Standards are prescribed. The AQI categories and health breakpoints for the eight pollutants are given in Table 4.

Table 4: Air quality index categories and health breakpoints

AQI	Associated impacts
Good (0–50)	Minimal impact
Satisfactory (51–100)	May cause minor breathing discomfort to sensitive people
Moderate (101–200)	May cause breathing discomfort to the people with lung disease such as asthma and discomfort to people with heart disease, children and older adults
Poor (201–300)	May cause breathing discomfort to people on prolonged exposure and discomfort to people with heart disease with short exposure
Very poor (301–400)	May cause respiratory illness to the people on prolonged exposure. Effect may be more pronounced in people with lung and heart diseases
Severe (401–500)	○ May cause respiratory effects even on healthy people and serious health impacts on people with lung/heart diseases. ○ The health impacts may be experienced even during light physical activity

OTHER MEASURES

Other measures to improve air quality were taken by the government for improvements in energy efficiency and air pollution control in India. Some of these are cited here:

- Advanced vehicle emission and fuel quality standards—BSIV from 2017 and BSVI from 2020.
- Plan to introduce a voluntary fleet modernization and an old-vehicle scrappage programme in India.
- Introducing a National Electric Mobility Mission Plan 2020.
- Introducing gas as an automotive fuel in many cities.
- Introduction and enhancement of the metro rail-based public transport and bus-based public transport systems in selected cities.
- Pradhan Mantri Ujjwala Yojana (PMUY) to accelerate the LPG penetration programme for cooking in households.
- Electrification to reduce kerosene consumption for lighting.
- Introducing an energy-efficiency labeling programme for energy-intensive home appliances such as air conditioners.
- Notifying new stringent standards for diesel generator sets for standby power generation.

ANNEXURE 1: CHILDBIRTH CHECKLIST (WORLD HEALTH ORGANIZATION)

BEFORE BIRTH

WHO Safe Childbirth Checklist

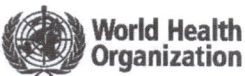 **World Health Organization**

1	**On Admission**

Does mother need referral?
- ☐ No
- ☐ Yes, organized

Check your facility's criteria

Partograph started?
- ☐ No, will start when ≥4cm
- ☐ Yes

Start plotting when cervix ≥4 cm, then cervix should dilate ≥1 cm/hr
- Every 30 min: plot HR, contractions, fetal HR
- Every 2 hrs: plot temperature
- Every 4 hrs: plot BP

Does mother need to start:

Antibiotics?
- ☐ No
- ☐ Yes, given

Ask for allergies before administration of any medication
Give antibiotics to mother if any of:
- Mother's temperature ≥38°C
- History of foul-smelling vaginal discharge
- Rupture of membranes >18 hrs

Magnesium sulfate and antihypertensive treatment?
- ☐ No
- ☐ Yes, magnesium sulfate given
- ☐ Yes, antihypertensive medication given

Give magnesium sulfate to mother if any of:
- Diastolic BP ≥110 mmHg and 3+ proteinuria
- Diastolic BP ≥90 mmHg, 2+ proteinuria, and any: severe headache, visual disturbance, epigastric pain

Give antihypertensive medication to mother if systolic BP >160 mmHg
- Goal: keep BP <150/100 mmHg

☐ **Confirm supplies are available to clean hands and wear gloves for each vaginal exam.**

☐ **Encourage birth companion to be present at birth.**

☐ **Confirm that mother or companion will call for help during labour if needed.**

Call for help if any of:
- Bleeding
- Severe abdominal pain
- Severe headache or visual disturbance
- Unable to urinate
- Urge to push

Completed by _____

BEFORE BIRTH

WHO Safe Childbirth Checklist

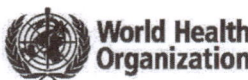 **World Health Organization**

2 Just Before Pushing (Or Before Caesarean)

Does mother need to start:

Antibiotics?
☐ No
☐ Yes, given

Ask for allergies before administration of any medication
Give antibiotics to mother if any of:
• Mother's temperature ≥38 °C
• History of foul-smelling vaginal discharge
• Rupture of membranes >18 hrs
• Caesarean section

Magnesium sulfate and antihypertensive treatment?
☐ No
☐ Yes, magnesium sulfate given
☐ Yes, antihypertensive medication given

Give magnesium sulfate to mother if any of:
• Diastolic BP ≥110 mmHg and 3+ proteinuria
• Diastolic BP ≥90 mmHg, 2+ proteinuria, and any: severe headache, visual disturbance, epigastric pain

Give antihypertensive medication to mother if systolic BP >160 mmHg
• Goal: keep BP <150/100 mmHg

Confirm essential supplies are at bedside and prepare for delivery:

For mother
☐ Gloves
☐ Alcohol-based handrub or soap and clean water
☐ Oxytocin 10 units in syringe

Prepare to care for mother immediately after birth:
Confirm single baby only (not multiple birth)
1. Give oxytocin within 1 minute after birth
2. Deliver placenta 1-3 minutes after birth
3. Massage uterus after placenta is delivered
4. Confirm uterus is contracted

For baby
☐ Clean towel
☐ Tie or cord clamp
☐ Sterile blade to cut cord
☐ Suction device
☐ Bag-and-mask

Prepare to care for baby immediately after birth:
1. Dry baby, keep warm
2. If not breathing, stimulate and clear airway
3. If still not breathing:
   • clamp and cut cord
   • clean airway if necessary
   • ventilate with bag-and-mask
   • shout for help

☐ **Assistant identified and ready to help at birth if needed.**

WHO Safe Childbirth Checklist   Completed by _____

AFTER BIRTH
WHO Safe Childbirth Checklist

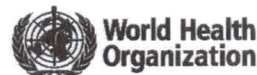
World Health Organization

3 Soon After Birth (Within 1 Hour)

Is mother bleeding abnormally?
☐ No
☐ Yes, shout for help

If bleeding abnormally:
• Massage uterus
• Consider more uterotonic
• Start IV fluids and keep mother warm
• Treat cause: uterine atony, retained placenta/fragments, vaginal tear, uterine rupture

Does mother need to start:
Antibiotics?
☐ No
☐ Yes, given

Ask for allergies before administration of any medication
Give antibiotics to mother if placenta manually removed or if mother's temperature ≥38 °C and any of:
• Chills
• Foul-smelling vaginal discharge

If the mother has a third or fourth degree of perineal tear give antibiotics to prevent infection

Magnesium sulfate and antihypertensive treatment?
☐ No
☐ Yes, magnesium sulfate given
☐ Yes, antihypertensive medication given

Give magnesium sulfate to mother if any of:
• Diastolic BP ≥110 mmHg and 3+ proteinuria
• Diastolic BP ≥90 mmHg, 2+ proteinuria, and any: severe headache, visual disturbance, epigastric pain

Give antihypertensive medication to mother if systolic BP >160 mmHg
• Goal: keep BP <150/100 mmHg

Does baby need:
Referral?
☐ No
☐ Yes, organized

Check your facility's criteria.

Antibiotics?
☐ No
☐ Yes, given

Give baby antibiotics if antibiotics given to mother for treatment of maternal infection during childbirth or if baby has any of:
• Respiratory rate >60/min or <30/min
• Chest in-drawing, grunting, or convulsions
• Poor movement on stimulation
• Baby's temperature <35 °C (and not rising after warming) or baby's temperature ≥38 °C

Special care and monitoring?
☐ No
☐ Yes, organized

Arrange special care/monitoring for baby if any:
• More than 1 month early
• Birth weight <2500 grams
• Needs antibiotics
• Required resuscitation

☐ **Started breastfeeding and skin-to-skin contact (if mother and baby are well).**

☐ **Confirm mother / companion will call for help if danger signs present.**

WHO Safe Childbirth Checklist

Completed by _____

AFTER BIRTH
WHO Safe Childbirth Checklist
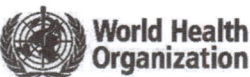
World Health Organization

4   Before Discharge

☐ **Confirm stay at facility for 24 hours after delivery.**

Does mother need to start antibiotics? ☐ No ☐ Yes, given and delay discharge	Ask for allergies before administration of any medication Give antibiotics to mother if any of: • Mother's temperature ≥38 °C • Foul-smelling vaginal discharge
Is mother's blood pressure normal? ☐ No, treat and delay discharge ☐ Yes	Give magnesium sulfate to mother if any of: • Diastolic BP ≥110 mmHg and 3+ proteinuria • Diastolic BP ≥90 mmHg, 2+ proteinuria, and any: severe headache, visual disturbance, epigastric pain Give antihypertensive medication to mother if systolic BP >160 mmHg • Goal: keep BP <150/100 mmHg
Is mother bleeding abnormally? ☐ No ☐ Yes, treat and delay discharge	If pulse >110 beats per minute and blood pressure <90 mmHg • Start IV and keep mother warm • Treat cause (hypovolemic shock)
Does baby need to start antibiotics? ☐ No ☐ Yes, give antibiotics, delay discharge, give special care	Give antibiotics to baby if any of: • Respiratory rate >60/min or <30/min • Chest in-drawing, grunting, or convulsions • Poor movement on stimulation • Baby's temperature <35°C (and not rising after warming) or baby's temperature ≥38°C • Stopped breastfeeding well • Umbilicus redness extending to skin or draining pus

Is baby feeding well?

☐ No, establish good breastfeeding practices and delay discharge
☐ Yes

☐ **Discuss and offer family planning options to mother.**

☐ **Arrange follow-up and confirm mother / companion will seek help if danger signs appear after discharge.**

Danger Signs

Mother has any of:
- Bleeding
- Severe abdominal pain
- Severe headache or visual disturbance
- Breathing difficulty
- Fever or chills
- Difficulty emptying bladder
- Epigastric pain

Baby has any of:
- Fast/difficult breathing
- Fever
- Unusually cold
- Stops feeding well
- Less activity than normal
- Whole body becomes yellow

WHO Safe Childbirth Checklist   Completed by _____

Introduction: Concepts of Health, Community Health and Community Health Nursing

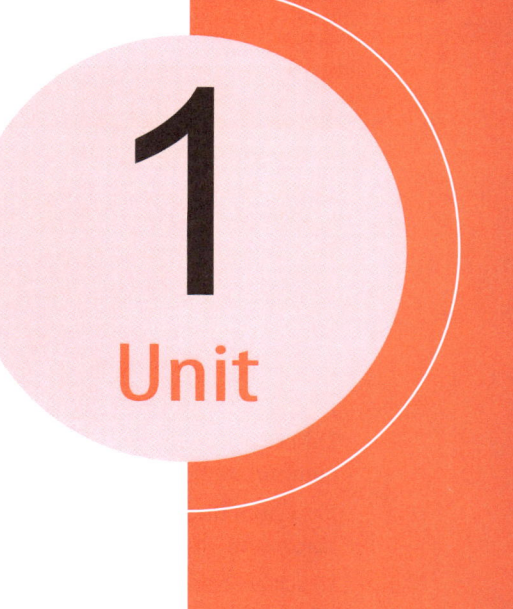

1 Unit

Unit Outline

Learning Objectives

At the end of this unit the learners will be able to:

○ Define health, public health, community, community health, community health nursing, public health nursing and population health

○ Describe the scope of community health nursing

○ State the various roles of community health nurses

○ List down the principles of community health nursing practice

○ Describe briefly on the historical development of community health in the world

○ Describe briefly on the historical development of community health nursing in the world

○ Describe briefly on the development of community health in India during pre and post-independence

○ Describe briefly on the development of community health nursing in India during pre and post-independence

KEY TERMS

- Health
- Public health
- Clinician
- Educator
- Advocate
- Manager
- Collaborator
- Leader
- Researcher
- Ripple effect
- Health education
- American Red Cross Society
- National organization for public health nursing
- Frontier nursing
- Indian Nursing Service (INS)
- Indian Nursing Association
- TNAI

There is always a common way of interpreting the word "*public*" to "*population*". According to Cambridge-dictionary, "*public*" means relating to or involving people in general rather than being limited to a group of people. Meaning and usage of the word, "*health*" is well explained in "Textbook of Community Health Nursing-I." The terms "*public health*" and "*community health*" are interpreted differently or used interchangeably to describe the health of a specific community or population at large. As per the literature, there is always an evidence that the term "*public health*" was in use from beginning and the use of the term "*community health*" emerged into practice in recent decades. Learning the definitions of specific terms

like health, public health, community, community health and community health nursing become vital to provide a greater platform of our understanding of this unit. Students and other readers need to read the first unit of author's first volume of community health nursing to have a better understanding on the concept of "health".

IMPORTANT DEFINITIONS

Health

Health is a concept with multiple determinants.

World Health Organization (WHO) defines health as on April 7, 1948 "Health is a state of complete physical, mental, and social well-being and not merely the absence of disease or infirmity".

Right to Health

Universal Declaration of human rights established a declaration in 1948, "Everyone has the right to a standard of living adequate for the health and well-being of himself and his family". The preamble to the WHO constitution also affirms that it is one of the fundamental rights of every human being to enjoy "the highest attainable standard of health".

The concept "Right to health" encompasses

○ Right to medical care

○ Right to responsibility for health

○ Right to healthy environment

○ Right to food

○ Right to procreate or not

○ Right of the deceased persons (determination of death, autopsies, abortion, etc.)

○ Right to die.

Changing Concepts of Health

Biomedical Concept

Perception of the concept of health differs from one individual to another, one professional community to another. Traditionally health was considered as "absence of disease".

An individual was considered healthy, if he was free from diseases. This concept was referred to as biomedical concept. Medically human body was equated to a machine and disease was looked as breakdown of machine while doctor was considered as the repairer of the machine. Thus, health became the ultimate goal of medicine.

Criticism

Biomedical concept minimized the role of other determinants of health namely social, environmental, psychological and cultural. Thus, it was found inefficient in solving major health-related problems (drug abuse, accidents, malnutrition, etc.).

Ecological Concept

○ Human ecology is a part of the science of ecology. Human ecosystem includes all dimensions of man-made environment—physical, chemical, biological and psychological in addition to natural environment.

○ According to the ecologists, health is viewed as a dynamic equilibrium between man and environment, and disease is viewed as an imbalance between the two. Human ecological and cultural adaptations determine not only the occurrence of disease, but also food security and population explosion.

○ The ecological concept revolves around two issues: man and environment. Adaptation of man to natural environment can result in prolonged life expectancies and better quality of life even in the absence of modern health amenities.

○ Man has created new health problems by altering the environment in terms of various activities like urban-ization, industrialization, deforestation, construction of dams and canals.

Psychological Concept

○ Developments in social sciences revealed the fact that health is not only absence of disease but also is a social, economic, psychological, cultural and political entity.

○ These factors should be considered while measuring health.

Holistic Concept

○ This concept corresponds to the view of ancient population that health implies sound mind in a sound body in a sound family and in a sound environment.

○ This concept encompasses all the other concepts. The influence of social, economic, political and environment on health has been well identified.

○ It has been described as unified or multidimensional process of achieving well-being of a person in the context of environment.

○ The holistic approach indicates that all sectors of the society have an influence on health.

○ Sectors include agriculture, animal husbandry, food, industry, education, housing, public works, communication and alike, with emphasis on promotion and protection of health.

○ Environmental factors and ecological considerations must be built into the total planning process. Prevention of disease through ecological or environmental is much cheaper, safer and sustainable rational approach than other means of control.

Public Health

Winslow (1923) defined public health as "the science and art of preventing disease, prolonging life, and promoting physical health and efficiency through organized community efforts for the sanitation of the environment, the control of community infections, the education of the individual in principles of personal hygiene, the organization

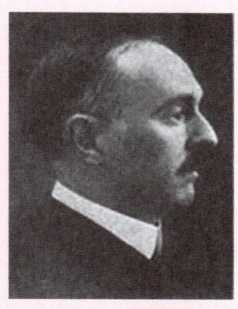

Prof. CEA Winslow

of medical and nursing services for the early diagnosis and preventive treatment of disease, and the development of social machinery, which will ensure to every individual in the community a standard of living adequate for the maintenance of health."

The IOM defines public health as "organized community efforts aimed at the prevention of disease and promotion of health."

Public health is defined as the process of mobilizing local, state, national and international resources to solve the major health problems affecting communities and to achieve Health for All by 2000 AD.

Public Health Nursing

According to American Nurses Association (ANA, 1999) public health nursing is a population-focused community nursing practice with the goal of prevention of disease and disability by creating the conditions where people can be healthy.

Public health nursing (PHN) involves working with communities and populations as equal partners, and focusing on primary prevention and health promotion (ANA, 2007).

Public health nursing is the practice of promoting and protecting the health of populations using knowledge from nursing, social, and public health sciences (American Public Health Association, Public Health Nursing Section, 1996).

Community

"Community" implies people acting together in some way as a group, and the whole meaning more than the sum of its parts. A community is not just a collection of individuals; those individuals are part of something bigger, which has meaning for them and for others. The function of any community includes its members' collective sense of belonging and their shared identity, values, norms, communication, and common interests and concerns (Bruce and McKane, 2000; Clark, 2002).

Communities are "systems composed of individual members and sectors that have a variety of distinct characteristics and interrelationships." They can be defined by the characteristics of its people; geographic boundaries; shared values, interests, or history; or power dynamics (CDC, 1998).

> The definition of a community should take into account "opportunity for interpersonal and networking interactions within the unit" (Hancock et al., 1997).

The term community refers to a collection of people who interact with one another and whose common interests or characteristics form the basis for a sense of unity or belonging.

Community Health

> Community health refers to the health status of a defined group of people and the actions and conditions, both private and public (government), to promote, protect, and preserve their health.

Community Health Nursing

> Community health nursing is a synthesis of nursing practice and public health practice, applied to promoting and preserving the health of populations.

Health promotion, health maintenance, health education and management, coordination, and continuity of care are used in a holistic approach in the management of the health care of individuals, families, and groups in a community (ANA, 1986).

Community health nurses are on the front lines of health care and prevention of diseases and promotion of health. Community health nursing is the synthesis of nursing and public health practice applied to promote and protect the health of population. It combines all the basic elements of professional, clinical nursing with public health and community practice. Community health nursing is community based and most importantly, it is population focused. Operating within an environment of rapid change and increasingly complex challenges, this field of nursing holds the potential for positively shaping the quality of community health services and improving the health of the public.

Community health nursing, as a field of nursing, combines nursing science with public health science to formulate a community-based and population-focused practice (Williams, 2000).

Population Health

> Population health refers to the health status of people who are not organized and have no identity as a group or locality and the actions and conditions to promote, protect and preserve their health.

The term population health, which is similar to community health, has emerged in recent years. The primary difference between these two terms is the degree of organization or identity of the people. The focus of the population-based practice is to identify the problems of the population under care. Here, again, the identified problems are approached based on the priority.

SCOPE OF COMMUNITY HEALTH NURSING

In the "health care system" of any given country, public health care delivery accounts for the major share. Qualified health care professionals of different fields work together as a team to provide comprehensive care to the public. The core knowledge "public health" makes foundation for public and community health nursing.

> The WHO recommends that "basic nursing education for community health practice should prepare nurses to identify, assess, plan, implement, and evaluate the population at risk (WHO, 1985)".

The major areas of work for nurses are at the bedside, in the community, in hospitals and in homes. Nurses are the largest group of health care professionals who are always placed on the front lines of work. They are the primary point of contact for individuals/families and they function at the first level of decision-making. Community health nursing emphasizes on promotion of the health and provision of care to the individuals, families, and communities. Institute of Medicine's (IOM) report 2010 says, "By virtue of its numbers and adaptive capacity, the nursing profession has the potential to effect wide-reaching changes in the health care system."

Community health nurses practice in many settings in hospitals, primary health centers, community health centers, schools, homes, health clinics, long-term care facilities, various clinics like—mother care clinics, well baby clinics, lactation clinics, mobile clinics, immunization clinics, counseling centers, hospice centers, etc. They possess varying levels of education and skills. This community nursing education starts from licensed practical nurses, who take up the major share in contributing direct patient care in homes and primary health centers, to nurse scientist who works in researching and finding effective ways of promoting health, preventing the disease and protecting and maintaining the health.

> World health organization states that the community health-care system of many of the developing nations includes five layers, which are represented as: Individual care, family care, care and support by neighbors and known groups, support from health care providers and healers and support by local governments and community welfare organizations.

The scope of practice of community health nurses includes having collaboration as well being sensitive to the changes occurring with each layer of the system.

The roles and responsibilities of the community health nurse vary as per the policies, practices, health care demands, norms of the statutory bodies and service settings in which she functions.

Community health nurses work in close proximity to individuals, families, community, and other health team members. They serve as real key players to make contracts and partnerships to provide quality care in the community. The community health nurses usually win the confidence of their clients and are considered trustworthy. This helps them in collecting appropriate client data, which facilitates in identifying strengths, weaknesses, and further needs of the individuals and families.

Community health nurses take up many roles in day-to-day practice. However, there is always one primary role.

ROLES OF COMMUNITY HEALTH NURSES (FIG. 1)

- Nurse clinician
- Nurse educator
- Nurse advocate
- Nurse manager
- Nurse collaborator
- Nurse leader
- Nurse researcher.

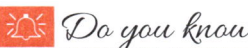 *Do you know*

In any setting, the role of community health nurse focuses on the prevention of illness, injury, or disability; the promotion of health; and maintenance of health.

Nurse Clinician

The most common and well-known role of the nurse is of a clinician or a care provider. However, in the context of

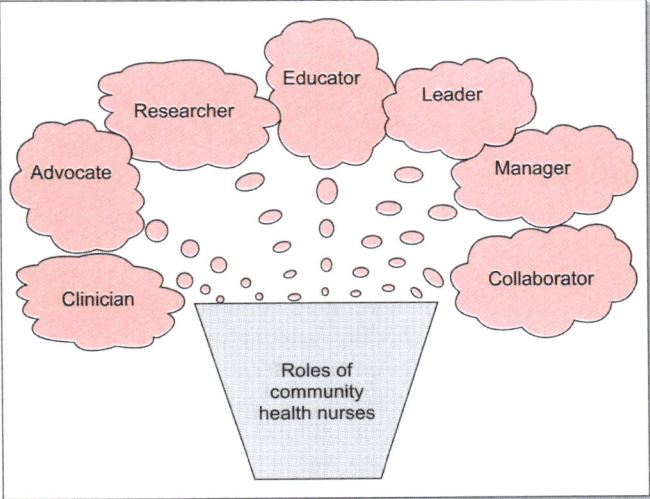

Figure 1: Role of community health nurses

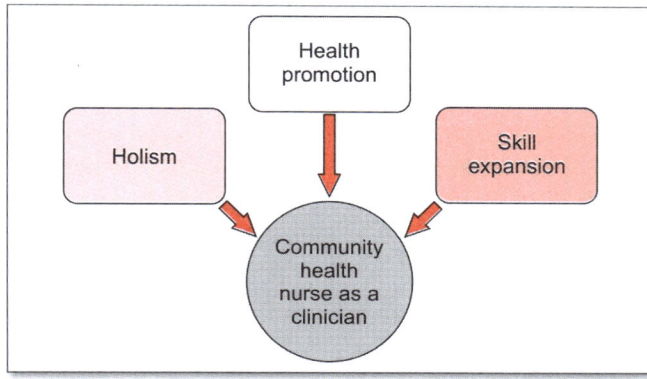

Figure 2: Roles of community health nurse as a clinician

community health nursing, the role of a clinician comes with various practical challenges. The **clinician** role in community health appropriates the health services to individuals and families, to groups and populations. A nurse's role as a clinician in the hospital focuses only on individuals and their families.

The clinician role of a nurse in community is differentiated from the clinician role in a hospital with a specific emphasis on holism, health promotion and skill expansion (Fig. 2).

Nurse Educator

The most important and popular role of the community health nurse is that of an educator or nurse-health teacher. Nurses act as educators to individuals or groups and community. Health teaching is a well-known component of community health nursing practice and a basic weapon in preventing behavior-oriented communicable diseases and noncommunicable diseases. Community health nurses in the capacity of health educators facilitate client's learning and create awareness on health matters. Client receives information both formally and informally. Considering the concept of self-care, clients are oriented to use appropriate health resources and seek out health information for themselves. The process of health teaching focuses on disease prevention and health promotion throughout.

Nurse Advocate

Community health nurses are the most easily available and approachable guides for people's advocacy. They explain about the health care system, advice on diseases, provide referrals, and guide them for follow-up. In community, people need someone to guide them through the complex system and assure the satisfaction of their needs.

The nurse advocate role sets certain criteria like being assertive, willing to take risks, communicating and negotiating, and identifying resources and obtaining results.

Nurse Manager

As a manager, the nurse exercises administrative direction towards the accomplishment of specified goals by assessing clients' needs; planning and organizing to meet those needs; directing and leading to achieve results; and controlling and evaluating the progress to ensure that goals are met.

Nurse Collaborator

Community health nurses take up the role of **collaborator**, in which they work together with others toward a common goal or purpose.

Community health nurses work in government or private firms in collaboration with other nurses, physicians, teachers, health educators, social workers, physical therapists, nutritionists, occupational therapists, psychologists, epidemiologists, biostatisticians and legislators.

Nurse Researcher

Literature provides the base for evidence-based community health nursing practice. Active questions relating to current knowledge and practice and finding an answer through research will contribute to the existing knowledge of community health nursing.

Nurse Leader

Community health nursing is purely a matter of knowing people; their needs and problems, and working in collaboration to find solutions for the problems. Community health nurse needs to be an able leader and administrator to tackle people from various religion castes, culture and backgrounds.

According to WHO, new nurse graduates should be trained as generalists with strengths in community health nursing interventions to meet the challenges of community health care rather than specialists in community health care.

WORK SITES OF COMMUNITY HEALTH NURSE

Home Care

Community health nurses provide care in the houses of people since time immemorial. The services may include preventive, promotive, curative and rehabilitative. Present days, community health nursing concentrates more on family centered care. Basically the very structure, functions, and processes of the family predisposes the individual family member's health or illness leading to overall health status of the family (Fig. 3).

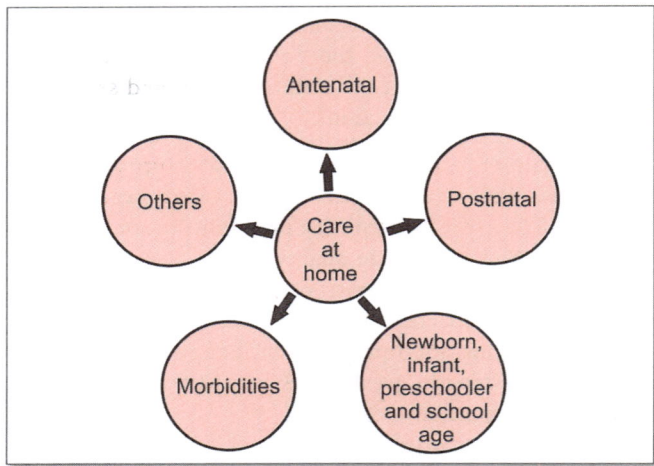

Figure 3: Care at home by community health nurse

Family refers to two or more individuals, who depend on one another for emotional, physical, and economical support. The members of the family are self defined.
(Hanson, 2005)

Family health is a dynamic changing state of well-being, which includes the biological, psychological, spiritual, sociological, and cultural factors of individual members and the whole family system. *(Hanson, 2005)*

Family meets the basic needs of the family members. Some of them may include identity, affection, food, shelter, clothing and protection. Community health nurses have focussed on family care role even during yester years. It is easy to understand the "ripple effect" when you observe and work amidst the family. Ripple effect refers to "the changes in individual member of the family are reflected as changes in the family." Community health nurse provides care at home to newborn, infants, preschoolers, school aged, antenatal, postnatal mothers, and persons with acute and chronic illnesses. Apart, health promotion, health protection and health maintenance and rehabilitation are the most prominent roles of the community health nurses at home.

School Health Nurse

School is the most popular work site of community health nurse. Health promotion, periodical health checkup, immunization, nutrition, screening for diseases and treatment of minor ailments and referrals are the functions of the school health nurse. In previous decades, community health nurses performed periodical checkup, health promotion and disease prevention activities in government-schools of India. Primary health centers are responsible to conduct screening and periodical checkups in their assigned areas and community health nurses take significant role in it. In addition, in recent years, many private owned schools appoint community health nurses in the designation of health officer to take care of health activities in the school. In recent years, some corporate hospitals in India also have started to concentrate on school health by appointing BSc and MSc nursing graduates as nursing health officers.

In Industries

Western countries offer masters degree in occupational health nursing. Nevertheless, in most developing countries community health nurses play the role. They work in factories and industries to perform health promotion, disease prevention, health protection, and maintenance activities among the workers. Occupational health nursing also extends the care to members of the family. Reviewing the folders of the family members would help in knowing the family's strength and stressors of the individual and plan his care accordingly.

Occupational health nurses actively participate in:

- Promotion of nutrition
- Personal hygiene and health maintenance
- Prevention of communicable diseases and environmental sanitation
- Promotion of mental health
- Promotion of small family norm
- Health education
- Counseling and training programs.

COMMUNITY HEALTH NURSES AND THEIR EDUCATION IN INDIA

Indian Nursing Council took great interest in providing higher-level importance for community health nursing in curriculum. Community health nursing is found as a core subject in all the basic courses like multipurpose health workers (MPWs), diploma in general nursing and midwifery (DGNM), basic BSc nursing and post basic BSc nursing India, holding the second most populous country of the world needs more number of community health nurses to tackle the challenges in the community. In India, the "primary level care" in the community is mostly shouldered by the MPWs whose educational preparation is minimum to meet the challenges of community.

There are different educational levels with which community health nurses function in the field of community: Diploma in General Nursing and Midwifery (DGNM) and Bachelor of Science in Nursing (BSc) nurses work in primary health centers and community health centers and community clinics. BSc nursing degree holders can work as tutors in nursing schools and colleges and as "public health nursing tutors" in community training centers. Master degree holders in community health nursing specialty are eligible to function from "tutor" to "professor cum principal level" based on their experience and

norms set by "Indian Nursing Council". Nurses with "MSc in community health nursing specialization" are eligible to pursue PhD and later post-nursing doctoral education.

> As per Indian Nursing Council, PhD is the desirable qualification to function as principal or vice principal in nursing colleges.

PRINCIPLES OF COMMUNITY HEALTH NURSING

In community health nursing practice, nurses build their expertise in a specialty area and demonstrate skills using following principles:

- Promote, protect and preserve health, prevent disease and injury.
- Promote, protect and preserve the environment that contributes to health.
- Advocate for healthy public policy.
- Lead in the integration of comprehensive and multiple health promotion approaches that build the capacity of patients.
- Respect the diversity of clients and caregivers, focus on the linkages between health and illness experiences and enable the clients to achieve health.
- Provide evidence-based informed care in a variety of settings such as the patient's home, school, office, clinics, on the street, communal living settings or workplace.
- Cooperate, coordinate and collaborate with a variety of partners, disciplines, and sectors.
- Recognize that healthy communities and systems that support health and contribute to health for all. Engage a range of resources to support health by coordinating care, and planning services, and programs.
- Work with a high degree of autonomy to initiate strategies that will address the determinants of health and positively impact people and their community.

HISTORY OF DEVELOPMENT OF COMMUNITY HEALTH—GLOBALLY

Modern public health system started to take a shape some 150 years ago. The major factors that contributed to the community development are knowledge on causes and control of diseases and cooperation extended from the public to accept the process of disease prevention and control. Scientific knowledge provided a platform to public health authorities to initiate various activities like educating mass on various aspects of health to enhance individual responsibility on personal health. Public sanitation, immunization and health regulations were given large attention to perpetuate the human life.

Advancing technology, high expectations of people and increasing burden of elderly population resulted in escalating costs on health care in industrial countries. Further, people of developing countries live amidst of poverty with unmet needs.

Ancient Societies

Archaeological research activities at sites of some of the earliest civilizations indicated the evidences for community health activities.

Archaeological findings from the Indus Valley of Northern India, dating from about 2000 BC, reveal the evidence of bathrooms and drains in homes and sewers below street level.

It was evident from ruins of ancient Egypt (2700–2000 BC) that drainage facilities were in place in houses and streets. The Mycenaean who lived in 1600 BC had the facilities like toilets, flushing systems, and sewers. They had the practice of burying famous people in large, circular tombs with possessions to go along with them in the next world. Egyptians were aware of more than 700 drugs in 1500 BC itself.

It is hard to trace most community practices of early communities due to the missing records or evidences. They were strict in insisting people not to defecate near the drinking water sources. Herbal use was prominent to cure the diseases. Shared roles within a family and the community helped the mothers in labor and child rearing practices. They followed specific customs and practices related to burial of the dead.

Hippocrates (460 BC) highlighted the importance of environment and human behaviors in health.

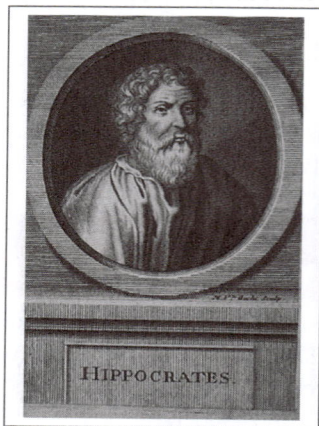

Classical Cultures (500 BC to AD 500)

It is widely accepted fact that basic sciences like anatomy, physiology and psychology were of importance to identify the cause of the diseases as well to promote health. Medical schools started and the popular philosophy noted was "Methodists" that equals medical thinking. **Asclepius** was the founder of Methodist medical school that stressed on health maintenance and understanding the patient and his health.

The Greeks showed interest in community sanitation. They had the practice of meeting the water requirements of the city by storing water in huge cisterns placed high above the sea level. Hippocrates believed practicing medicine in a scientific way based on the natural sciences. Hippocrates is the founder of ancient Greek medicine. Hippocrates wanted physicians to study anatomy, especially that of the spine and its relationship to the nervous system that controlled all functions of the body. He advised to keep wound dry after cleaning with wine or water for quick healing. The ancient Greeks believed that body and mind should be in harmony to maintain good health. Physical activity was considered as a vital component of the training in schools to promote physical and mental health. **Galen** was one of the great physicians after Hippocrates.

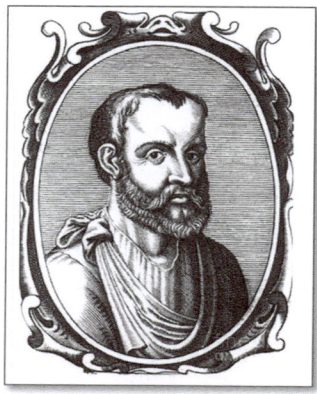

Galen

Romans outperformed Greeks in promoting the evolution of nursing. Roman armies developed war-nursing units in which nurses took care of injured soldiers. Initially these nurses were selected from family members, servants or slaves. However, Roman era gave importance to nursing discipline and nursing grew as a separate discipline. Initially the hospitals were set in corridors and dormitories, which were later converted into hospitals.

Middle Ages (500–1500 AD)

Before the Eighteenth Century

Communicable diseases that ended up in epidemics were identified as a threat to humanity. Public health system of the nations tried to protect the people from diseases like smallpox, cholera, etc. Strict practices on isolation of ill and quarantine of travellers were adopted to protect people from dreadful communicable diseases. European cities enforced isolation, quarantine practices related to communicable diseases and advised to report the deaths from plague. People gradually accepted to take up inoculations administered from smallpox scab to prevent smallpox.

Decline of Roman dynasty pulled down the developments in community health organization.

Though there were some developments in the field of health care man showed interest in believing superstitions, his brain went empty. People started to construct big houses to get the feel of "safe home". Big buildings and huge wall around the house invited overcrowding, poor sanitation and poor hygiene.

There was no provision for clean water, waste disposal and sanitation. People threw the garbage on the street and no health behavior seen in people. People did not show interest in their health and environment. People seldom bathed since they believed it was immoral to look at their bodies. Though people lacked knowledge on health, hospitals emerged to take care of needy like sick, old and neglected individuals. Emergent of many monasteries and convents to take care of sick provided a strong foundation for the development of nursing activities.

Practice of nurses joining military orders during the time of Crusades started between 1091 and 1291.

Initially, Christian services started through churches to care only sick, poor and fatherless. Crusaders came up with hospitals with a gained knowledge from Arabs. During this era, many nuns came forward to care patients. Health education gained importance to enhance personal hygiene. Christianity took interest in inculcating the concept of responsibility for self and others which taught people to show positive attitude in caring sick people. Some books written on health promotion created awareness among people. A changed philosophy on community health and personal health emerged with Christian era.

Renaissance (1500 AD to 1700 AD)

People gradually changed their attitude toward health. People with superstitious beliefs slowly took a transition to make intellectual inquiries. There was a growing interest advancing science and technology that facilitated the developments in medicine and public health field.

In 1601 the Church of England introduced, "Elizabethan poor law" and made it compulsory.

This made people care for poor, blind, orphans and lame. Wealthy people took care of the sick at home by paying nurses. Poor did not have means to do so. Under the directions of "Poor law", sick poor were taken care in hospitals or alms houses. Many people arrived hospital with advanced sickness/ diseases. So most often they died in the hospital itself. Graunt was the first person who analyzed the bills of mortality, which documented the weekly counts of births and deaths in London. **Graunt published** the results of his findings in the year 1662 in "*Natural and Political Observations...Made upon the Bills of Mortality*".

Eighteenth Century

Many cities like New York, Boston came forward to enforce quarantine and isolation measures. Initially the neighbors in local communities cared people with physical and mental illnesses. Later this became official in England by adoption of "1601- poor law". Due to the increase in number of sick people, the demand for care also went high where poor law practices could not help it. As a result in 1752 the first American voluntary hospital was established in Philadelphia for people who were physically ill. The first public mental hospital was established in Williamsburg, Virginia in 1773. (Turner, 1977).

During 18th century James Lind, a surgeon from British navy strengthened the foundations of epidemiology through his contribution on *scurvy.*

Based on Lind's findings British navy made lemon juice as a compulsory one in sailors' diets. This strategy had helped to eradicate scurvy from the British navy. In late 18th century (1760) industrial revolution began in England. Government took no efforts to improve health care system until 18th century.

Nineteenth Century

Due to increased urbanization people of London suffered many diseases like smallpox, cholera, typhoid, and tuberculosis to reach unimaginable numbers. Survey of 16th ward of New York identified more than 1,200 cases of smallpox and more than 2,000 cases of typhus. (Winslow, 1923). In Massachusetts in 1850, deaths from tuberculosis were 300 per 100,000 populations, and infant mortality was about 200 per 1,000 live births. (Hanlon and Pickett, 1984).

Toward mid-19th century there was tremendous advancement in public health. During this period filth was identified as the reason for disease and its transmission. This provided a basic platform for change in people's perception and thought about health. Illness, considered as the reflection of poor moral, spiritual, living and environmental conditions. Hygiene, faithfulness and isolation were recognized measures to prevent the disease. This period was referred to "**The great sanitary awakening**." (Winslow, 1923). Sanitation and public health became the focus to protect public health from diseases and maintain sound health.

The huge cholera epidemic of 1832 grabbed the attention of Edwin Chadwick, a London lawyer to show a great interest in the "**sanitary reform movement**".

As a basic step Chadwick assessed the health status of people with a view to improve people's living conditions. The "Poor law commission" of London conducted studies of the life and health of the working class in 1838 and that of the entire country in 1842 under the head of Chadwick. This study documented the poor working conditions of industrial towns and rural areas of the United Kingdom that have compelled their deaths.

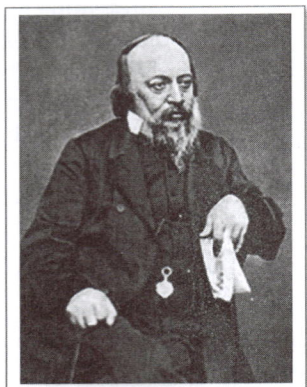

Sir Edwin Chadwick

Chadwick assumed that the diseases occurred by bad air from the decomposed waste; **Chadwick** proposed to build a drainage network to remove sewage and waste. He also recommended that to local national board of health. His suggestions adopted in the **Public Health Act of 1848** and his work influenced later developments in public health in England and the United States. After Chadwick's report, many cities showed interest in conducting surveys.

Lemuel Shattuck, a Massachusetts bookseller and statistician published a survey *Report of the Massachusetts Sanitary Commission* in 1850. Shattuck's report highlighted the importance of adopting various measures to improve health conditions.

Shattuck's recommendations are as follows:

Establishment of state health departments, sanitary surveys, cleanliness, morality, personal responsibility, surveys of local health conditions, supervision of water supplies and waste disposal, census and vital health statistics were some measures included in the report to control the diseases. He also expected services to public under the names: well childcare, school age children's health, immunization, mental health, health education for all and health planning.

Shattuck's report was very much revolutionary toward public health mission and scope. Unfortunately, his report was accepted and recognized only after his death. After much contradiction, Shattuck's report was considered as one of the most farsighted and influential documents in the history of the American public health system.

Edward Jenner of Berkeley found that persons who developed cowpox never got smallpox, a deadly disease. He had saved many lives with his discovery of **"smallpox vaccination."** With his wonderful discovery in 1980 the smallpox disease was declared as eradicated.

William Farr (1839) stressed the importance of vital statistics for studying health problems. This century started to have many successful events in controlling communicable diseases.

John Snow, English physician, a specialist in obstetric anesthesiology, was interested to find the cause and spread of cholera epidemics that occurred periodically in London. In 1854, Snow started his inquiries during the third cholera epidemics. While most physicians attributed the disease to miasma (bad air) Snow, held the deep-seated view that cholera was caused by contact with germ contaminated matter, particularly bad water. Snow's collected details revealed that the cholera spreads through contaminated water. After resolving the cholera epidemics in London, **John Snow** was given the title of **"Father of modern epidemiology".**

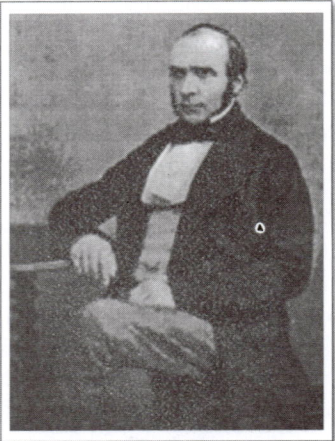

John Snow

In **1877 Louis Pasteur**, a French chemist, proved that anthrax is caused by bacteria. In 1884, with his untiring efforts he could develop an artificial immunization against anthrax. The germ theory of disease took a lead role in providing scientific foundation for public health.

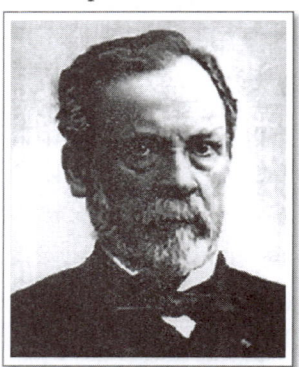

Louis Pasteur

Laboratory research revealed exact causes and specific methods for preventing every single disease. The fact that disease had single, specific cause was brought to light. Science also revealed that both the environment and people could be the agents of disease. In 1891, WT Sedgwick, biologist for Massachusetts, identified the presence of fecal bacteria in water as the cause of typhoid fever and voluntarily developed the first sewage treatment techniques. His work focussed on improving environmental sanitation.

Twentieth Century

During 20th century, people started looking beyond the traditional concept of protecting people from polluted environment and communicable diseases. More attention was paid to preventive behavior and lifestyle-oriented diseases and its prevention and reduction. In this period, people started to understand the relationship between bacteria and communicable diseases. After the initial few decades of 20th century, there was a great planning among the health experts to provide significant importance on provision of safe water and sanitation, nutrition, control of communicable diseases and specific immunizations.

🔔 *Do you know*

One of the biggest challenges of 20th century was HIV/AIDS. According to UNAIDS, there were 30 million HIV-related deaths globally during this period.

In the early 20th century, home visits offered by public health nurses in New York and Baltimore. School health clinics were established in Boston (1894), New York (1903) and in Rhode Island (1906) to support and promote the health of school going children. In 1906, Food and Drug Act passed to control the manufacture, labeling, and sale of food. An expert like Winslow exclaimed at the improved work of sanitary engineering and bacteriology in preventing people from diseases. Contemporary diseases like obesity, hypertension, and accidents grabbed the attention of health professionals and health system. One of the biggest challenges that emerged during late 20th century was HIV/AIDS.

According to UNAIDS there were 30 million HIV related deaths globally during this period. In 1923, CEA Winslow defined public health as the science not only preventing contagious disease, but also "prolonging life, and promoting physical health and efficiency." Federal Board of Maternity and Infant Hygiene was established by Sheppard-Towner Act(1922) to provide funds to the Children's Bureau and states to establish maternal and child health programs. This act was the first to assist personal health services through federal funding.

Twenty First Century

We are in the second decade of 21st century. There are many developments occurring in the field of community health and community health nursing. Community partnership research is a greatly encouraged methodology to place people's health in their hands and sensitizing their personal accountability on health.

DEVELOPMENT OF COMMUNITY HEALTH NURSING—GLOBALLY

In ancient period, nursing care was rendered in home setting. This is evident from the new testament that there was a practice of visiting sick people at home to speed up their recovery.

Nursing care in 20th century was mainly associated with hospital settings.

In ancient days, family members only provided nursing care to each other. The first nurse was the first mother. Elders of the families who had lived in experiences on handling health-related issues provided consultation to their own family members and guided them.

DEVELOPMENT OF PUBLIC HEALTH NURSING: SIGNIFICANT EVENTS WORLDWIDE

In the **middle Ages**, family members only took care of the sick and ill. Few hospitals run by monks and nuns could be affordable only by the wealthy. Overcrowding, lack of sanitation and increasing population caused persistent epidemics. Black Plague of 14th century killed about one-fourth of the population of Europe. From the 1500s through the 1700s, the renaissance in **Europe** stimulated the rise of scientific thought and social consciousness.

The Sisters (or Daughters) of Charity or "Grey Sisters," was founded in 1617 in **France**, with the aim of providing care to the sick poor.

The mission was successful and taken from the rural districts to Paris. In 1633, a training program established for young women to serve needy people. By 19th century, this nursing community had established itself throughout the world for providing care to the poor sick. The motherhouse "Sisters of Charity" is located in Paris.

With many reforms by 1825, **England** had established around 154 hospitals; but it was not possible to bring down the fatality rates. Many deaths occurred among newborns and people with open wound.

People were afraid to go to hospitals and addressed hospitals as, "death houses".

The main reason indicated was the caregivers in the hospitals were only "ward maids" means housekeepers.

In **Holland**, women appointed by churches to care for the poor called as deaconess-groups.

In 1836, Theodor Fliedner, a German Lutheran pastor, started 3 years training school for Deaconesses, following which parish districts founded to provide care to residents.

Florence Nightingale, daughter of Wealthy English family, committed to prevent illness and death. In 1851, she attended **Theodor Fliedner's** program for Deaconesses—for nurse training—in Kaiserswerth, **Germany**. Florence took a lead role with a team of nurses and assisted soldiers during the **Crimean War** (1854–1856). This is a recorded historical event saved lives through prevention of infections and improving.

During Victorian era, poorhouses accommodated chronically ill poor people, who were often elderly and did not have family or any other support. Some "pauper nurses" assigned were poor, illiterate, intoxicated and were cruel to residents.

In 1859, William Rathbone, a Quaker merchant and philanthropist of England hired **Mary Robinson**, a nurse (who later named as the **first district nurse**) to take care of people in one of the poorest parish districts in Liverpool. Soon the mission of district nursing started disseminated from Liverpool to other places. Rathbone took assistance from Florence Nightingale one who attended Theodor Fliedner's nurse training program for deaconesses in Kaiserswerth, Germany. Nightingale with her team of nurses assisted soldiers during the Crimean War (1854–1856) and promptly recorded her successes with necessary statistical diagrams. In 1860, following the war, Nightingale started the first school of nursing, and Rathbone hired several graduates as district nurses. Two years later, with Nightingale's assistance, he established a nursing school in Liverpool.

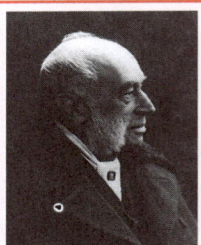

William Rathbone showed great concern and interest in nursing which "... occupied more than half his life ... he was the founder of district nursing ... [and] he recognized the importance of effective training for all nurses. He was also largely responsible for improved workhouse conditions ..." (Gwen Hardy William Rathbone and the Early History of District Nursing, 1981, p. 5).

William Rathbone

During mid-20th century (1930–1970), there was great expansion in the roles of the government in encouraging personal health. **National League for Nursing** (NLN) has predicted 10 trends in health care that will affect nursing in forthcoming decades:

1. Population dynamics
2. Proliferating technology
3. Globalization of the world's economy and society
4. Educated consumers, alternative therapies and genomics, and palliative care
5. Focus on population-based care
6. Rise in health care costs and challenges of managed care
7. Impact of health policy and regulation
8. Growing necessity for interdisciplinary education and collaborative practice
9. Nursing shortages, opportunities for lifelong learning, and workforce development
10. Significant advances in nursing science and research.

Initiatives in United States

At the beginning of 19th century people were well aware about the then existing health care system and were in need of an organized system. In 1809, the **Sisters of Charity** (also called Daughters of Charity) founded by **Elizabeth Ann Seton** came up with many hospitals, orphanages, and educational institutions to help people. In 1813, the **Ladies' Benevolent Society of Charleston**, South Carolina, started to provide organized home care services to the sick.

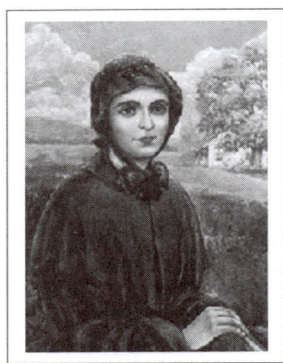

Elizabeth Ann Seton

In 1836, Dorothea Dix met William Rathbone in Liverpool, England. During that time, the "lunacy reform movement of England" published detailed investigations on madhouses resulted in legislative changes. After returning from England in 1840, Dix also visited jails and insane asylums in Massachusetts. After a compelling report from Dix funds allocated to establish the first hospitals for the mentally ill.

Clara Barton widely recognized for her social interest during the Civil War; she distributed supplies, cared for the injured soldiers and casualties with a team of nurses. She served as a major cause for establishing American Red Cross Society to provide aid for natural disasters.

In the 1880s, 20 years after the establishment of district nursing in England, a similar movement began in the United States to combat the challenges caused by unsanitary conditions and infectious diseases.

Lillian Wald was a nurse passed out from New York Hospital School of Nursing. In 1893, Wald and her classmate Mary Brewster founded the Henry Street Settlement and they considered the affordability of patients while fixing fee. In addition to care they also delivered classes on health and hygiene. Wald addressed her services as "public health nursing." Soon many other settlement houses developed in American cities. Lillian Wald known as the founder of public health nursing. Gradually the Henry Street Settlement developed a team of 20 nurses and offered array of innovative and effective social, recreational, and educational services. Later, the Henry Street Settlement changed its name as the Visiting Nurse Association of New York City.

In 1912, Wald assisted to find the **National Organization for Public Health Nursing**.

The first professional standards for the practice of public health nursing were set by this organization. These standards served as a precursor to ANA's *Public Health Nursing: Scope and Standards of Practice*, which guides the practice of public health nursing today. Wald insisted to appoint first professor of nursing in institutions of higher learning that laid the foundation for higher nursing education.

During 20th century, there was a tremendous growth in the field of public health nursing. Federal governments recognized public health nursing as one of the most vital area. Initially the focus of public health nurses were to render care at the bedside, but later changed their idea thinking that it may not yield good results in unsanitary and poor houses which had no food. Public health nurses functioned as role models to others to care for the sick, instructing them on how to prevent illness, and promoting maternal and child health.

Mary Breckinridge the founder of "Frontier nursing" traveled on horseback, and assessed the health situations and needs of the mountain people.

In 1939, she helped to establish the Frontier Graduate School of Midwifery, one of the first midwifery programs in the country. The number of public health nurses employed by industry almost doubled during this time. The discipline of public health nursing expanded in rural areas after World War I and II where many countries were involved.

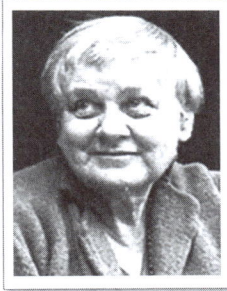
Mary Breckinridge

CHALLENGES OF 21ST CENTURY FOR COMMUNITY HEALTH NURSING

Many unexpected changes may occur in this 21st century all over the world in the field of health/nursing/community health nursing. There are chances for serious transformation that may dominate the environment along with the changes in other areas like culture, beliefs, practice, technology, and economy.

Evidence-based Practice

In this fast growing customer, oriented quality driven world the major weapon to be used in practice is "Evidence-based practice" Evidence-based public health is a public health venture in which there is cautious use of evidence derived from variety of sciences and social sciences research. Most often community health nurses use the evidences from the field of epidemiologic research to assess their clients and for planning and implementing care in the community. Evidence based practice helps in updating of knowledge and skill to function as a real-time clinician.

Growing Cultural Interaction

This is one of the issue in the front line which seeks the nurses to be culturally competent as well recognize the assessment needs pertaining to increasing interaction among different cultures.

COMMUNITY HEALTH IN BRITISH INDIA

It is evident from the history that the ancient people of India focused on birth, health, illness, and deaths and no religion or culture was ignorant of these factual events. Though the early society did not own much technology base they still adapted efficient practices like choosing the burial place and waste disposal areas away from the living areas. They also developed sewage systems, and draining marshes to control communicable disease. The family and community attended the sick people on most occasions. The main caregivers of ancient time were usually women. These early caregivers practiced heat and cold applications to relieve pain, immobilized fractures for better healing, dressed the wounds with herbs cultivated by them, delivered babies and took great work to attend dead bodies. Knowing the genesis of the profession would help us with the background knowledge for better understanding the characteristics of nursing profession and activities of today.

The British Company gained footing in India in 1612 after Mughal emperor Jahangir granted the rights to establish a factory (a trading post) in Surat to Sir Thomas Roe, a representative diplomat of Queen Elizabeth-I of England.

Bengal became the first victim of the British rule in India. The war at the field of Plassey, located in south of Murshidabad on June 23, 1757 made the foundation for British rule in India. The Battle of Plassey helped the English to grab the wealth of Bengal. The victory of British in the battle of Plassey changed the fate of a mere trading company into a political power. Following the Government of India Act in1858, the British government took up the administration of India. British rule in India lasted from 1757 to 1947 for the period of about 190 years.

DEVELOPMENT OF COMMUNITY HEALTH NURSING IN INDIA— PREINDEPENDENCE (TABLE 1)

Community nursing has been continuously growing and changing in response to government policy and ever changing needs of the communities. Prior to independence colonial British officials and missionaries took bigger efforts to design and construct the framework for nursing. During British rule India received funds and help from both Britain and USA. This had a great influence in giving directions to the development of nursing profession in India. British officials inculcated the image of a professional nurse that may include but not limited to high professionalism, noble dedication, and decorum.

Caring for the sick people confined to bed was the realm of the family. People perceived woman as selfless caregiver for her family members. And again, nursing care of the family members was the extended duty of her household work. The *Susruta Samhita*, (600–350 BCE) described four types of midwives and among which one was "good at giving birth to a child (*prajananakusalah*)". The text also recommends that the midwife should be a female who assisted with childbirth. The indigenous, rural midwife, "*dai*" the female who rendered the care giving services in India. *Dais*, were from low-caste, primarily worked in villages, conducted deliveries and engaged in midwifery services. In order to reach the aim of having a professional modern Indian nurse, caste was a great challenge to British colonial officials.

British officials wanted to admire idealized cleanliness and rationality whereas the *dai* was an ignorant, superstitious lady who never gave importance for cleanliness or hygiene in her care practices. Efforts to develop modern midwifery in India started in 19th century and concentrated on training Indian *dais*. The Government of Madras sanctioned a training school for midwives in the year 1854 which offered a diploma in midwifery. Missionaries started to train "*dais*" in the field midwifery in late 1860s. St Stephen's Hospital, Delhi, in 1867 started to provide training to Indian women in a systematic nursing training course.

Colonial British and American officials strongly believed that education would help Indian nurses to understand the profession and to surpass the perception of branding nursing as a as a low-caste profession.

During 19th century hospitals in England was equaled to death houses and the nurses were drunk and disordered as we discussed earlier. For Nightingale, it became important to make nursing an acceptable profession for women and she also felt that this was possible only by boosting the morale through necessary respect. Her very entry to nursing profession, improved the image and respect of nurses in England since Nightingale was from a wealthy family. Nightingale's model of nursing recognized women nurses and the practice of paying for their services introduced. This enhanced the professional image of nurses all over the world. Nursing model of Nightingale was adopted by other countries United States and Australia. British colonial officials adopted and replicated the same ideas to develop the nursing profession in India. These modern nursing thoughts developed from **Florence Nightingale** played a significant role in professionalizing and inculcating nursing culture in India.

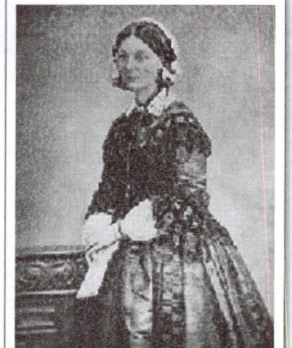
Florence Nightingale

According to a historian British officials in India did not show much interest to the health of Indian women prior to 1885. Though Florence Nightingale never visited India, her ideas stood front in influencing the creation of the Royal Sanitary Commission in 1859 on the Health of the British Army stationed in India. Consequent to the report of Royal Sanitary Commission in 1863, **the Indian Nursing Service (INS)** was created in 1888 to provide proper nursing care for British soldiers. The INS was renamed as the **Queen Alexandra's Military Nursing Service for India (QAIMNS)** in 1903. Nurses of QAIMNS served during World War I.

The Vicereine, **Lady Dufferin**, in 1883 established "**Dufferin Fund**" at Queen Victoria's request to supply medical aid to Indian women. This fund also extended financial support to provide tuition to doctors and nurses and midwives. The Vicereine, Lady Minto, launched the Indian Nursing Association in 1906. The Minto Nurses' were mainly trained to provide nursing care primarily to European families.

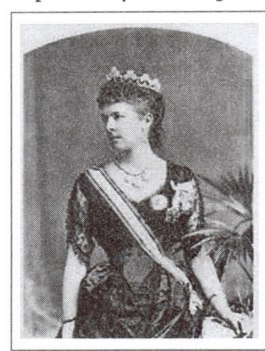
Lady Dufferin

The Trained Nurses Association of India (TNAI) formed in 1908 at the conference held for Association of Nursing Superintendents in Bombay (now Mumbai).

There was an evergrowing focus on maternal and child health in India. From 1920, it was believed that the community health nurses role is significant to bring changes in health and politics. In 1918 **Lady Chelmsford** provided great support in starting training courses for health visitors and maternity supervisors. A "Health school" was opened in Delhi with the grants from government, which was later named as "Lady Reading School".

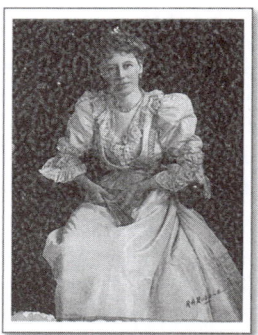
Lady Chelmsford

In the Indian history of development upper class British women had significant importance because they always stood forefront for developing Indian women's education and training. In addition, upper class Indian women entered the political field during the 1920–30 following their participation in the nationalist movement. Witnessing collectivism and unity among Indian and British women, both British and Indian nurses developed unity about "global sisterhood."

In 1920–30 British and American officials showed strong interest in establishing professional organizations. As influenced the provincial governments legislated nurse registration acts in late 1920s and Tamil Nadu Nurses and Midwives Act for registering nurses introduced in 1926. In 1922 **Griffin** launched a new wing for health visitors under TNAI in the name of **"health visitors league"**. This was renamed as "association for ANMS" from 1970 onwards.

By 1931 health schools started in Punjab and Calcutta for training health visitors. The Red Cross Society also started health schools in Nagpur, Chennai and Calcutta. But involvement of nurses in India those days was not paradoxically balanced between hospitals and community, the focus was primarily in the hospitals. Major proportion of nurses worked in hospitals rather than in community health programs. However, nursing leaders of India considered community health as an important branch of nursing. In 1938, Florence Nightingale memorial scholarship to pursue further training in England announced. This obligated nurses to write on public health titles like maternal and child health, nutrition, school health, etc.

With the support from the **Rockfeller Foundations,** seven health centers were established from 1931 to 1939 in the cities of Delhi, Madras, Bangalore, Luknow, Trivandrum, Pune and Calcutta. In 1942 there were severe "shortage of trained nurses. Following which the Auxiliary Nursing Service (ANS) was established. Auxiliary nurses were given 6 months training in civil hospitals and appointed as assistant nurses to serve the colonial army.

Diana Hartley, a British nurse , the editor of "Nursing Journal of India" between 1935 and 1944 in her writings stated that the Indian nurses sick and lived in poor conditions. In 1944 TNAI strongly suggested and recommended to include "Public health nursing" nursing in nurse's basic training.

Four years bachelor program for nursing was first established in India in 1946 at the Colleges of Nursing in Delhi and christian medical college and hospital (CHCH) Vellore.

The Rajkumari Amrit Kaur College of Nursing, New Delhi, under Ministry of Health and Family Welfare established in 1946 with the aim of developing model programs in nursing education.

College of Nursing in New Delhi, CMC Hospital Vellore and the Government General Hospital Madras started to offer Post-certificate courses in nursing administration, supervision and teaching even prior to 1947.

All the above educational foundations helped in developing qualified and skillful nursing graduates who could use scientific rationale while practicing in hospital as well in community.

Table 1: Significant milestones of public health development in British India

Year	Events
1757	The British had established the civil and military services sooner they captured the power to rule India.
1825	**Quarantine Act:** A public health policy emerged in 14th century following "Black Death." Under this quarantine system traveler and merchandise who came from known infected places or regions were isolated to protect people.
1829	**Royal Commission** appointed in India. It served to find out the reasons for the poor health status of British Army. This commission had recommended to establish "Commission of Public Health" mainly to protect water sources, and provide drainage facilities with a view to prevent epidemics and maintain the health of the civilians thereby protect their army.
1864	Establishment of **sanitary commissions** at Bombay, Madras and Bengal. The Civil Surgeons/District Medical Officers became ex-officio District Health Officers.
1869	A **Public Health Commissioner** and a **Statistical Officer** appointed by government of India.
1873	A **Birth and Death Registration Act came in to force** to register and maintain the birth and death data all over India
1880	The **Vaccination Act** introduced. This act had the power to prohibit inoculation and to make the vaccination of children compulsory.
1881	The **Indian Factories Act** introduced. This Act was designed to protect children from child labor and to develop necessary measures to promote health and safety of the workers.
1885	The **Local Self-Government Act** launched.
1888	The **Government of India assigned local bodies** responsible for sanitation. Though they were assigned for sanitation no public health staff was brought into look after sanitation
1896	The **Plague Commission** was appointed.
1897	The **Epidemic Diseases Act** was passed. The epidemic disease act focused on protecting people from dangerous epidemic diseases.
1904	The **Plague Commission report** submitted. Plague commission suggested to reorganize, expand public health departments with facilities for research and production of vaccines.

Contd…

Year	Events
1909	The **Central Malaria Bureau** founded at **Kasauli**. Initially concentrated only on malarial activities. Later, shifted to Delhi, on July 30, 1963 and named as **"The National Institute of Communicable Diseases"** to cover all other communicable diseases under its umbrella.
1911	The **Indian Research Fund Association** formulated to promote research and now this functions in the name of ICMR.
1918	The **Lady Reading Health School, Delhi**, established to train health visitors to work in the community.
1918	The **Nutrition Research Laboratory established at Coonoor in 1918** at Pasteur Institute of South India. The Institute was shifted to Hyderabad in 1959 and renamed as **National Institute of Nutrition (NIN) in 1978.**
1919	The **Montague-Chelmsford** Constitutional Reforms initiated: Provinces took care of public health, sanitation and vital statistics under the direction of an elected minister. Decentralization of health administration began in India.
1920–21	**Municipality and Local Board Act** passed. This helped for further advancement of public health in most provinces with legal provisions.
1930	The **All India Institute of Hygiene and Public Health, Calcutta** was established. The Rockefeller Foundation provided the aid to start this.
1930	The **Child Marriage Restraint Act (Sarda Act)** introduced: Minimum age of marriage for girls and boys fixed as 14 and 18 respectively.
1931	A **Maternity and Child Welfare Bureau** was established. This was set to function under the Indian Red Cross Society
1935	The **Government of India Act, 1935 revitalized** the 1919 Act: Provinces gained greater autonomy. Health activities were grouped under the names of federal, concurrent and provincial lists and controlled by Central, Central-cum-Provincial and Provincial Governments respectively.
1937	Establishment of the **central advisory** board for health: Public Health Commissioner appointed as Secretary and representatives from the provinces appointed as members. This is mainly to coordinate the public health activities of the country.
1939	The **Madras Public Health Act** was passed. Under this the first Rural Health Training Center at Singur (near Calcutta) established with the aid from the Rockefeller Foundation.
1939	**Tuberculosis Association of India** was established. This association aims at the prevention, control, treatment, relief and research activities of tuberculosis.
1940	The **Drugs Act** was passed, the main purpose was to bring all the drugs under control.

Contd…

Year	Events
1943	The **Health Survey and Development Committee (Bhore Committee)** appointed. This focus was to survey the existing position concerning health conditions and health organization in the country and to provide recommendations for further development in future.
1946	**Bhore committee submitted** its report after making a thorough observation on existing public health, medical relief, professional education, research and international health. The committee also set short and long-term programs to attain realistic health services that match concept of modern health practice.

Sir Joseph William Bhore

Note: Calcutta is now Kolkata, Bombay is now Mumbai, Bangalore is now Bengaluru, Madras is now Chennai.

DEVELOPMENT OF COMMUNITY HEALTH NURSING—POSTINDEPENDENCE (TABLE 2)

In 1935, **Hartley** wrote that nurses' quarters were more sordid than pigsties. In **1947**, survey conducted by **CMAI** revealed that the nurses were in poor living conditions with low salaries; only 40% of the nurses had the salary of above ₹30/month. In the beginning couple of decades of 19th century "caste and purdah system" of India denied entry into nursing profession.

In **1946**, **Bhore committee** gave the recommendations on nurse to population ratio. One of the recommendations of Bhore committee was to staff PHC with 2 doctors, one nurse, four public health nurses, four midwives, four trained *dais*, two sanitary inspectors, two health assistants, one pharmacist and fifteen other class IV employees.

In **1947, nurse leaders from the Nurses' Auxiliary of the CMAI** openly conveyed about the fact that nursing is not publicly accepted as a profession but looked upon as a lower menial service; stressed the urgent need to get students from 'higher cultural and social backgrounds' to make them know and understand about nursing (CMAI 1947).

In 1947, greater concentration on community development and expansion of hospital service have created huge demand for nurses, auxiliary nurse midwives (ANMs), health visitors, midwives, nursing tutors and nursing administrators. On December 31, 1947, an ordinance passed to start **"Indian Nursing Council"** and constituted in the year **1949. In 1956, Ms TK Adranwala became the Nursing Advisor** to Government of India. The development of community health nursing in India was highly influenced by

World War and British rule. Apart from these the Christian missionaries made enormous contribution toward the development of community health nursing. International agencies like World Health Organization, United Nations Children's Fund (UNICEF), Red Cross, and United States Agency for International Development (USAID) were also the significant contributors of community health nursing development in India.

Exercise:

Learners may take up some of the significant roles (leaders/pioneers/Vicereine) from the historical development of community health nursing and make a role play.

In 1952, international tutors (4 in number) were appointed in Calcutta to train nurses in general nursing, nursing arts, midwifery and pediatric nursing. A certificate course in Public Health Nursing (CPHN) that included comprehensive health nursing services was introduced in 1953.

Twenty-four students joined in certificate course of public health nursing in All India Institute of Hygiene and Public Health (Calcutta) in **1953** which was a big number compared to 3 of the previous year.

Ms TK Adranvala in one of her articles of Nursing Journal of India (NJI) mentioned about the initiation of a midwifery tutor course in Delhi in the year 1956. In **1959 the first Master's degree** course for 2 years of duration was developed in India at the University of Delhi. Further, some specialization courses started in different specialties like public health nursing, Psychiatric Nursing, and Pediatric Nursing, etc.

In 1959, Rock feller provided 2 nursing fellowships and the Colombo plan sent 29 Indian nurses to abroad to pursue higher education.

1959–1961, World Health organization offered 9 fellowships to Indian nurses.

During post-independence many popular Indian nursing leaders were sent abroad one or the other form of higher education in nursing to enrich nursing education in India. In addition, time spent on nursing educational certificates or degrees abroad, gave respect and benefit to Indian nurses.

Overseas education of Indian nurses provided current updates and novel ideas in the area of public health education.

In 1960 international seminar on "nursing research" was hosted by the joint efforts of TNAI and INC.

In 1962, USAID sponsored 45 Indian nurses to pursue public health education from USA.

In 1962, Mudaliar committee reported that primary health centers were understaffed and most of the workload was shouldered by ANMs or public health nurses and the PHCs should be strengthened.

Chadha Committee, 1963 recommended 1 basic health worker per 10,000 populations to carry out NMEP National Malaria Eradication Program (NMEP) vigilance activity as well to function as MPWs.

Mukherjee Committee, 1965 recommended separate staff for the family planning program and delink the staff from NMEP.

In 1971, trained nurses of India sponsored conference at Chandigarh stressed the need on taking up nursing education to university system. From 1990s TNAI highlighted the need for phasing out of general nursing program.

Kartar Singh Committee, 1973 had recommended converting auxiliary nurse midwives into MPW (F) and the basic health workers to MPW (M); in addition, the designation of "health visitor" was changed into "health supervisor."

In 1975, Adranvala stated that nurses have responsibility to speak on behalf of ANMs and Health visitors.

Shrivastav Committee, 1975 served as a cause for **establishment of "Rural Health Service"** in the year **1977**. A foremost important health strategy by this committee was bringing in the concept of cadre of village-based health auxiliaries called the **Community Health workers**. The program was started in 777 Primary health centers where MPWs were already in place. The community health workers got training for 3 months in simple promotive and curative skills and supervised by MPWs.

In the year **1987** succession of nursing leaders started "College of Nursing Community Health Services" (CONCH) at Vellore, Tamil Nadu. This program functions under Community Health Nursing Department—College of Nursing CMCH, Vellore. This was mainly to serve the rural and semiurban population through regular home visits, nurse run clinics with standing orders and referral system.

In 1991, the Baby-Friendly Hospital Initiative (BFHI) was launched by WHO and UNICEF promote and support breastfeeding.

In 2005, INC decided to advice on upgrading all nursing schools to college. In 2007, INC initiated National Florence Nightingale Award to recognize the services of nurses.

In 2008, the Global Fund to Fight AIDS, Tuberculosis and Malaria (GFATM) project was taken up by INC in coordination with National AIDS Control Organization (NACO) in order to strengthen 55 nursing institutes and to train 90,000 nurses of India on HIV/AIDS and ARV. From 2009 onward INC and NACO started to train nurses under this project.

In **2010**, World Health Organization published "A framework for community health nursing education."

In **2012**, Directorate General of health services Ministry of Health and Family Welfare revised the Indian Public Health Standards (IPHS) Guidelines for community health centers, PHCs and health subcenters.

In **2016**, INC has drafted **"primary health care practitioner"** course in order to develop nurses with advanced skills to function efficiently in community.

Since the time of independence, the nursing education has grown rapidly with a significant rise in the infrastructure and manpower.

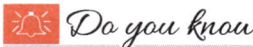

Do you know

Indian nursing council initiated National Florence Nightingale award for nurses since the year 2007 that carries a certificate of merit and cash award of ₹ 50,000.

Table 2: Developmental milestones of public health in independent India

1947	**Ministers for health** appointed. The new post of Director to the Union Government on both medical and public health matters introduced.
1948	○ India became a member state in **World Health Organization (WHO).** WHO addresses the most important public health concerns of populations around the world and responds to the needs of member states. ○ The **Employees State Insurance Act**, passed. This applies to all employees in factories or establishments and they shall be insured as per the regulations of this Act. ○ The report of the **Environmental Hygiene Committee** was published. The central government appointed this committee to assess the prevailing problems related to environmental hygiene and make necessary recommendations for the welfare of the nation and people.
1949	○ The **Constituent Assembly** adopted the Constitution of India on November 26, 1949. The Constituent of assembly of India met in total 11 sessions. The first session was held in December 1946 and the eleventh session took place between 14 and 26 November, 1949. ○ Post of Registrar General of India introduced ○ World Health Organization's "South East Asia Regional Office established in New Delhi. ○ The **Indian Research Fund Association** reconstituted into Indian Council of Medical Research to strengthen the medical research.
1950	○ The **Planning Commission** was set up. ○ **India became a Republic** in the Commonwealth. ○ Drafting of the **First Five-Year Plan** began for the period between 1951 and 1956.
1951	The **BCG vaccination** program implemented in the country to prevent tuberculosis by vaccinating babies.
1952	○ **The Community Development Program** was launched on October 2, 1952. The main focus was all-round development of the rural areas with a provision of medical relief and preventive health services. ○ **The Central Council of Health** was constituted: Central health council coordinated health policies between the central and state governments.
1953	○ The **central council** of health accepted to set one **primary health center in each block**: It was planned to set up primary health centers in a phased manner with community participation. ○ The **national malaria control program (NMCP)** started. It was one of the major components of the first Five Year Plan to control malaria. ○ The **national extension service program** started in many states as a permanent organization to bring about rural development. ○ **Family planning program** introduced throughout the nation. This was considered as a measure to control population and to bring up nation's health and economic status. ○ **Model Public Health Act** India appointed a committee to draft a Model Public Health Act for the country.
1954	○ Central government launched **Contributory Health Service Scheme at Delhi**. Government provided free medical service or reimbursement to employees. ○ India set up the **Central Social Welfare Board**. ○ **National leprosy control program** started. ○ **VDRL antigen** production started in Calcutta. ○ Parliament passed **"The Prevention of Food Adulteration Act"**.
1955	○ **National Filaria control program** was initiated under first five year plan. ○ **Filaria training center** was established in Ernakulam. ○ **The Hindu Marriage Act** set the age for marriage: 18 years for boys and 15 years for girls were set as acceptable age for marriage.

Contd…

1956	○ India launched its **Second Five-Year Plan** (1956–61). ₹4,800 crores in allocated in general; ₹225 crores, earmarked for health programs.
	○ **The Model Public Health Act,** published.
	○ Union Health Ministry established **"The Central Health Education Bureau."** This was started with the primarily for educating the people about health plans and programs. But, currently, it also concentrates on training, supplying of health education (IEC) materials and research.
	○ Union health ministry appointed a **Director to direct Family Planning services** to strengthen the family planning services.
	○ The Government of India and the Sir Dorabji Tata Trust sponsored jointly **"The Demographic Training and Research Center"** in Bombay. It was known as the **International Institute for Population Studies (IIPS)** till 1985. This was primarily established to train persons from India and other countries in demography and family planning and develop research. Now recognized as premier institute for training and research in population studies for developing countries in the Asia and Pacific region. Now functioning as Deemed university.
	○ **The Tuberculosis Chemotherapy Center** established in **Madras**. This was setup by the joint venture of ICMR, Madras government, WHO and British Medical Research council.
	○ The Indian Government, initiated the **"Trachoma Control Pilot Project"** with the assistance from the WHO and UNICEF to prevent communicable eye diseases through primary health care approach, training and research.
	○ Union health ministry started the R-C-A projects.
	○ Ford Foundation provided the aid for **RCA projects**.
1957	○ **Influenza pandemic** swept the country and subcontinent within 12 weeks.
	○ Influenza attacked India with an initial entry to Madras.
	○ **The Demographic Research Centers** were established in **Calcutta, Delhi** and **Trivandrum** to strengthen the research in demography.
1958	○ **The National Malaria Control Program (NMCP)** converted into National Malaria Eradication Program. Remarkable accomplishment of NMCP motivated to change it to "National Malarial Eradication Program (NMEP)" in 1958.
	○ **The Leprosy Advisory Committee of India** was set up to provide advice and guide the leprosy control activities.
	○ **The National Development Council** approved the recommendations of Balwantrai Mehta Committee on Panchayati Raj. A **three-tier structure** of local self-governing bodies from the village to the district has been recommended for dispersal of power and responsibilities in the future.
	○ The **National TB Survey** was conducted to obtain the baseline data on tuberculosis for further planning and management.
1959	○ Government of India appointed **Mudaliar Committee** to review the improvement in the field of health. Mainly to review the improvement took place in health services following the submission of the Bhore Committee's report, and make recommendations for further action.
	○ A Central Expert Committee appointed under the **ICMR** specifically to **study the problems of cholera and smallpox.** The committee had strongly recommended on measures to adopt to eradicate cholera and smallpox.
	○ Introduction of "Panchayati Raj System" to state in India. **Rajasthan was the first** State to introduce Panchayati Raj.
	○ The **National Tuberculosis Institute at Bangalore** was established.
1960	○ The **"School Health Committee"** constituted by the Union Health Ministry of India. This was constituted to assess the existing standards of health and nutrition on school children and suggest ways and means to improve them.
	○ A **"National Nutrition Advisory Committee"** constituted to provide advice regarding the nutritional policies that the government should adopt.
	○ **Pilot projects** for the **eradication of smallpox** were initiated. This helped in strengthening the eradication measures.
	○ Ministry of Home Affairs was assigned the work of maintenance of vital statistics Accordingly Registrar General of India, Ministry of Home Affairs, took over the responsibility of vital statistics from the Directorate General of Health Services.
1961	○ **The Third Five-Year Plan (1961–66)** was launched and ₹7,500 crores assigned. Out of which ₹342 crores (4.3%) were provided for health programs.
	○ The **"Report of the Mudaliar Committee"** published.
	○ The **Central Bureau of Health Intelligence** was established.
1962	○ The **Central Family Planning Institute** was established in Delhi.
	○ This helped to combine Family Planning Training Center, family Planning Communications and action Research Center.
	○ The **National Smallpox Eradication Program** was launched.
	○ The **School Health Program** was initiated.
	○ The **National Goitre control program** was launched.
	○ The **District Tuberculosis Program** started.

Contd...

1963	○ The **Applied Nutrition Program** was launched by the Government of India with aid from UNICEF, FAO and WHO.
	○ The **Defence Institute of Physiology** and Allied Sciences was set up.
	○ The **National Institute of Communicable Diseases** (formerly Malaria Institute of India) was set up.
	○ The **National Trachoma Control Program** was launched.
	○ Contributory Health Service Scheme was renamed as **"Central Government Health Scheme".**
	○ **Extended Family Planning Program** was launched. There was a shift from the clinic approach to "Extension approach" in family planning services.
	○ The **Chadha committee** set a norm as one basic health worker to 10,000 population to provide efficient services at basic level in the community.
	○ A **Drinking Water Board** was set up.
1964	○ The **National Institute of Health Administration and Education** was instituted.
	○ This had the collaboration with the Ford Foundation.
	○ A Committee was set up by the Union Government under the chairmanship of Shantilal Shah, to study the question for **legalizing abortions.**
1965	○ Director, ICMR, recommended **Lippes Loop as a safe** and effective method for a mass program.
	○ Reinforced Extended Family Planning was launched.
	○ **'Direct' BCG vaccination** with prior tuberculin test, on a house to house basis, was introduced.
1966	○ India constituted a **committee of Health Secretaries headed by Mukherjee,** Secretary, Ministry of Health, Government of India to give special attention into the minimum additional staff required for the primary health centers to take up the maintenance work of malaria and smallpox.
	○ The Minister of Health was also appointed Minister for Family Planning.
	○ A separate department of Family Planning in the Union Ministry of Health advised to coordinate family planning program at the Center and States by paying extra attention.
	○ The Population Council initiated the **"International Postpartum Family Planning Program"** in 25 hospitals in 15 countries.
	○ Two of these hospitals were located in India—Delhi and Trivandrum.
1967	○ The **Modhok Committee** was constituted. To review the working of the **National Malaria Eradication Program** and recommend measures for improvement.
	○ **A Small Family Norm Committee** was set up to recommend suitable incentives to the people who accept the small family norm and practicing family planning.
	○ The Central Council of Health recommended the **levy of a health cess** on patients attending hospitals. A minimum charge of 10 paise per patient and a minimum charge of 25 paise per day of hospital stay.
1968	○ The **"Small Family Committee"** submitted its report.
	○ "A Bill of **"Registration of Births and Deaths"** passed by the Rajya Sabha.
	○ The Government of India appointed the **Medical Education Committee** to review all aspects of medical education in relation to the needs and resources of India.
1969	○ **The Fourth Five-Year Plan** (1969–74)
	○ The Nutrition Research Laboratories renamed as National Institute of Nutrition.
	○ **The Central Births and Deaths Registration Act (1969)** was submitted.
	○ **The Medical education** Committee submitted its **report.**
	▫ According to this committee the total period for MBBS course was set to 4½ years with 1 year of internship during which students to be posted in a rural center for a period of at least 3 months.
	▫ The medical training should prepare basic doctors who are aware of problems of the community and take up an efficient role in preventive and curative health services.
1970	○ The **Drugs (Price Control) Order**, promulgated.
	○ **All India Hospital (Post-partum) Family Planning Program** was started.
	○ **The Population Council of India** was formed in April 1970.
	○ **Chittaranjan Mobile Hospitals** (mobile training-cum-service unit) were installed on the birth centenary (November 5, 1970) of Late CR Dass. The scheme stressed the importance of attachment of a mobile hospital to a suitable medical college in each State.
	○ The name of the Demographic Training and Research Center, Bombay was changed into **International Institute for Population Studies.**
1971	○ **The Family Pension Scheme (FPS) for industrial workers** came into force.
	○ National Service Bill that authorized the Government to compel medical personnel below 30 years of age to take up work in the countryside came into force.
	○ The National Nutrition Monitoring Bureau under the Indian Council of Medical Research, with headquarters at the National Institute of Nutrition, Hyderabad was set up. Regional units established in the States.

Contd…

1972	○ The **National "Minimum Needs program"** has been incorporated in the Fifth Year Plan. A sum of ₹2,803 crores allotted for this program, to cover elementary education, rural health, nutrition, rural roads and water supply, housing, slum improvement and rural electrification.
	○ The Government has envisaged a scheme for setting up 30-bedded rural hospitals and one such hospital for every 4 primary health centers.
	○ The **Kartar Singh Commitee** reommended that a new cadre of health workers named **"Multi-purpose Health Workers"** to deliver health, family planning and nutrition services to the rural communities; in addition, this cadre will replace the basic health workers, family planning health assistants, and auxiliary nurse midwives in a course of time.
1974	○ The **Fifth Five-Year Plan** was launched on April 1, 1974 with a total outlay of ₹53,411 crores of which ₹37,250 crores for public sector and ₹16,161 crores for the private sector. A sum of ₹796 crores were allotted to health, and ₹516 crores to family planning.
	○ Reports on the National Malaria Eradication Program (NMEP) submitted. Evaluation and expert committees suggested "revised strategy" for malaria control.
	○ The United Nations designated **"the year 1974" as World Population Year**.
	○ Parliament enacted the Water (prevention and control of pollution) Act, 1974.
1975	○ India became **smallpox free on 5 July, 1975**
	○ The Government of India accepted the **Revised strategy for NMEP**.
	○ The country has embarked on a scheme of **"Integrated Child Development"** from October 2, 1975.
	○ A high powered **National Children's Welfare Board** was set up.
	○ The **ESI Act** was amended.
	○ The Cigarettes Regulation (of Production, Supply and Distribution) Act, 1975 was passed by parliament.
	○ The Group on **Medical Education and Support Manpower (Shrivastav Committee)** submitted its report.
1976	○ **Indian Factories Act** of 1948 amended.
	○ The **Prevention of Food Adulteration April 1, (Amendment) Act** came into force on 1976.
	○ The **Equal Remuneration Act, 1975** was promulgated providing for equal wages for men and women for the same work of a similar nature. The Union Health Ministry announced a **'new population policy'**.
	○ The Central Council of Health proposed a **3-tier plan for medical care in villages.**
	○ The Indian Center of **Japan Leprosy Mission for Asia** at Agra was handed over to the Indian authorities.
	○ **National Program for Prevention of Blindness** was formulated.
1977	○ **Eradication of smallpox** declared in April by the International commission.
	○ **National Institute of Health and Family Planning** formed.
	○ **Rural Health Scheme** was launched. Training of community health workers was taken up.
	○ **Revised Modified Plan of malaria eradication** was put into operation.
	○ WHO adopted the goal of Health for All by 2000 AD.
	○ **Reorientation of medical education (ROME) scheme** was launched.
1978	○ **Bill on Air Pollution** introduced in the Lok Sabha. Parliament approved the Child Marriage Restraint (Amendment) Bill, 1978 fixing the minimum age at marriage 21 years for boys and 18 years for girls. **Expanded program on Immunization (EPI)** was launched.
	○ The Charter for Health Development in South East Asia was finalized and endorsed.
	○ **Declaration of Alma-Ata** and introduction of primary health care approach.
1979	○ World Health Assembly endorsed the Declaration of Alma-Ata on primary health care.
	○ The offices of family welfare and NMEP were merged and named as Regional Office for Health and Family Welfare.
1980	On May 8, 1980, World Health Assembly declared officially on eradication of smallpox from the entire world. **Sixth Five-Year Plan** (1980–85) was launched.
1981	○ The 1981 census was taken.
	○ WHO and Member Countries adopted the Global strategy for Health for All.
	○ Report on Health for All, was published by working committee formed by planning commission India is committed to the goal of providing safe drinking water and adequate sanitation for all by 1990, in view of Sanitation Decade 1981–90.
	○ The Air (Prevention and Control of Pollution) Act of 1981 was enacted.
1982	○ The New 20 Point Program was announced. India announced its National Health Policy.
1983	○ India launched a National Plan of Action against avoidable Disablement, known as **"IMPACT India"**. National Leprosy Control Program renamed as National Leprosy Eradication Program.
	○ Medical Education Review Committee submitted its report.
	○ National Health Policy was approved by the Parliament. Guinea-worm eradication Program was launched.

Contd...

1984	o **Bhopal gas tragedy**, the worst ever industrial accident happened due to leakage of gas on the night of December 2–3 took a toll of at least 2500 people and no fewer than 50,000 affected.
	o The ESI (Amendment) Bill, approved
	o The Workmen's Compensation (Amendment) Act, came to force in July 1, 1984.
1985	o **Seventh Five-Year Plan** (1985–90) was launched. Universal Immunization Program was launched. Women and Child Development was set up as a separate department under the newly established "Ministry of Human resource Development."
1986	**The Environment (Protection) Act**,1986 promulgated 20-point plan restructured.
1987	o **New 20-point program** was launched Indian Standards institution (ISI) was renamed as **"Bureau of Indian Standards"**.
	o **"Safe motherhood"** campaign- launched by World Bank throughout the world.
	o **National Diabetes Control Program** and National **AIDS Control** Program initiated.
	o **The Factories (Amendment) Act 1987** operated - with inclusion of aims to protect employees exposed to hazardous processes.
1989	o **Blood Safety Program** was launched.
	o **The ESI (Amendment)Act** 1989 operated. This had the modifications in dependent, employee, family, factory and seasonal factory definitions and provisons on orginal Act.
1990	**Acute Respiratory Infection (ARI) control program** launched as in 14 districts as a pilot measure to reduce the mortality rates among under five children.
1991	India conducted the **decadal census** to count and update the population of the country.
1992	o The **Eighth Five-Year Plan** (1992–97) launched.
	o **Child Survival and Safe Motherhood Program (CSSM)** started on 20th August considering mother and child as one unit.
1993	o **Revised tuberculosis program** was introduced with "Directly Observed Short course Treatment **(DOTS)."**
	o **National nutrition policy** introduced.
1994	Plague disease re-emerged after 28 years.
1995	o **ICDS** changed into **IMCD** (Integrated mother and child development services).
	o Guidelines set for malaria action plan.
1996	o **Pulse polio immunization for all children** on pre-announced days began to eradicate polio:
	o First phase: 9th Dec (1995) and 20th Jan (1996) were chosen as Pulse Polio Immunization days; Second phase: 7th Dec 1996 and 18th Jan 1997.
	o **Family planning program** started to use **target-free approach** from April 1, 1996 onwards.
	o **Prenatal diagnostic technique act** was implemented from 1996.
	o Eradication program for Yaws launched.
1997	**Ninth Five-Year Plan** implemented (1997–2002).
1997	**Reproductive and child health program** launched.
1998–99	o **National family health survey** conducted for 90000 women of reproductive age (15–49 years) group.
	o National malaria eradication program was renamed as **National anti-malaria program.**
2000	o **National population policy-2000** was launched.
	o India was declared as **"guinea worm free country."**
	o India signed UN millennium declaration.
	o **National population commission** constituted.
2001	o **First census of 21ˢᵗ century** carried out.
	o India launched **women empowerment policy** on 20th March 2001.
2002	o India introduced **National health policy 2002**.
	o **Tenth Five-Year Plan** implemented (2002–2007).
	o **National AIDS prevention and control policy** announced.
	o **Severe Acute Respiratory Syndrome (SARS)** appeared
2003	**Control of cigarettes** and other to tobacco products act amended.
2004	o **Vandemataram scheme** launched.
	o **Midday meal scheme** launched.
	o **Low osmolarity oral rehydration salt** replaced the formula existed for oral rehydration during that period.
	o Feeding guidelines for infant and children introduced.

Contd…

2005	○ **Reproductive and child health phase II** launched.
	○ **Janani suraksha yojana** launched: India provided onetime cash assistance to pregnant women for undergoing institutional/ home births through skilled assistance.
	○ **National rural health mission** launched.
	○ **Indian public health standards for community health centers** formulated.
	○ India achieved leprosy elimination target.
	○ **Plan of action for children** formulated.
2006	○ **New pediatric growth chart** based on breast fed children introduced by WHO.
	○ National family health survey 3 conducted.
	○ **Integrated Management of Neonatal and Childhood Illnesses (IMNCI)** was launched in 16 states.
2007	**Eleventh Five-Year Plan** launched (2007–2012).
2007	**Indian public health standards for primary health centers** and sub-centers formulated.
2007	Bill passed maintenance and **welfare of parents and senior citizens** bill passed.
2009	**Influenza A(H₁N₁) pandemic** occurred.
2011	India conducted the **second census of the century.**
2011	India launched **"National Program for the Health care of Elderly (NPHCE)"** scheme to ease the access to primary health care for elderly people.
2011	**Janani-Shishu Suraksha Karyakram** (JSSK) introduced. JSSK launched on 1st of June, 2011 to assure free services to all pregnant women and sick neonates accessing public health institutions.
2012	○ All India Institute of Medical Sciences **(AIIMS) launched new hospitals** additionally in seven places (Bhopal, Bhuvaneshwar, Jodhpur, Patna, Raipur and Rishikesh).
	○ **Twelfth Five-Year Plan** launched for the period 2012–2017.
2013	○ National health mission launched.
	○ **RMNCH+A approach** launched in 2013 with prime attention on **R**eproductive, **M**aternal, **N**ewborn, **C**hild and **A**dolescent Health.
2014	○ Ministry of health and family welfare launched **"Mission Indradhanush"** to immunize all children against seven major vaccine preventable diseases, namely diphtheria, pertussiss, tetanus, poliomyelitis, tuberculosis, measles and hepatitis b by the year 2020.
	○ India launched **TB-Mission 2020 to eliminate tuberculosis** from the country by the year 2020.
	○ Ministry of Health and Family Welfare launched **"Rashtriya Kishor Swasthya Karyakram (RKSK)"** on January 7, 2014 to reach and serve adolescents with a special interest on marginalized and undeserved groups.
	○ The **India Newborn Action Plan** (INAP).
	○ India was declared as **"Polio free country".**
	○ **Swachh Bharat Abhiyan** initiated by Prime Minister Modi to provide total sanitation to every household by the year 2019.
2015	**NITI Aayog** replaces Yojana Aayog on January 1, 2015.

Note: Calcutta is now Kolkata, Bombay is now Mumbai, Bangalore and is now Begaluru and Madras is now Chennai.

TWENTY-FIRST CENTURY AND CHALLENGES FOR COMMUNITY HEALTH NURSING

Many unexpected changes may occur in this 21st century all over the world in the field of health/nursing/community health nursing. There are chances for serious transformation that may dominate the environment along with the changes in other areas like culture, beliefs, practice, technology and economy.

○ In this fast growing customer, oriented quality driven world the major weapon to be used in practice is "evidence-based practice"

Evidence-based public health is a public health venture in which there is cautious use of evidence derived from a variety of science and social science research. Most often community health nurses use the evidences from the field of epidemiologic research to assess their clients and for planning and implementing care in the community. Updating of knowledge and skill to function as a real time clinician.

○ **Growing cultural interaction:** This is one of the issue in the front line which seeks the nurses to be culturally competent as well recognize the needs pertaining to increasing interaction among different cultures.

○ **Media that causes awareness:** One of the health educational principles is "known to unknown." Traditionally we follow it however, in present days' world we need to be extra cautious in allotting more time to the individual/family before we step our health talk, instructions, or guidelines on any health-related issues. Even your opposite end may know or collected more information than you are about to convey. This is mainly the effect of taking responsibility on personal care that motivates people to seek more information.

Exercise:

Having learnt the developmental perspectives of community health nursing learners can have a discussion about the happenings of community health nursing in 21st century.

○ **Consumer first:** Anything that is purchased gives ownership to the consumer. Here again, patients pay for their health, become consumers. There is no surprise consumer (patient) looks for "quality" in the care delivered to them.

○ **Societal needs and growing specializations:** Curriculum planning needs to show higher concentration on societal needs and job opportunities. Redesigning the general specialties into more specific ones and providing some crash courses as an addition in each specialty will be an expected change in the curriculum to meet the present and future challenges.

○ **Primary health care nurse practitioners:** To shoulder the huge health care load and responsibilities in community "master level qualified primary health care nurse practitioners" are the right choice.

○ **Interdisciplinary approach:** Community health nurse never practice in isolation. But still giving a strong identity to interdisciplinary care through interdisciplinary research works will be complementing practice of in community health nurses.

○ **Healthy lifestyle—a slogan that is "must for children":** Inculcation of "Healthy behavior" among children equals healthy future nation. It is a mandatory challenge on community health nurses to grow and nurture healthy India.

Summary

Health is a state of complete physical, mental and social well-being and not merely the absence of disease or infirmity. The IOM defines public health as "organized community efforts aimed at the prevention of disease and promotion of health." "Community" implies people acting together in some way as a group, and the whole meaning more than the sum of its parts. According to ANA (1999), public health nursing is a population-focused community nursing practice with the goal of prevention of disease and disability by creating the conditions where people can be healthy. Community health nurses are on the front lines of health care and prevention of diseases and promotion of health. The term population health, which is similar to community health, has emerged in recent years.

Community health nurses play various roles like clinician, educator, advocate, manager, collaborator, leader, and researcher. Community health nurses' work in various settings like home, school, industry, clinics, community health centers, maternity homes and primary health centers and as educators in nursing schools and colleges and in training centers.

After much contradiction, Shattuck's report was considered as one of the most farsighted and influential documents in the history of the decline of Roman dynasty pulled down the developments in community health organization. There was no provision for clean water, waste disposal and sanitation. People threw the garbage on the street and no health behavior seen in people. Practice of nurses joining military orders during the time of Crusades started between 1091 and 1291.

In 1601, the Church of England introduced, "Elizabethan poor law" and made it compulsory. This made people care for poor, blind, orphans and lame. Initially the neighbors in local communities cared people with physical and mental illnesses. Later this became official in England by adoption of "1601- poor law". Toward mid-nineteenth century there was tremendous advancement in public health. This period was referred to "**the great sanitary awakening.**"(Winslow, 1923). **Chadwick** proposed to build a drainage network to remove sewage and waste. **Lemuel Shattuck**, a Massachusetts bookseller and statistician published a survey *Report of the Massachusetts Sanitary Commission* in 1850. The Greeks showed interest in community sanitation.

American public health system: Edward Jenner of Berkeley had saved many lives with his discovery of "**Smallpox Vaccination. William Farr** (1839) stressed the importance of "vital statistics" for studying health problems. In **1854, Snow** discovered that the cholera epidemics occurred due to polluted water. **John Snow** was given the title of "**father of modern epidemiology."** In **1877 Louis Pasteur**, a French chemist, proved that anthrax is caused by bacteria.

During 20th century, people started look beyond the traditional concept of protecting people from polluted environment and communicable diseases. People started to understand the relationship between bacteria and communicable diseases. In the early 20th century, home visits offered by public health nurses in New York and Baltimore. School health clinics were established in Boston (1894), New York (1903) and in Rhode Island (1906) to support and promote the health of school going children.

Elders of the families who had lived in experiences on handling health-related issues provided consultation to their own family members and guided them.

In the **middle ages**, family members only took care of the sick and ill. From the 1500s through the 1700s, the renaissance in **Europe** stimulated the rise of scientific thought and social consciousness. The Sisters (or Daughters) of Charity or "Grey Sisters," was founded in 1617 in **France,** with the aim of providing care to the sick poor. People were afraid to go to hospitals and addressed hospitals as, "death houses". In **Holland**, women appointed by churches to care for the poor called as deaconess-groups. **Florence Nightingale**, daughter of Wealthy English family, committed to prevent illness and death. Florence took a lead role with a team of nurses and assisted soldiers during the **Crimean War** (1854–1856).

In 1859 William Rathbone, a Quaker merchant and philanthropist of England hired **Mary Robinson**, a nurse (who later named as the **first district nurse**) to take care of people in one of the poorest parish districts in Liverpool. Nightingale started the first school of nursing, and Rathbone hired several graduates as district nurses. Two years later, with Nightingale's assistance, he established a nursing school in Liverpool. In 1813, the **Ladies' Benevolent Society of Charleston**, South Carolina, started to provide organized home care services to the sick. In 1912, Wald assisted to found the **National Organization for Public Health Nursing.** Mary Breckinridge the founder of "Frontier nursing" traveled on horseback, and assessed the health situations and needs of the mountain people. In 1939, she helped to establish the Frontier Graduate School of Midwifery, one of the first midwifery programs in the country.

Many unexpected changes may occur in this 21st century all over the world in the field of health/nursing /community health nursing. There are chances for serious transformation that may dominate the environment along with the changes in other areas like culture, beliefs, practice, technology and economy.

Development of Community health nursing in India—Pre-independence

Caring for the sick people confined to bed was the realm of the family. The Susruta Samhita, (600–350 BCE) described four types of midwives and among which one was "good at giving birth to a child (prajanana kusalah)."British officials wanted to admire idealized cleanliness and rationality whereas the *dai* was an ignorant, superstitious lady who never gave importance for cleanliness or hygiene in her care practices. The Government of Madras sanctioned a training school for midwives in the year 1854. These modern nursing thoughts developed from Florence Nightingale played a significant role in professionalizing and inculcating nursing culture in India. Consequent to the report of Royal Sanitary Commission in 1863, **the Indian Nursing Service (INS) was** created in 1888 to provide proper nursing care for British soldiers. The Vicereine, **Lady Dufferin**, in 1883 established "**Dufferin Fund.**" The Vicereine, Lady Minto, launched the Indian Nursing Association in 1906. **The Trained Nurses Association of India (TNAI)** formed in 1908.

In 1918 **Lady Chelmsford** provided great support in starting training courses for health visitors and maternity supervisors. A "Health school" was opened in Delhi with the grants from government, which was later named as "Lady Reading School". In 1922 **Griffin** launched a new wing for Health visitors under TNAI in the name of **"Health visitors league"**. This was renamed as "association for ANMS" from 1970 onward. In 1938, Florence Nightingale memorial scholarship to pursue further training in England announced. **Diana Hartley**, a British nurse, the editor of "Nursing Journal of India." With the support from the **Rockfeller Foundations,** seven health centers were established from 1931 to 1939 in the cities of Delhi.

Development of community health nursing–Post-Independence

In 1946 **Bhore committee** gave the recommendations on nurse to population ratio. In **1947, nurse leaders from the Nurses' Auxiliary of the CMAI** openly conveyed about the fact that nursing is not publicly accepted as a profession. On December 31, 1947, an ordinance passed to start **"Indian Nursing Council"** and constituted in the year **1949.** Christian missionaries made enormous contribution toward the development of community health nursing. **In 1952** international tutors (4 in number) were appointed in Calcutta to train nurses in general nursing, nursing arts, midwifery and pediatric nursing. In **1959 the first Master's degree** course for 2 years of duration was developed in India at the University of Delhi. **In 1959 Rockfeller** provided 2 nursing fellowships and the Colombo plan sent 29 Indian nurses to abroad to pursue higher education. **Kartar Singh Committee in 1973** had recommended converting auxiliary nurse midwives into MPW (F) and the basic health workers to MPW (M); in addition, the designation of "health visitor" was changed into "health supervisor."

In 2008, the Global Fund to Fight AIDS, tuberculosis and malaria (GFATM) project was taken up by Indian Nursing Council (INC) in coordination with National AIDS Control Organization (NACO). **In 2016 –INC has drafted "Primary Health Care** practitioner" course in order to develop nurses with advanced skills to function efficiently in community. Many unexpected changes may occur in this 21st century all over the world in the field of health/nursing /community health nursing. There are chances for serious transformation that may dominate the environment along with the changes in other areas like culture, beliefs, practice, technology, and economy.

Assess Yourself

I. Multiple Choice Questions (Choose the Correct Answer)

1. Which of these following years "Royal Commission" appointed in India?
   a. 1829   b. 1839
   c. 1849   d. 1859

2. Which of these following years the "Vaccination Act" introduced in India?
   a. 1870   b. 1880
   c. 1890   d. 1900

3. Which of these following years the "Indian Factories Act" introduced?
   a. 1861   b. 1871
   c. 1881   d. 1891

4. Which of these years the "Local Self-Government Act" launched?
   a. 1885   b. 1895
   c. 1905   d. 1915

5. Which of these years the "Epidemic Diseases Act" passed?
   a. 1867   b. 1877
   c. 1887   d. 1897

6. The "Lady Reading Health School" at Delhi, established to train
   a. Health visitors   b. Staff nurses
   c. Village health nurses   d. Doctors

7. The All India Institute of Hygiene and Public Health, was established in
   a. Delhi   b. Chennai
   c. Calcutta   d. Mumbai

8. Which of these following years the "Child Marriage Restraint Act" launched?
   a. 1920   b. 1930
   c. 1940   d. 1960

9. Which of these following years the "Tuberculosis Association of India" established?
   a. 1939   b. 1949
   c. 1959   d. 1969

10. Which of these following years the "Health Survey and Development Committee (Bhore Committee)" appointed?
    a. 1943   b. 1953
    c. 1963   d. 1973

11. Which of these following years the "Drugs Act" passed?
    a. 1930   b. 1940
    c. 1950   d. 1960

12. India became a member state in World Health Organization (WHO) in the year
    a. 1948   b. 1958
    c. 1968   d. 1978

13. The Employees State Insurance Act, passed in the year
    a. 1948   b. 1958
    c. 1968   d. 1978

14. The Planning Commission of India set up in the year
    a. 1940   b. 1950
    c. 1960   d. 1970

15. India became a Republic from the Commonwealth counties in the year
    a. 1930   b. 1940
    c. 1950   d. 1960

16. The BCG vaccination program implemented in the country to prevent tuberculosis in the year
    a. 1951   b. 1961
    c. 1971   d. 1981

17. The Community Development Program launched in the year
    a. 1952   b. 1962
    c. 1972   d. 1982

18. The first district nurse appointed by William Rathbone is
    a. Clara   b. Mary Robinson
    c. Minto   d. Mary Williams

19. Which of these nursing leaders found the "National Organization for Public Health Nursing"?
    a. Wald   b. Clara Barton
    c. Florence Nightingale   d. Diana Hartley

20. An ordinance passed to start "Indian Nursing Council" in the year
    a. 1929   b. 1939
    c. 1949   d. 1959

21. The Population Council initiated the "International Postpartum Family Planning Program" in the year
    a. 1946   b. 1956
    c. 1966   d. 1976

22. Indian Nursing Association launched in the year 1906 by
    a. Lady Minto   b. Lady Dufferin
    c. Lady Chelmsford   d. Queen Victoria

23. The Global Fund to Fight AIDS, Tuberculosis and Malaria (GFATM) project in India was initiated by
    a. UNICEF and NACO   b. INC and NACO
    c. USAID and NACO   d. USAID and INC

24. The Trained Nurses, Association of India (TNAI) formed in the year
    a. 1908   b. 1918
    c. 1928   d. 1938

25. The Baby-friendly Hospital Initiative (BFHI) was launched by WHO and UNICEF promote and support breastfeeding in the year
    a. 1971   b. 1981
    c. 1991   d. 2001

26. "The great sanitary awakening" took place in
    a. 17th century
    b. 18th century
    c. 19th century
    d. 20th century

27. World Health Organization published "A framework for community health nursing education" in the year
    a. 1980
    b. 1990
    c. 2000
    d. 2010

28. Which of these committees had recommended on converting auxiliary nurse midwives into MPW (F)?
    a. Mudaliar committee
    b. Bhore committee
    c. Bajaj Committee
    d. Kartar Singh committee

29. "Swatchh Bharat Abhiyan" initiated by Prime minister Modi in the year
    a. 2011
    b. 2012
    c. 2013
    d. 2014

30. NITI Aayog replaced Yojana Aayog on first Jan
    a. 2012
    b. 2013
    c. 2014
    d. 2015

II. Short answer questions (Answer in one or two sentences)

1. Define health
2. Define public health
3. Define community health
4. Define community health nursing
5. What is GFATM?

III. Write short notes on:

1. Role of community health nurse
2. Work settings for community health nurse

IV. Essay or long answer questions:

1. Explain briefly on significant events of community health development in the world
2. Briefly describe the significant events of development of community health in India
3. Describe in detail about the scope of community health nursing
4. Explain the various roles of community health nurse
5. Describe various work settings of community health nurses
6. Describe the development of community health nursing in India during pre-Independence
7. Describe the development of community health nursing in India during post-Independence
8. Write an essay on historical milestones in the development of community health nursing in India.

ANSWERS

I.
1. a	2. b	3. c	4. a	5. d	6. a	7. c	8. b
9. a	10. a	11. b	12. a	13. a	14. b	15. c	16. a
17. a	18. b	19. a	20. c	21. c	22. a	23. b	24. a
25. c	26. c	27. d	28. d	29. d	30. d		

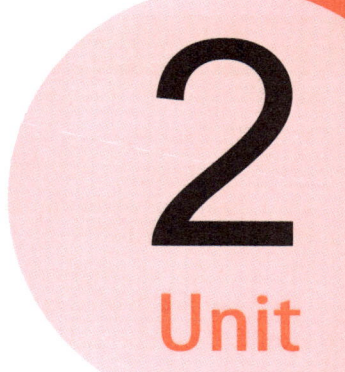

Health Planning, Policies and Problems

Unit Outline

- ■ Health Planning in India
- ● Contributions of Various Committees and Commissions on Health
  - ■ Health Committees
  - ■ Health Commissions
  - ■ National Institution for Transforming India (NITI) Aayog
  - ■ Summary of Investment During Annual and Five-Year Plan
- ● Central Council for Health and Family Welfare
- ● National Health Policy 1983
- ● National Health Policy (NHP) 2002
- ● National Population Policy 2000
- ● National Health Problems in India
  - ■ Communicable Disease
  - ■ Noncommunicable Disease (NCD) Problems
  - ■ Environmental Sanitation Problems
  - ■ Medical Care Problems
  - ■ Population Problems

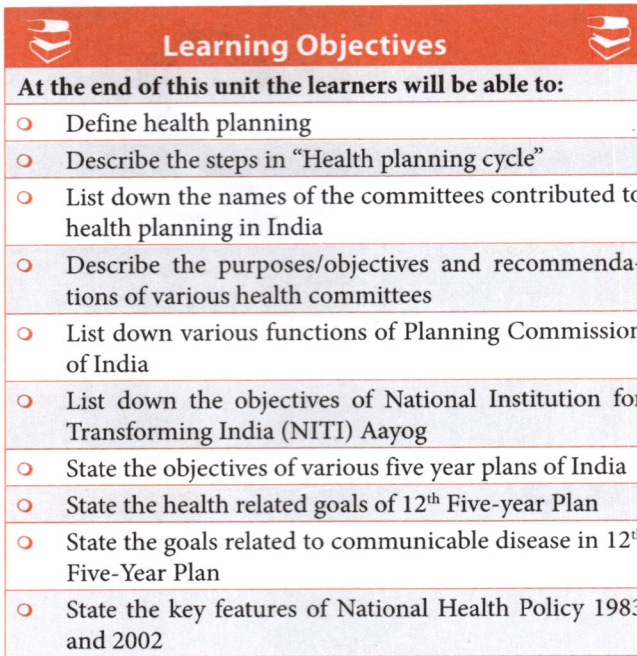

Learning Objectives

At the end of this unit the learners will be able to:

○ Define health planning
○ Describe the steps in "Health planning cycle"
○ List down the names of the committees contributed to health planning in India
○ Describe the purposes/objectives and recommendations of various health committees
○ List down various functions of Planning Commission of India
○ List down the objectives of National Institution for Transforming India (NITI) Aayog
○ State the objectives of various five year plans of India
○ State the health related goals of 12th Five-year Plan
○ State the goals related to communicable disease in 12th Five-Year Plan
○ State the key features of National Health Policy 1983 and 2002
○ Describe the National Population Policy 2000
○ Describe the National Health Problems in India

KEY TERMS

- Monitoring
- Social physicians
- Auxiliary nurse midwives (ANMs)
- Universalization
- Net Reproduction Rate
- Total fertility rate (TFR)
- Malaria
- Filaria
- Tuberculosis
- Leprosy
- AIDS
- Protein Energy Malnutrition
- Nutritional Anemia
- Low birthweight

HEALTH PLANNING IN INDIA

There is a universal say, **"failing to plan is planning to fail."** Planning is the word used from gross level to the topmost plans. In our daily life, planning takes its place with no alarm or alert. Yes, many of us make "mental plans" on our daily routines and special tasks consciously or unconsciously. The plan of individual or a family do not have the schedule or record but lies tacit and helps implementing our tasks. However, we happen to see family members make their monthly budgets sitting with a paper and pen. This is one of the typical examples of planning consciously to control the expenses within their capacity to spend. Therefore, planning is the most important task of individual, family and the country.

India the second most populous country of the world, tries the effective means and measures to utilize its men, money, material and time, since many years now. Indian government appointed many committees from time to time to provide advice on huge number of health problems. The reports of these committees have served important platform of "health planning in India."

Health planning in India and a brief account on various committees and their significant recommendations are explained below.

Definitions

○ Planning is the orderly process of defining health problems, identifying unmet needs and surveying the resources to meet them, establishing priority goals that are realistic and feasible, and projecting administrative action, concerned not only with the adequacy, efficacy and efficiency of health services but also with those factors of ecology and of social and individual behavior that affect the health of the individual and the community
—WHO, 1975

○ It is the process of organizing decisions and actions to achieve particular ends, set within a policy. **—WHO, 1988**

○ It is a code word for public decision making towards the future. **—WHO, 1984**

Steps in Health Planning Cycle

Health planning runs in systematic cyclical steps (Fig. 1)

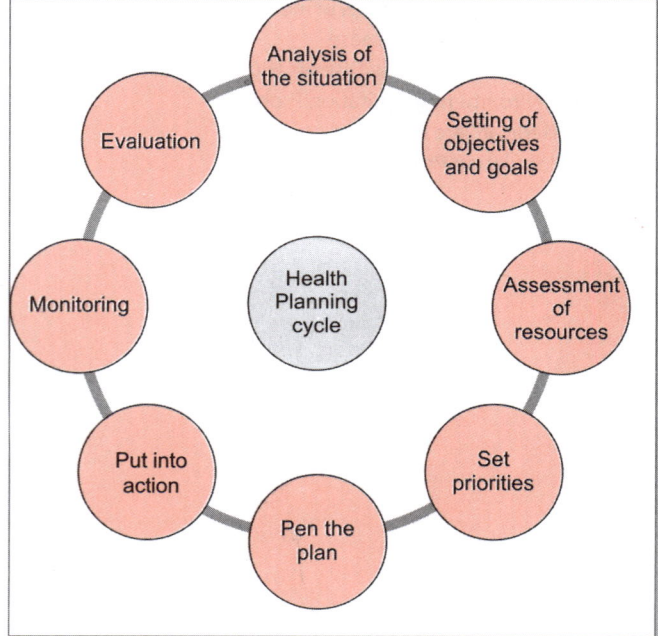

Figure 1: Health planning cycle

- **Analysis of the situation:** The first and foremost step in health planning process is the analysis of the existing health situation of a given region or country.

  The various aspects to be studied include:
  - Population, age and sex composition
  - Morbidity and mortality data
  - Distribution pattern of the diseases
  - The available facilities like hospitals, health centers, etc.
  - Availability of technical manpower
  - Available training facilities for staff
  - Community awareness on concerned disease

- **Setting of objectives and goals:** Setting clear goals and objectives will guide the planning process in an efficient manner. At the beginning of the planning process, objectives at the central level are more broader and general and the objectives at later levels are more specific. Objectives help in measuring and assessing the work undertaken.

- **Assessment of resources:** The available resources like money, material, human resources should be assessed; in addition, the knowledge, skill and technical expertise should also be assessed.

- **Set priorities:** Not all problems can be attended at the same time. The planners should list and rank the problems based on their priority considering the availability of the resources, magnitude and urgency of the problem.

- **Pen the plan:** After setting the priorities a neat systematic plan should be drawn including the resources needed and the result expected.

- **Put into action (implementation):** Here actually the rubber meets the road, that is to put the actual plan into action. Improper implementation may collapse the entire program. A careful implementation itself based on guiding administration.

- **Monitoring:** One should show a keen interest in monitoring the work on day-to-day basis and take necessary action whenever needed. Keep the record of all activities based on your observation and give necessary feedback on continuous basis.

- **Evaluation:** Outcome measurements with the set objectives help in knowing how far the program process has done. Justice at all the steps should be done for good end result and outcome. Any program planning must have an inbuilt evaluation system.

CONTRIBUTIONS OF VARIOUS COMMITTEES AND COMMISSIONS ON HEALTH

HEALTH COMMITTEES

Bhore Committee (1946)

This committee, popularly known as the "Health Survey and Development Committee" appointed in 1943 under the Chairmanship of **Sir Joseph William Bhore**, an Indian civil servant.

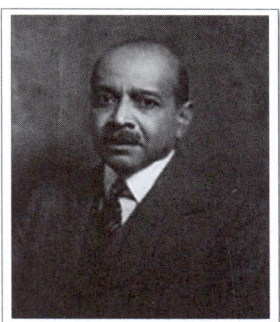

Sir Joseph William Bhore

Major Purposes

- To survey the existing conditions and organization and to give suggestions for future development
- Primarily to review those activities within the scope of health administration

Bhore committee submitted its **report in 1946**. The report consisted of four volumes: I—A survey of the State of the Public Health and the Existing Health Organization, II—Recommendations, III—Appendices and IV—Summary.

Recommendations

It stressed on the importance of integration of curative and preventive medicine at all levels.

The committee recommended short- and long-term plans towards setting up of primary health centers.

Short-Term Plan

- To be implemented within 5–10 years.
- Each primary health center in the rural area to cater to a population of 40,000.
- It should have a secondary health center to serve as a supervisory, coordinating and referral institution.
- For each PHC: 2 medical officers, 4 public health nurses, 1 nurse, 4 midwives, 4 trained *dais* and 15 class IV employees.

Long-Term Plan

- Health care system in three tiers (Fig. 2).
- Three months training in preventive and social medicine to prepare "social physicians"
- Special emphasis on preventive work (Integration of curative and preventive services)
- Village health committee consisting of 5–7 individuals for procuring the active participation of the people in the local health program.

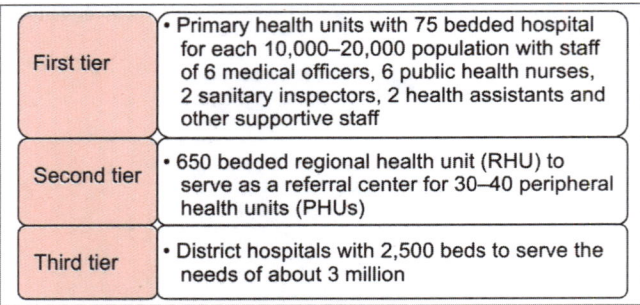

First tier	• Primary health units with 75 bedded hospital for each 10,000–20,000 population with staff of 6 medical officers, 6 public health nurses, 2 sanitary inspectors, 2 health assistants and other supportive staff
Second tier	• 650 bedded regional health unit (RHU) to serve as a referral center for 30–40 peripheral health units (PHUs)
Third tier	• District hospitals with 2,500 beds to serve the needs of about 3 million

Figure 2: Three tiers health care system

o   Intersectoral coordination

o   The Bhore committee focused on many issues however, it was failed to include any component towards comprehensive national socioeconomic development. In spite of this criticism, no one denies the fact that the recommendations of Bhore committee provided a major platform for further health planning and development in India.

Mudaliar Committee (1962)

Government of India constituted Mudaliar Committee in the year 1959 under Chairmanship of Dr A Lakshmanaswamy Mudaliar, Vice Chancellor, Madras University. The committee is popularly known as "Health Survey and Planning Committee." The committee submitted its report in 1962.

Objectives

o   To make an assessment about the implementation of Bhore Committee's recommendations in the field of medical relief and public health since the time of submission of the report

o   To review the first and second five-year plan—health projects

o   To make further recommendations for health and development of the country.

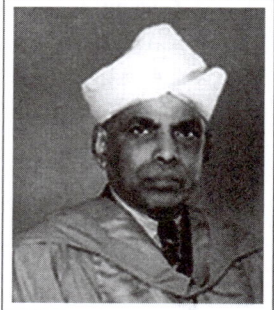

Dr AL Mudaliar

Major Observations

o   It was found that the basic health facilities had not reached at least half of the nation

o   Gross mal distribution in allocating hospitals and beds that favored urban areas

o   Poor functioning of primary health centers with lack of referral system and gross under-staffing due to insufficient resources.

Recommendations

o   To consolidate the advances made in the period of first two five-year plans

o   To strengthen district hospitals to function as central base for providing specialist services

o   Each primary health center should cover the population non-exceeding 40,000 and should 1 basic health worker per every 10,000 population

o   To improve the quality of health services at primary health centers

o   Improve secondary level services

o   Integration of medical and health services.

Chadha Committee (1963)

Initially, the health administrators and malariologists who reviewed the National Malaria Eradication Program suggested to appoint a special committee to study and plan the activities required to be adopted in the maintenance phase of malaria. The government of India constituted Chadha committee in the year 1963 under the chairmanship of Dr MS Chadha, the then Director General of Health Services.

Recommendations

o   Maintenance phase of malaria should be carried by general health services at block level and district level through basic health workers (BHW) (1 per 10,000 population)

o   Basic health workers should make home visits once in a month to perform malaria activities.

o   Apart from malaria vigilance activities, the BHWs are envisaged as multipurpose health workers (MPHWs) to work for family planning and collection of vital statistics

o   Each family planning health assistant (FPHA) to supervise 3–4 BHWs.

Mukherjee Committee (1965)

After 2 years of implementation of Chadha committee's recommendations, it came to the light that the BHWs could not function effectively in the designation of MPHWs. As a result the family planning program and the malaria vigilance operations both were disturbed and failed to bring desired outcome. Following a meeting with central council of health, a committee was constituted in 1965 under the chairmanship of Shri Mukherjee, the then Secretary, Ministry of Health and Family Planning, India.

Recommendations

○ To setup strong executive agency in health directorate of each state government to exclusively deal with family planning

○ Approval of existing urban family welfare planning center

○ Basic health workers to be utilized as MPWs for general services

○ Family planning health assistants to undertake only their duties and no need to supervise BHWs

○ Delink malarial activities from family planning activities.

Mukherjee Committee (1966)

States were discussed their difficulties in taking up the burden of maintenance phase of malaria and other programs like small pox, leprosy, family planning and trachoma during the meeting of the Central Council of Health held at Bangalore (now Bengaluru) in June, 1966. Following this government of India constituted a committee in 1966 under Shri B Mukherjee the then Union Health Secretary.

Recommendations

○ Basic health services at block level.

○ Any attempt to give more work to the BHW would endanger malaria vigilance work or would need large numbers of BHWs than recommended.

○ Health workers at the lower levels should become increasingly oriented to multipurpose

○ Adopt integrated approach in the entire health field.

Jungalwalla Committee (1967)

Jungalwalla Committee was constituted under the chairmanship of Dr N Jungalwalla, additional director general of health services and referred as "Committee on Integration of Health Services." This committee had submitted its report in 1967.

Objectives

○ To study the problems of the health services and its conditions.

○ Integrate health services

○ Eliminate private practice by government doctors.

Recommendations

○ Use unified approach instead of segmented approach in serving for all the problems.

○ Medical care and health programs to function under a single administrator.

○ Operating in unified manner at all levels of hierarchy with due priority for each program.

○ The integration of services from the lowest to the highest level should include:
  ❑ Unified cader
  ❑ Common seniority
  ❑ Recognition of extra qualifications
  ❑ Equal pay for equal work
  ❑ Special pay for specialized work
  ❑ No private practice among government doctors and good service conditions
  ❑ States were permitted to work out their own strategy

Kartar Singh Committee (1973)

In 1972, the government of India during Central Family Planning Council meet, appointed a committee called "the committee on multipurpose workers under Health and Family Planning" under the chairmanship of Kartar Singh the then additional secretary of health and family welfare. This committee had submitted its report in 1973.

This committee was given the following terms of reference to initiate the study:

○ The structure of integrated service at the peripheral and supervisory levels

○ The feasibility of having multipurpose and bi-purpose workers in the field or each worker

○ The training requirements for such workers

○ The utilization of mobile service units operating in the field.

Recommendations

○ Multipurpose workers—feasible and desirable

○ Re-designation:
  ❑ Auxiliary nurse midwives (ANMs) should be replaced by female health workers (FHWs)
  ❑ Basic health workers, Malaria surveillance workers, vaccinators, FPHAs should be replaced by male health workers (MHWs)
  ❑ Lady health visitors (LHV) should be designated as female health (FH) supervisor

○ These MPHWs should be initially introduced in malaria maintenance phase areas and small pox controlled areas

○ Clearly spelt out the job responsibilities of HWs and Supervisors

○ One primary health center (PHC) per 50,000 population

- One primary health center will have 16 health subcenter. Each health subcenter to provide service to 2,000–3,500 population
- One health sub center will have one MPHW one male and one female MPHWs
- One male supervisor for every four MHWs male
- One female supervisor for every four FHWs female
- Doctor will be in charge of all supervisors
- All these to be implemented in 5th five-year plan.

Shrivastav Committee (1975)

In 1974, government of India assigned a group named "group on medical education and support manpower" known as Shrivastav Committee. The group had submitted its report in 1975.

Recommendations

- Organization of the basic health services (including nutrition, health education and family planning) within the community to impart training to the personnel required for these purposes.
- Introduction of paraprofessional and semi-professional health workers like teachers, postmasters, gram sevaks who can provide comprehensive health services as paraprofessionals.
- Placing the health in community's hands by involving the people within the community.
- Organization of economically efficient health services to link the community with the first level referral center—the PHC.
- Creation of MPHWs and health assistants (HA) in between the village health guides (VHG) and medical officer (MO) in charge of PHC.
- One male and one female health worker for every 5,000 population.
- Reorganization of the of medical program and health education.
- Establishment of 'The Medical and Health Education Commission'
- Based on these recommendations **"Rural Health Scheme"** was launched by the government of India in the year 1977–78.

Rural Health Scheme (1977–78)

The major steps taken under this scheme are as follows:

- Involvement of medical colleges in health care was assessed with the objective of reorienting medical education according to rural population need called **"Reorientation of Medical Education"** (ROME).

- Under this scheme train all the undergraduate students and interns at PHCs.
- Reorientation training to all multipurpose workers and training of **Village Health Guides** and utilizing their services in the general health service system.

Bajaj Committee (1987)

The Bajaj committee constituted under Dr JS Bajaj, Professor of Medicine. The committee was popularly known as "**health manpower planning, production and management**."

Following areas were emphasized by the committee:

- Procedures relating to admissions to undergraduate courses
- Procedures relating to admissions to the postgraduate course
- Duration of the undergraduate course and internship
- Duration of the postgraduate courses and thesis
- Review of the residency scheme
- Measures to bring about overall improvement in the undergraduate and postgraduate education.

Krishnan Committee Health Report 1992

This committee worked under the chairmanship of Dr Krishnan to review the recommendations and achievements of previous health committees and comment on any deficits. Consequent to this the committee devised the health post scheme for urban slum areas.

Recommendations

The committee had recommended one voluntary health worker (VHW) per 2,000 population with an honorarium of ₹100. Its report specifically outlines which services have to be provided by the health post. These services have been divided into outreach, preventive, family planning, curative, support (referral) services and reporting and record keeping. Outreach services include population education, motivation for family planning, and health education. In the present context, very few outreach services are being provided to urban slums.

HEALTH COMMISSIONS

National Commission on Macroeconomics and Health (2005)

National commission was formed under the chairmanship of P Chidambaram, the than Finance Minister and Dr Anbumani Ramadoss, the then health minister with the objectives of:

- Promoting equity by reducing household expenditure on total health spending and experimenting with alternate models of health financing

- Restructuring the existing primary health care system to make it more accountable
- Reducing disease burden and the level of risk
- Establishing institutional frameworks for improved quality of governance of health
- Investing in technology and human resources for a more professional and skilled workforce and better monitoring.

Planning Commission of India

Primarily the economic planning of India that gave authority to state began in 1930s during British period. Initially the formal planning board of colonial government of India existed from the year 1944 to 1946. India became "independent country" on August 15, 1947 and became "Republic India" on January 29, 1950. Following which **"Planning commission"** was established **on March 15, 1950** adopting a formal functioning model under the Chairmanship of Prime Minister **Jawaharlal Nehru.** After the establishment of the formal planning commission (Fig. 3) it started to report directly to the Prime Minister of India.

Structure

Planning commission included a chairman, deputy chairman, and five members and functioned through program advisors, general secretariat and technical divisions. A senior officer headed each of this division. The major task of planning commission was formulation of five year plans to guide the country in a developing path. Planning commission adopted "decentralized approach" in planning process in view to achieve decentralized district planning.

Functions

The 1950 resolution on establishment of the Planning Commission framed its functions as given below:

- Assessment on existing resources of the country like manpower, money and material and augment these resources in areas of deficiencies.

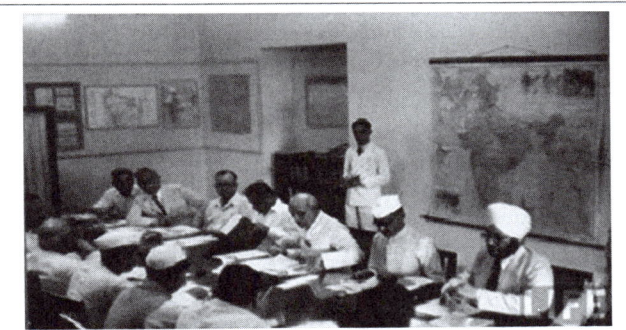

Figure 3: Planning Commission of India—under the chairmanship of Prime Minister Jawaharlal Nehru

- Formulates plan for the appropriate and balanced use of resources of the country.
- Sets priorities and allocates resources in a phased manner for fulfilling the work at each phase.
- Alerts the factors that may impede the process of economic growth of the country and identifies suitable conditions for successful implementation of the plan.
- To decide upon the equipment and technology required for the implementation of plan.
- Continuous monitoring, assessment and feedback on each stage with appropriate changes and modifications in the policies.
- Make interim plans and recommendations to make appropriate changes in the existing policies and to seek advice from Central and State government.
- Planning Commission plays a mediatory and facilitating role in the best interest of all state and central government.

NATIONAL INSTITUTION FOR TRANSFORMING INDIA (NITI) AAYOG

Government of India dissolved the "Planning Commission" that was in function since 1950 and formulated "National Institution for Transforming India (NITI) Aayog" on January 1, 2015 by the Prime Minister Narendra Modi. NITI Aayog has been assigned the role to coordinate **'Transforming our world: the 2030 Agenda for Sustainable Development."**

Objectives of NITI Aayog

- To have a shared vision in developmental priorities of the nation by involving state governments and other sectors in achieving national objectives
- To encourage accommodating federalism through structured support initiatives
- To build practical ways to draw realistic plans initially at the village level and implement the same at higher levels of government
- To pay special attention to the weaker sections of our society in view of economic progress of the country
- To pay attention on inter-sectoral and inter-departmental issues to gear up the execution of the development agenda
- To adopt best practices that would promote sustainable and equitable development and help their dissemination to stakeholders
- To monitor continuously on the execution of programs and initiatives and receive feedback for planning.
- To focus on capacity building through necessary technology upgradation.

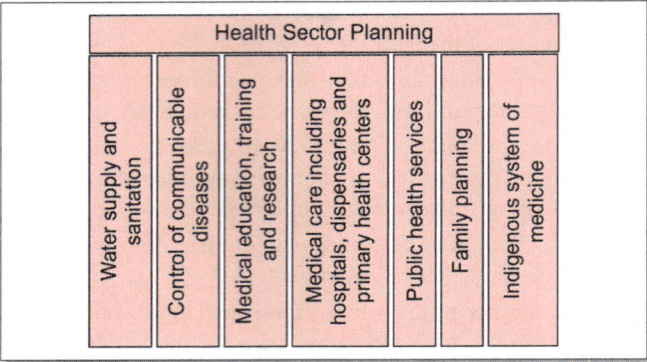

Figure 4: Health sector planning

Table 1: Budget allocation during first five-year plan

A total of 206.8 billion allocated during first-five year plan
○ Irrigation and energy—27.2%
○ Agriculture and community development—17.4%
○ Transport and communications—24%
○ Industry—8.4%
○ Social services—16.64%
○ Land rehabilitation—4.1%
○ Others—2.5%

Planning Commission and Health Sector Planning

Health is the major phenomenon of interest in the developmental representation of the country. Consequently, planning commission of India gave significant importance in including and allocating the resources on various health programs across five-year plans. A Planning Bureau under **"Ministry of Health"** was introduced in the year 1965 to enhance coordination between central and state governments and to compile five-year plans. The planning commission divided the priority areas of health for the purposes of planning and providing specific attention on each (Fig. 4).

Five-Year Plans

The five-year plans provide a basic framework and helps in providing overall directions for making policies, procedures, and programs that lead to the development of the country.

First Five-Year Plan (1951–1956)

Since the time of independence, India concentrated mainly on bringing about a fast and balanced economic development. Shri Jawaharlal Nehru, the first Indian Prime Minister presented the first five-year plan to the Parliament of India on December 8, 1951. A total of 206.8 billion allocated in first five year plan for developing and modifying various sectors (Table 1).

The first plan initiated in the year 1951 with the focus on primary sector.

Objectives

○ To reinstate the financial system and overcome the pressures of inflation, establish the transport system and enhance the state of availability of food and raw material

○ To promote the progress by activating substantial development programs.

○ To initiate measures of social justice on a wider scale.

To establish relevant administrative changes for development purposes.

Various aspects considered to enhance health

○ Water supply and sanitation

○ Control/Eradication of common communicable diseases

○ Maternal and child health services and health education

○ Strengthening rural health facilities by establishing health subcenters and primary health centers and develop health manpower resources

○ Preventive health care of the rural population through health units and mobile units

○ Family planning

○ Self-sufficiency in drugs and equipment.

Second Five-Year Plan (1956–1961)

The second five-year plan was more ambitious with twice the budget provision for development than the first five year plan. Second five-year plan was concentrated on development of public sector.

Aims

○ National annual income to increase 5%

○ Additional employment facilities for 10 million people

○ Rapid industrialization with specific attention to the production of iron and steel

○ Empowerment of people by reducing inequalities in income and wealth.

Objectives

○ Establishment of institutional facilities to serve people

○ Development of technical manpower through training programs and provision of employment for those trained

○ Measures to control communicable diseases prevalent in community

○ Create awareness on environmental hygiene, family planning and other supporting programs.

Third Five-Year Plan (1961–1966)

The third five-year plan gave larger importance to the development of agriculture to improve production of rice, but due to the economic threat caused by Sino-India War (1962) the focus of the country was shifted towards defence. During 1965–1966, the Green Revolution in India boosted agriculture development in India. As a measure to disseminate democracy Panchayat elections were conducted. Sino-India War (1962) and Indo-Pakistan War (1965) brought down the gross domestic product rate to 2.7%. Third plan initiated with a total outlay of about ₹342 crores, about ₹297 crores to States and the rest to the Center.

Aims

- To maintain 5–6% annual increase in national income and to sustain the same in further plans
- To become self-sufficient and increase agricultural production in order to meet the needs of industry and the growing population
- To increase major industries like steel, fuel, power and chemical thereby enhance the use of our resources for industrialization
- To utilize manpower effectively and substantiate employment opportunities
- To bring down the disparities in income and wealth to create economic power among people.

Aims for health sector

- Improvement of environmental sanitation, and safe water supply.
- Control of communicable diseases.
- Organization of institutional facilities for providing care and for the training of medical and health personnel.
- Provision of services like maternal and child welfare, health education and nutrition.
- High priority to family planning.

Fourth Five-Year Plan (1969–1974)

Fourth five-year plan deferred for three years because of the operational difficulties faced and inadequate growth of the economy. A total of 433.53 crores was the outlay assigned for health and family planning in fourth five-year plan.

General objectives

- To enhance stability and self-reliance in various productive activities of the country.
- To emphasize on productive activity, principally on agricultural production.

- To enhance technological advancement in industrial activity and enterprise.
- To extend help to small producers and increase job opportunities for present and future.
- To make supplies available evenly.
- To include "Panchayati Raj Institutions" for planning towards integrated cooperative structure and building social and economic democracy.

Health-related objectives

- To eradicate communicable diseases.
- To establish primary health centers in each community development block.
- Family planning program.
- Expand medical and nursing education and training of paramedical personnel to meet the technical manpower requirements.

Fifth Five-Year Plan (1974–1978)

Fifth five-year plan focused on employment, poverty alleviation, and justice. The plan continued to pay attention on self-reliance in agricultural production and defense. The Morarji Desai government took over in the year 1978 following which the plan was rejected.

Major objectives

- Elimination of poverty
- Realization and attainment of self-reliance

Sixth Five-Year Plan (1980–1985)

Sixth five-year plan was started on April 1, 1980, which continued till March 31, 1985. Sixth plan aimed at rapid industrial development specifically in the area of information technology. Family planning activities geared up in order to prevent overpopulation.

General objectives

- To bring down poverty and unemployment rate progressively
- Saving and development of indigenous sources of energy with efficiency
- Progressive reduction of regional disparities to enhance technological benefits
- Population control policies and procedures towards voluntary acceptance of the small family norm
- Promote, protect and improve ecological and environmental assets through harmonious short- and long-term goals

○ Promote the involvement of people from all sections of the society through education, communication and other strategies of the institutions.

Health-related objectives

○ Increasing the accessibility of health services to rural areas
○ Correcting regional imbalances
○ Further development of referral services by removal of deficiencies in District/Subdivisional hospitals
○ Intensification of the control/eradication of communicable diseases especially malaria and smallpox
○ Qualitative improvement in the education and training of health personnel
○ Development of referral services by providing specialist attention to common diseases in rural areas.

Seventh Five-Year Plan (1985–1990)

Seventh five-year plan was focused on steady growth with significant importance to self-reliance and improved efficiency in productivity. Equity and social justice were the elements used for distributing the benefits yielded. The total outlay for the health sector was ₹3392.89 crores.

General objectives

○ To support and speedup the production of food grains
○ To implement various programs that would facilitate meeting the basic requirements
○ To boost self-reliance and increase job opportunities to people
○ To gear up the process of expansion of scientific and technological capabilities.

Health-related objectives

○ Coordination and coupling of health and health-related services and activities, e.g. nutrition, safe drinking water, etc.
○ Special efforts on urban health services, school health services and mental and dental health services to ensure comprehensive coverage
○ Community participation and intersectoral coordination
○ Control and eradication of communicable diseases
○ Training and education of doctors and paramedical personnel
○ Rural health programs.

Annual Plans (1990–1992)

There were no five-year plans between the years 1990 and 1992 due to disturbed political situation. The country had only annual plans for the years 1990–1991 and 1991–1992. Following to that the eighth five-year plan was launched in 1992. Dr Manmohan Singh gave greater attention on India's free market reforms that brought about the economic stability. During this plan period privatization and liberalization began in India.

Eighth Five-Year Plan (1992–1997)

Eighth five-year plan was started on April 1, 1992 with major concern of modernizing the industries. The major components of eighth plan include strengthening the infrastructure, check on population growth, poverty reduction and people's participation.

General objectives

○ Creation of adequate job opportunities to achieve near full employment by the turn of the century
○ Universalization of elementary education and eradication of illiteracy among the age group of 15–35 years
○ Control population growth by voluntary acceptance of family planning and through incentives and disincentives
○ Provision of safe drinking water and primary health care to the entire population
○ Develop and strengthen the areas like communication infrastructure, irrigation and energy production to enhance the growth of the country.

Health-related objectives

○ Containing population growth with the goals:
  ▫ Reducing the birth rate from 29.9 per thousand in 1990 to 26 per thousand by 1997
  ▫ The infant mortality rate (IMR) will also be brought down from 80 per thousand live births in 1990 to 70% by 1997.
○ Convergence of health services provided by various sectors, e.g. welfare, human resource development, nutrition, etc.
○ Consolidation and operationalization of sub-centers, PHCs and CHCs so that their performance is optimized
○ The health for all (HFA) paradigm must take into account not only high risk but also vulnerable groups, i.e. mothers and children.

Ninth Five-Year Plan (1997–2002)

The ninth plan came to act from April 1, 1997.

Main objectives

○ Agriculture and rural development
○ Generate adequate employment and eradicate poverty

- Increase economic growth rate with stable prices
- Ensuring food and nutritional security for all
- Provision of basic services like safe drinking water, primary health care, universal primary education, etc.
- Containing the growth rate of population
- Empowerment of women and socially disadvantaged
- Promotion of people's participation through Panchayati Raj Institutions and self-help groups.

Health-related objectives

- Ensure existing SC, PHC are fully operational
- Fill the gaps in CHCs through re-structuring existing block level PHC, Taluk, and Sub-divisional hospital
- Establish functional referral linkages
- Local recruitment of doctors, if necessary on part-time basis
- Provide adequate diagnostics, consumables and drugs
- Strengthen emergency services.

Tenth Five-Year Plan (2002–2007)

Apart from economic growth, the "tenth five year plan" (2002–2007) also aimed at improving the quality of life of the people.

Main objectives

- Reduction in poverty ratio 5% by 2007
- Providing gainful high quality employment to the additional labor force
- All children to be enrolled in schools and complete 5 years of schooling
- Reduction of gender gaps in literacy and wage rates by at least 50%
- Reduction in decadal rate of population growth between 2001 and 2011 to 16.2%
- Increase in literacy rate to 75% within the plan period
- All villages to have sustained access to potable drinking water within the plan period
- Cleaning of major polluted rivers and other notified stretches
- Reduction in IMR and maternal mortality rate (MMR).

Health-related objectives

- Reorganization and restructuring of the existing government health care system with appropriate referral linkages

- Efficient and effective logistics system for the supply of drugs, and consumables based on need and utilization
- Improving content and quality of education for health professionals
- Skill upgradation of all health care providers
- Promotion of the rational use of diagnostics and drugs
- Research and development
- Strengthening and sustaining civil registration and sample registration system.

Eleventh Five-Year Plan (2007–2012)

Objectives

- To accelerate GDP growth from 8% to 9%
- To create 70 million new work opportunities
- To reduce educated unemployment to below 5%
- To raise real wage rate of unskilled workers by 20%
- Attain WHO standards of air quality in all major cities by 2011–2012
- Attention on taking care of the older persons
- Reducing disability and integrating disabled

Health-Related Objectives

- Reducing maternal morality ratio (MMR) to 1 per 1,000 live births.
- Reducing infant mortality rate (IMR) to 28 per 1,000 live births.
- Reducing total fertility rate (TFR) to 2.1.
- Providing clean drinking water for all by 2009 and ensuring no slip-backs.
- Reducing malnutrition among children of age group 0–3 to half from its present level.
- Reducing anemia among women and girls by 50%.
- Raising the sex ratio for age group 0–6 to 935 by 2011–12 and 950 by 2016–17.
- Improving medical, paramedical, nursing, and dental education and then availability.
- Reorienting AYUSH education and utilization.

Twelfth Five-Year Plan (2012–2017)

The twelfth five-year plan is a centralized and integrated national economic program depicted its broad vision and aspirations in the subtitle: "Faster, sustainable, and more inclusive growth". Initially, the planning commission estimated to register an average growth rate of 8.2% in the twelfth plan (2007–12) but later fixed at 8% target that was more feasible.

Goals related to energy and production

- Increasing green cover by one million hectare every year and adding 30,000 MW of renewable energy generation capacity in the plan period.

- To reduce emission intensity of the GDP in line with the target of 20–25 reduction by 2020 over 2005 levels.
- Raising agriculture output to 4% for the full plan.
- Manufacturing sector growth to 10% for the full plan.
- Target of adding over 88,000 MW of power generation capacity in the 12th five-year plan.

Planning commission has constituted a high level expert group (HLEG) on universal health coverage, seven working groups and two steering committees to define the appropriate strategy for the health sector for the XII plan.

Goals Related to Health Sector

- Reduction of infant mortality rate (IMR) to 25 per 1,000 live births
- Reduction of maternal mortality ratio (MMR) to 100 per 100,000 live births
- Reduction of total fertility rate (TFR) to 2.1
- Prevention and reduction of under-nutrition in children under 3 years to half of NFHS-3 (2005–06) levels
- Prevention and reduction of anemia among women aged 15–49 years to 28%
- Raising child sex ratio in the 0–6 year age group from 914 to 950
- Prevention and reduction of burden of communicable and noncommunicable diseases (including mental illnesses) and injuries
- Reduction of poor households' out-of-pocket expenditure.

National Health Goals for Communicable Disease in 12th Five-Year Plan are given in Table 2

Table 2: National health goals for communicable disease in 12th five-year plan

Diseases	Goals
Tuberculosis	Reduce annual incidence and mortality by half
Leprosy	Reduce prevalence to <1/10,000 population and incidence to zero in all districts,
Malaria	Annual malaria incidence of <1/1000
Filariasis	<1% microfilaria prevalence in all districts
Dengue	Sustaining case fatality rate of <1%
Chikungunya	Containment of outbreaks
Japanese encephalitis	Reduction in JE mortality by 30%
Kala-azar	<1% microfilaria prevalence in all districts

Contd...

Diseases	Goals
HIV/AIDS	Reduce new infections to zero and provide comprehensive care and support to all persons living with HIV/AIDS and treatment services for all those who require it.

SUMMARY OF INVESTMENT DURING ANNUAL AND FIVE-YEAR PLAN (TABLE 3)

Table 3: Investment during annual and five-year plan periods

Period	Total plan investment (Crore)	Health investment (Crore)
First Plan (1951–1956)	1960.00	65.20
Second Plan (1956–1961)	4672.00	140.80
Third Plan (1961–1966)	8576.00	225.00
Annual Plans (1966–1969)	6625.40	140.20
Fourth Plan (1969–1974)	15778.80	335.50
Fifth Plan (1974–1978)	39322.00	682.00
1979–1980 (outlay)	11650.00	268.20
Sixth Plan (1980–1985)	97500.00	1,821.05
Seventh Plan (1980–1985)	180000.00	3,392.00
Annual Plan (1990–1991)	61518.10	960.90
Annual Plan (1991–1992)	72316.80	1,185.50
Eighth Plan (1992–1997)	79800.00	7,575.92
Ninth Plan (1997–2002)	859200.00	10,818.00
Tenth Plan (2002–2007)	1,484,131.00	31,020.30
Eleventh Plan (2007–2012)	2,156,571.00	136,147.00
Twelfth Plan (2012–2017)	7,66,9807.00	1,93,405.00

CENTRAL COUNCIL FOR HEALTH AND FAMILY WELFARE

On August 9, 1952 "Central Council of Health and Family Welfare" (CCHFW) was set up under article 263 as per the Presidential order to enhance the relationship and better coordination between the center and state governments in health-related program, planning and implementation. Central council of health and family welfare functions with the union health minister as its chairman and ministers of states and union territories as its members.

Functions of the Council

- To enhance good coordination and working relationship between the health organizations at the central and state level

- Development and proposal of policies relating to medical relief, health care and training of health care professionals
- Proposing suitable ethical and legal guidelines in matters relating to public health
- Recommends allocation of the funds to states for health-related matters and makes periodical review on utilization of the same.

NATIONAL HEALTH POLICY 1983

It was not until 1983 that India adopted a formal or official National Health Policy with commitment to attain the goal of "Health for all by 2000 AD." Prior to that states were working within the framework set through the five-year plans and recommendations from various committees appointed time to time. During the five-year plans the constituted health schemes worked with set targets. Recurring global debates on new approach required for health systems, Alma Ata declaration on primary health care and ICMR-ICSSR Joint Panel report, the government of India sought a new healthcare approach—"It is felt that an integrated, comprehensive approach towards the future development of medical education, research and health services requires to be established to serve the actual health needs and priorities of the country. It is in this context that the need has been felt to evolve a National Health policy," (MoHFW, 1983, p 1)

Key Features

- Provision of comprehensive integrated health services relevant to the actual needs of the people at a cost that the community can afford
- Encourage community participation
- Promotion of family planning as a "people's program", on a voluntary basis
- Strengthening of welfare programs for women and children
- Medical and health education
- To restructure the health services through comprehensive primary health care services, linked with health education
- The decentralization of services with the inclusion of community participation and established of working referral system
- Access to urgent specialist case for all irrespective of the people living in urban and rural areas
- Reorientation of the existing health personnel.

NATIONAL HEALTH POLICY (NHP) 2002

National health policy 2002 evolved by considering the changes took place in factors that revolve around the health sector and in other determinants of health. National health policy 2002 has laid down specific goals to be attained by the years 2005, 2007, 2010 and 2015 (Table 4).

Table 4: National health policy goals to be achieved by 2015

Eradication of polio and Yaws	2005
Elimination of leprosy	2005
Elimination of kala-azar	2010
Elimination of lymphatic filariasis	2015
Achieve zero level growth of HIV/AIDS	2007
Reduction of mortality by 50% on account of tuberculosis, malaria, other vector and water borne diseases	2010
Reduce prevalence of blindness to 0.5%	2010
Reduction of IMR to 30/1000 and MMR to 100/lakh	2010
Increase utilization of public health facilities from current level of <20% to >75%	2010
Establishment of an integrated system of surveillance, National Health Accounts and health statistics	2005
Increase health expenditure by government as a % of GDP from the existing 0.9%–2%	2010
Increase share of central grants to constitute at least 25% of total health spending	2010
Increase state sector health spending from 5.5%–7% of the budget	2005
Further increase of state sector health spending from 7% to 8 %	2010

Objectives

- Attaining an acceptable standard of good health to population of India by decentralizing public health system and upgrading the infrastructure in existing institutions.
- Ensuring a more equitable access to health service across the social and geographical expansion of India.
- Encouraging the contribution of private sector in providing health services for people who can pay.
- Giving primacy or prevention and first line curative initiative.
- Emphasizing rational use of drugs.
- Increasing the access to traditional medicine system.

NATIONAL POPULATION POLICY 2000

In 1951, India has the proud to say that it is the first in 1951 country in the world to launch a family planning program to battle the population growth. India had formed its first national population policy in the year 1976 and it had increased the legal minimum age for females from 15 to 18 years and for males 18 to 21 years. Modified policy of 1977 stressed on "small family norm" without compulsion and simultaneously changed the title of the program as "Family welfare program." The "Net Reproduction Rate" (NRR) of 1 set by National health policy 1983 to achieve by 2000AD. There was a criticism considering NRR as a goal and the NHP 2000 goal (replacing the fertility level by 2010) was much appreciated over the earlier one.

National Population Policy: Sociodemographic Goals

National Population Policy 2000 was set to achieve following Sociodemographic goals by 2010:

- Address the unmet needs for basic reproductive and child health services, supplies and infrastructure.
- Make school education up to age of 14 free and compulsory, and reduce drop outs at primary and secondary school levels to below 20% for both boys and girls.
- Reduce infant mortality rate to below 30 per 1000 live births.
- Reduce maternal mortality ratio to below 100 per 100,000 live births.
- Achieve universal immunization of children against all vaccine preventable diseases.
- Promote delayed marriage for girls, not earlier than age 18 and preferably after 20 years of age.
- Achieve 80% institutional deliveries and 100% deliveries by trained persons.
- Achieve universal access to information/counseling, and services for fertility regulation and contraception with a wide basket of choices.
- Achieve 100% registration of births, deaths, marriage and pregnancy.
- Contain the spread of acquired immunodeficiency syndrome (AIDS), and promote greater integration between the management of reproductive tract infections (RTI) and sexually transmitted infections (STI) and the National AIDS Control Organization.
- Prevent and control communicable diseases.
- Integrate Indian Systems of Medicine (ISM) in the provision of reproductive and child health services, and in reaching out to households.
- Promote vigorously the small family norm to achieve replacement levels of TFR.
- Bring about convergence in implementation of related social sector programs so that family welfare becomes a people-centered program.

  On May 11, 2000 population of India reached 100 crore or 1 billion or 1000 million. The estimated current trends of population of India alarms that India will become "the most populous country" in the world by 2045. Population in India increased nearly five times from 23 crore to 100 crore, during the 20th century while world's

population increased nearly three times from 200 crore to 600 crore during the same period. There is difference found between TFR rates at urban and rural areas of India (Table 5).

- The percent decadal growth rate of the country declined significantly from 21.5% for the period 1991–2001 to 17.7% during 2001–2011.
- Total fertility rate (TFR) was 3.2 when "National Population Policy 2000" was adopted and the same has declined to 2.3 (SRS-India, 2013).
- India is yet to achieve TFR replacement level of 2.1.

Table 5: Total fertility rate in India

Indicator	Total	Rural	Urban	Differential
TFR (2012)	2.4	2.6	1.8	44%

Strategies Adopted to Promote "Small Family Norm" in National Population Policy

- Rewards towards the exemplary performance of Panchayats and Zila Parishads
- Under the scheme of **"Balika Samridhi Yojana"** ₹500 is awarded at birth to the girl child of birth order 1 or 2 to enhance survival and care.
- **Maternity benefit scheme**—₹500 is awarded to mothers who have deliver their first child after 19 years of age.
- Family welfare - linked **Health insurance plan**.
- Reward to couples below poverty line if they **marry** and produce two children **after age of 21 years.**
- Establishing **crèches**/centers for children in rural and urban slums in view to **promote women employment.**
- Provision of wider and affordable choices of contraceptives
- Provision and expansion of **safe abortion facilities**.
- Creation of **vocational training schemes** for girls' self-employment.
- Provision of soft loans to villagers to run **ambulance services** for referrals.
- Establishing **self-help groups** at villages

NATIONAL HEALTH PROBLEMS IN INDIA

India has huge burden of health problems. In India, health problems are discussed under six major headings as commonly seen in the country. They are as follows (Flowchart 1):

COMMUNICABLE DISEASE

From ancient days, communicable disease served as the major cause of morbidity and mortality profile of the country.

Flowchart 1: National health problems in India

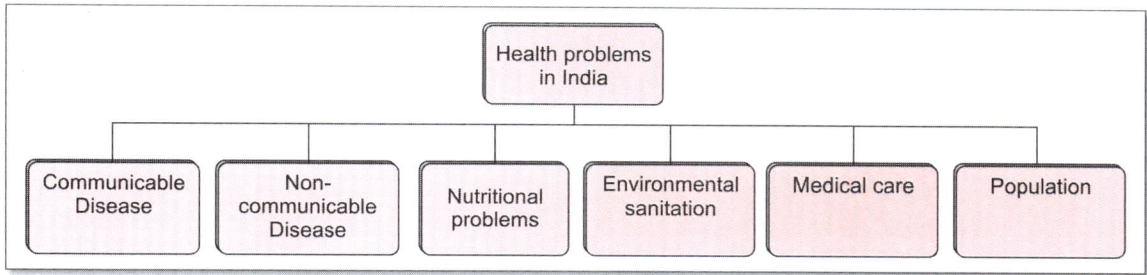

The introduction of vaccines against communicable diseases brought down the mortality rates largely. But still, the diseases cause public health burden.

Malaria

Overall, in the last 10 years in India, total malaria cases declined by 42%, from 1.92 million in 2004 to 1.1 million in 2014, combined with a 40.8% decline in malaria-related deaths from 949 to 562. Malaria cases seem to show increased incidence in North-East states of India. India accounts for 70% of malaria cases and 69% of malaria deaths in the South-East Asia region. Reduction in mortality and morbidity will not remain the same without continuous attention on the existing challenges of malaria.

Filaria

Around 1.1 billion people are at risk of getting lymphatic filariasis (LF) in 73 countries of the world. Among this 600 million Indian, who live in 250 districts of India, account for more than 40% of the global burden of LF. An estimated 50% of India's LF endemic population resides in northeastern India in areas of poverty. Historically, Odisha, identified as highly endemic and remains the same.

Acute Respiratory Infections

Southeast Asia stands first in number for ARI incidence accounting for >80% of all incidences. In India, pneumonia found to be accountable for 13–16% of all deaths occurring in the pediatric hospitals. Available statistics shows that on an average, every child has five episodes of ARI/year and 3.5% of the global burden of disease is due to ARI. Around 20% of deaths in children of <5 years are attributed to respiratory tract infections.

Tuberculosis

India alone accounts for 23% of the world's TB incidence and 21% of world TB deaths. The pattern and distribution of TB occurrence in 2013 in the region revealed that most cases found among young adults, particularly in 25–34 year age group and male female ratio of TB was 1:5. Tuberculosis is a leading cause of all HIV-related deaths. Around 38%

morbidity and 39% mortality of the world-tuberculosis burden is found in South-East Asia Region (SEAR) of world health organization.

Diarrheal Diseases

Diarrhea is most common in children under 5 years especially those between 6 months and 2 years. People with low immunity are prone for diarrheal infections. Diarrhea is more common in persons with malnutrition. Poverty, prematurity, reduced gastric acidity, immunodeficiency, lack of personal and domestic hygiene and incorrect feeding practices are all contribute to the occurrence of diarrheal diseases. About 1.2 lakh children under the age of 5 succumb to diarrhea every year. (2016, Health Ministry, India). This translates to 328 diarrhea deaths every day and 13 every hour.

Leprosy

Leprosy has been eliminated from 119 out of the 122 countries with the introduction of antileprosy treatment regimes. The prevalence rate (PR) of leprosy in India was 0.68 per 10,000 populations in 2014. Although, India achieved elimination of leprosy as a public health problem in 2005 still there are leprosy cases identified in high endemic states. The prevalence rates of states and districts vary. Mass chemotherapy used by India is brilliant strategy in reducing microfilaremia to very low levels among people who are on treatment.

AIDS

So far there is no treatment for curing HIV infection. However, the available antiretroviral (ARV) drugs can help effectively to control the virus so that people with HIV can enjoy healthy and productive lives. HIV is a life-threatening infection and claimed 34 million lives so far. Consent, confidentiality, counseling, correct test results and connection (linkage to care, treatment and other services) are the strategies recommended by World Health Organization to motivate people to come forward in using HIV testing facilities.

Others

Apart from the above communicable diseases there are other diseases that predominantly require attention from the government are: Dengue fever, enteric fever, meningitis, kala-azar and Japanese encephalitis, etc.

It is still a known challenge to India to modify the environment and to enhance the standards of living to battle these diseases.

NONCOMMUNICABLE DISEASE (NCD) PROBLEMS

Increased urbanization and industrialization, changing age structure and lifestyle of people has placed India at a critical position facing a continuous burden of NCDs.

Based on the prevalence rates cardiovascular diseases (CVDs), diabetes mellitus, chronic obstructive pulmonary disease (COPD) and cancer are the four leading chronic diseases in India. By 2030, the productivity loss due to noncommunicable diseases will be 17.9 million years lost.

Nonexistence of regular system for regular collection data on NCDs most often provides only estimates on approximation only. India had 46 million diabetes mellitus cases in 2015 compared to 38 million in 2010. Cases of coronary heart disease have gone up to 62 million in 2015 from 47 million in 2010. In 2015 there were around 23 million COPD (the second leading cause of death in India) compared to 21 million in 2010.

> **Do you know**
> India is the first country to develop specific national targets and indicators aimed at reducing the number of global premature deaths from NCDs by 25% by 2025.

One out of every 4 Indians risks dying from an NCD before reaching 70 years. There are about 1 million tobacco deaths occur each year in India. In 2012 an estimated 600,000–700,000 deaths in India were caused by cancer. Poor people die from cancer before the age of 70 years. The leading sites of cancers in males include lung, esophagus, larynx, mouth, tongue; in females breast and cervicouterine cancer. Oral health care is paid less attention, to that extent even the district hospitals do not have required machinery, material and equipment to provide oral health care to people.

Nutritional Problems

The Indian community has the mixed pattern of living styles which is influenced by specifically by poor and rich status of people who live in poor and rich living customs and practices respectively. The poor are largely undernourished and rich are over nourished contributing to major health problems. The problems of affluent groups of India mimic the problems of people of developed nations. In present context, rising food prices lead to lack of access to nutritious foods that ultimately ends up in malnutrition.

Protein Energy Malnutrition

Malnutrition is defined as insufficient, excessive or imbalanced consumption of nutrients. In developing countries, malnutrition is one of the indirect causes of 300,000 deaths that occur every year among children below the age of 5 years. Protein energy malnutrition is commonly found in all states of the country. Nutritional marasmus is more common than Kwashiorkor among under-five children.

Nutritional Anemia

Anemia is the most common morbidity occurs because of deficient or inadequately available micronutrients (iron, folic-acid and vitamin B_{12}) that affects health, education, productivity and entire development of the country. Anemia is a major health problem in India. Every second pregnant woman and 40% of preschool children in developing countries, estimated to be anemic. The timely treatment helps in restoring personal health and increasing the national productivity levels by as much as 20%.

Low Birthweight

The WHO has defined the term low birthweight (LBW) as birthweight less than 2500 g or 2.5 kg. In 2012, the World Health Assembly's Resolution- Comprehensive implementation plan sets to achieve 30% reduction of LBW by the year 2025. Concentrating on adolescent girls health and improving maternal nutrition would help in preparing healthy future mothers and bringing about healthy babies.

Xerophthalmia

Vitamin A deficiency is the major cause for blindness among children. About 0.04% of blindness in India is due to nutritional deficiency.

Iodine-Deficiency Disorders

The term "iodine-deficiency disorders" denotes many consequences that occur as a result of iodine deficiency. Goiter and iodine deficiency disorders have been endemic in sub Himalayan region. ICMR in its report revealed that the goiter is found in all parts of India. Out of 324 districts all over the country, 263 are found to be endemic with the prevalence of >10%. UNICEF, Indian Coalition for Control of Iodine Deficiency Disorders (ICCIDD), and World Health Organization (WHO) recommend iodine daily intake.

Others Problems

Now, problems like Lathyrism and Fluorosis have been found to be endemic in some parts of India. Another important and widely prevalent problem, which seeks attention, is food adulteration.

ENVIRONMENTAL SANITATION PROBLEMS

According to World Bank estimates, 21% of communicable diseases in India are due to unsafe water. Three "Ss" that are fundamental to global health include Safe water, Sanitation, and Safe water management. During 19th century, the "sanitary awakening" that took place in England had major share in changing and strengthening the environmental sanitation of many countries. But, India, which was under British rule then, lacks environmental sanitation even today. About 60% of this "toilet-less" population lives in India. This 60% equals 626 million people. Lack of safe water, old and improper methods of practice of excreta disposal, poverty and unemployment, increasing urbanization and industrialization and population increase are the major contributors of sanitation problems in India. It was recommended in the UN conference held in 1977 at Argentina that there should be provision of safe water supply and sanitation for all. Provision of safe water annually could prevent 1.4 million deaths among children due to diarrheal diseases. It was recommended in the UN conference held in 1977 at Argentina that there should be provision of safe water supply and sanitation for all.

MEDICAL CARE PROBLEMS

India has a good national policy but does not have "National Health Service." India is unable to run national health services due to inadequate financial resources. Eighty percent of health facilities of India are available in urban area where only 28% of population lives and the remaining 20% of the health facilities seen in rural area where 72% of population lives. Most hospitals, from small to high-tech are available in urban areas. Urbanization and migration from rural to urban areas have triggered urban health problems: overcrowding, poor housing, communicable diseases, shortage of health care professionals and other workers, inadequate supplies and high charges in the hospitals. Most villages depend upon indigenous practitioners available locally for meeting the health care needs; most often rural men and women end up in grave problems due to poor health practices by quacks and other unqualified practitioners. The basic problem in our health care is imbalanced distribution of health services to urban and rural. The "Primary health care approach" and "Health for all by 2000 AD" movement explicitly provided significant importance to equitable distribution of health care, community participation, and intersectoral coordination to combat the imbalances.

POPULATION PROBLEMS

India takes the share of 17.31% of the world's population. As a matter fact, 1 out of 6 people in the world is an Indian. The population density of India shows increasing trend. According to the records of population density (2011), population density of india has increased from 324 to 382 per square kilometer, which is higher than the average population density of the world (2011) i.e. only 46 per square kilometer. There are big differences found in the population density of the various states of India. Delhi had showed the highest population density in the year 2011 among all the states of India with 11,297 people per square kilometer. India had set the goal to attain 1% population growth rate by 2000 AD, but has not attained it yet. India's present population growth rate is 1.2%. Population explosion is everyone's problem, hence, it has become a social and economic hindrance. There is a need for a great coordination from all sectors as well among families to control population.

India became the signatory to the UN Millennium Declaration of the United Nations General Assembly in September 2000, and has consistently reiterated its commitment towards the eight "**Millennium development goals (MDGs)**" to achieve by the year 2015.

The Millennium Development Goals gave a strong influence globally on policy formulation and planning. MDGs mainly helped in bringing about a strong target-oriented agenda for development. Though India has been moving rightly in some areas, there are many areas that require more attention. The Millennium Development Goals (MDGs) were to be achieved by December 2015. The world is once again committed to adopt a new set of transformative and universal sustainable development goals (SDGs). The lessons learned from the MDGs are incorporated in planning the sustainable development goals to build upon the unfinished agenda of MDGs At this juncture, a critical to assessment is made on the achievements of the MDGs in India (Table 6).

Table 6: Millennium development goals (MDGs) and India's Achievements

Goals to achieve by year 2015	India's Achievements in 2015
MDG 1: Eradicate extreme poverty and hunger. Poverty Head Count Ratio (PHCR) level has to be 23.9%. To bring down Malnourishment 26%.	Moderately successful in reducing poverty. PHCR was 21.9%. Malnourishment declined to 40%. This is still below the target of reducing malnourishment to 26 percent.
Goal 2: Achieve Universal Primary Education	Significant progress shown in universalizing primary education,
Goal 3: Promote Gender Equality and Empower Women To achieve the proportion of 50% seats held by women in National Parliament	women's literacy rates are still lower than that of men Currently, the proportion of seats in National Parliament held by women is only 12.24%

Contd...

Goals to achieve by year 2015	India's Achievements in 2015
Goal 4: Reduce Child Mortality- to reduce mortality among children under five by two-thirds. To bring down child mortality as 42 per 1000 live births	India is moderately on way. It was only 49 per 1,000 live births in 201.
Goal 5: Improve Maternal Health-To reduce MMR to 109 per 100,000 live births by 2015	Maternal Mortality Rate (MMR), which has declined to 167 per 100,000 live births in 2009.
Goal 6: Combat HIV/ AIDS, Malaria and other Diseases	India is on track to achieving this goal, since HIV, malaria and tuberculosis prevalence have been declining. Adult prevalence of HIVhas come down from 0.45 percent in 2002 to 0.36 in 2009.
Goal 7: Ensure Environmental Sustainability	Made some progress. The overall proportion of households having access to improved water sources is 90.6 percent in 2011-12 which is greater than the previous.
Goal 8: Develop a global partnership for development	As of 2014 the Indian telecom network is the second largest network in the world. Telephone connections- Rural areas- 383.97 million; urban areas- 562.43

UN Member States adopted the 2030 Agenda for Sustainable Development during the " Sustainable Development Summit" on 25 September 2015. This include 17 Sustainable Development Goals (SDGs). These SDGs aims to end poverty, fight inequality and injustice, and tackle climate change by 2030. Sustainable Development Goals has 17 Goals and 169 Targets to achieve the goals. The goals try to do justice in all dimensions of development like economic, social and environmental

Sustainable Development Goals (SDGs)

Goal 1: No Poverty

Goal 2: Zero Hunger

Goal 3: Good Health and Well-being

Goal 4: Quality Education

Goal 5: Gender Equality

Goal 6: Clean water and sanitation

Goal 7: Affordable and clean energy

Goal 8: Decent work and economic growth

Goal 9: Industry, innovation, infrastructure

Goal 10: Reduced inequalities

Goal 11: Sustainable cities and communities

Goal 12: Sustainable Consumption and Production

Goal 13: Climate action

Goal 14: Life below water

Goal 15: Life on land

Goal 16: Peace, justice and strong institutions

Goal 17: Partnerships for the goals

Summary

Indian government appointed many committees from time to time to provide advice on a large number of health problems. The reports of these committees have served important platform of "health planning in India." Health planning runs in systematic steps.

The "Health Survey and Development Committee" was appointed in 1943 under the Chairmanship of **Sir Joseph William Bhore.** It stressed on the importance of integration of curative and preventive medicine at all levels. Government of India constituted Mudaliar committee in the year 1959 under chairmanship of **Dr A Lakshmanswamy Mudaliar**, Vice Chancellor, Madras University popularly known as "Health Survey and Planning Committee." This committee recommended that each primary health center's population coverage should not exceed 40,000 and there should be one basic health worker per every 10,000 population and stressed on improving the quality of health services at primary health centers.

Chadha committee was appointed in the year 1963 under the chairmanship of Dr MS Chadha, the then Director General of Health Services. According to this committee, apart from malaria vigilance activities, the basic health workers (BHW) were envisaged as multipurpose health workers (MPHW) to work for family planning and collection of vital statistics.

Following a meeting with central council of health, **Mukerjee committee** was constituted in 1965 under the chairmanship of Shri Mukherjee, the then Secretary, Ministry of Health and Family Planning, India. The committee was recommended to utilize basic health workers (BHWs) as multipurpose workers (MPW) for general services and delink malarial activities from family planning activities.

Jungalwalla Committee was constituted under the chairmanship of Dr N Jungalwalla, the than additional Director General of Health Services and referred as "Committee on Integration of Health Services." This committee advised to use unified approach in serving for all problems instead of segmented approach and medical care and health programs to function under a single administrator. The "Multipurpose workers under Health and Family Planning,"

Kartar Singh committee was under the chairmanship of Kartar Singh, submitted its report in 1973. This committee recommended to replace auxiliary nurse midwives (ANMs) by female health workers (FHWs) and basic health workers (BHWs), malaria surveillance workers and vaccinators, replaced by male health workers (**MHWs**). The job functions of MHWs **and supervisors** were clearly spelt out.

In 1974 Shrivastav Committee was appointed. This committee had recommended to reorganize the medical program and health education and establish 'The Medical and Health Education Commission." Based on these recommendations **"Rural Health Scheme"** was launched by the government of India in the year 1977–78. The **Bajaj committee** constituted under Dr JS Bajaj, Professor of Medicine. The committee popularly known as "**Health Manpower Planning, Production and Management.**" This provided recommendations on procedures relating to admissions to undergraduate and postgraduate courses. **Krishnan Committee, 1992** was setup under the chairmanship of Dr Krishnan to review the recommendations and achievements of previous health committees and comment on any deficits. The committee had recommended one voluntary health worker (VHW) per 2, 000 population with an honorarium of ₹100.

National Commission on Macroeconomics and Health (2005) was formed under the chairmanship of P Chidambaram the than Finance Minister and Dr Anbumani Ramadoss with the aims of promoting equity, restructuring the existing primary health care system and establishing institutional frameworks for improved quality of governance of health.

"Planning commission" was established **on March 15 1950** adopting a formal functioning model under the chairmanship of Prime Minister **Jawaharlal Nehru.** Planning commission adopted "Decentralized approach" in planning process in view to achieve Decentralized District Planning.

Government of India dissolved the "Planning commission" that was in function since 1950 and formulated "National Institution for Transforming India (NITI Aayog)" on January, 1 2015 by the Prime Minister Narendra Modi,. NITI Aayog has been assigned the role to coordinate '**Transforming our World: The 2030 Agenda for Sustainable Development.**" Planning commission of India gave significant importance in including and allocating the resources on various health programs across five-year plans. A Planning Bureau under **"Ministry of Health"** introduced in the year 1965 to enhance coordination between central and state governments and to compile five-year plans. Each five-year plan examined the previous five year plan and prioritize the old and new problems to be considered during the subsequent plans to use the resources of the nation in an effective manner.

The twelfth five-year Plan is a centralized and integrated national economic program depicted its broad vision and aspirations in the subtitle: "Faster, sustainable, and more inclusive growth".

Planning Commission has constituted a high level expert group (HLEG) on universal health coverage, seven working groups and two steering committees to define the appropriate strategy for the health sector for the XII Plan. Some of the important goals of 12th five year plan are to reduce "infant mortality rate (IMR)" to 25 per 1,000 live births, "maternal mortality ratio (MMR)" to 100 per 100000 live births and to achieve "total fertility rate (TFR)" of 2.1

On August 9, 1952, **"central council of health and family welfare" (CCHFW)** was set up. It functions with the union health minister as its chairman and ministers of states and union territories as its members. **National Health Policy 1983** was introduced to provide comprehensive integrated health services relevant to the actual needs of the people at a cost the community can afford and encourage community participation.

In 1951, India was the first country in the world to launch a family planning program to battle the population growth. The "net reproduction rate" (NRR) of 1 set by National health policy 1983 to achieve by 2000 AD. National Population Policy 2000 was set to achieve following Sociodemographic goals by 2010. On May 11, 2000 population of India reached 100 crores or 1 billion or 1000 million. India is yet to achieve TFR replacement level of 2.1.

India has huge burden of health problems. **Communicable disease** served as the major cause of morbidity and mortality profile of the country. **Malaria** cases seem to show increased incidence in North-East states of India. Around 1.1 billion people are at risk of getting **lymphatic filariasis** (LF) in 73 countries of the world, world. An estimated 50% of India's LF endemic population resides in northeastern India particularity in areas of poverty. In India, pneumonia found to be accountable for 13–16% of all deaths occurring in the pediatric hospitals.

*India alone accounts for 23% of the world's **TB** incidence and 21% of world TB deaths.*

Around 38% morbidity and 39% mortality of the world tuberculosis burden is found in South-East Asia Region (SEAR) of world health organization. **Diarrhea** is most common in children under 5 years especially those between 6 months and 2 years. About 1.2 lakh children under the age of 5 succumb to diarrhea every year. (2016, Health Ministry, India)

Leprosy has been eliminated from 119 out of 122 countries with the introduction of antileprosy treatment regimes. So far there is no treatment for curing **HIV** infection. However, the available antiretroviral (ARV) drugs can help effectively to control the virus so that people with HIV can enjoy healthy and productive lives.

Increased urbanization and industrialization, changing age structure and lifestyle of people has placed India at a critical position facing a continuous burden of **non-communicable diseases**.

Cardiovascular diseases (CVDs), diabetes mellitus, chronic obstructive pulmonary disease (COPD) and cancer are the four leading chronic diseases in India. One out of every 4 Indians risks dying from an NCD before reaching 70 years. The poor are largely undernourished and rich are over nourished which are contributing to major health problems. **Protein energy malnutrition** is commonly found in all states of the country. **Nutritional marasmus** is more common than **Kwashiorkor** among under-five children. Anemia is the most common morbidity occurs because of deficient or inadequately available micronutrients (iron, folic-acid and vitamin B$_{12}$) that affect health, education, productivity and entire development of the country. Concentrating on adolescent girls health and improving maternal nutrition would help in preparing healthy future mothers and bringing about healthy babies **vitamin A deficiency** is the major cause for blindness among children. The term **"iodine-deficiency disorders"** denotes many consequences that occur as a result of iodine deficiency.

According to World Bank estimates, 21% of **communicable diseases** in India are due to **unsafe water**. About 60% of this "toilet-less" population lives in India. Provision of safe water annually could prevent 1.4 million deaths among children due to diarrheal diseases.

India has a good national policy but does not have "National Health Service." **Eighty percent** of health facilities of India are available in urban area where as only **28% of population** lives and the remaining **20% of the health facilities** seen in rural area where **72% of population** lives.

The **"Primary health care approach"** and **"Health for all by 2000 AD"** movement explicitly provided significant importance to equitable distribution of health care, community participation, and intersectoral coordination to combat the imbalances. India takes the share of 17.31% of the world's population. As a matter of fact 1 out of 6 people in the world is an Indian There are big differences found in the population density of the various states of India. India had set the goal to attain 1% population growth rate by 2000 AD, but not attained it yet. India's present population growth rate is 1.2%. **Population explosion** is everyone's problem so it becomes a social and economic hindrance. There is a need for great coordination great coordination from all sectors as well among families to control population.

Assess Yourself

I. Multiple Choice Questions (Choose the Correct Answer)

1. Which of the following committee is popularly known as the "Health Survey and Development Committee"?
   a. Mudaliar committee
   b. Bhore committee
   c. Bajaj committee
   d. Chadha committee

2. Which of the following committee is popularly known as the "Health Survey and Planning Committee."?
   a. Mudaliar committee
   b. Bhore committee
   c. Bajaj committee
   d. Chadha committee

3. Bhore committee submitted its report in the year
   a. 1926
   b. 1936
   c. 1946
   d. 1956

4. Which of the population coverage recommended to primary health centers by Bhore committee?
   a. 20000
   b. 30000
   c. 40000
   d. 50000

5. Which of the committee had recommended the integration of medical and health services?
   a. Mudaliar committee
   b. Bhore committee
   c. Bajaj committee
   d. Chadha committee

6. Which of the committee had introduced the concept of "multipurpose health worker?"
   a. Mudaliar committee
   b. Bhore committee
   c. Bajaj committee
   d. Chadha committee

7. Which of the following committees had recommended delinking of malarial activities from family planning activities?
   a. Mudaliar committee
   b. Bhore committee
   c. Bajaj committee
   d. Mukerjee committee

8. Which of the following committee had recommended eliminating private practice by government doctors?
   a. Mudaliar committee
   b. Bajaj committee
   c. Mukerjee committee
   d. Jungalwalla Committee

9. Which of the following committee had recommended to replace Auxiliary nurse midwives (ANMs) by female health workers (FHWs)?
   a. Mudaliar committee
   b. Krishnan committee
   c. Chadha committee
   d. Kartar Singh committee

10. Which of the following committee was assigned the name of "Group on medical education and support manpower"?
    a. Mudaliar committee
    b. Bajaj committee
    c. Mukerjee committee
    d. Shrivastav committee

11. "Reorientation of Medical Education" (ROME) recommended by
    a. Mudaliar committee
    b. Krishnan committee
    c. Chadha committee
    d. Rural health scheme

12. The first five-year plan was implemented between
    a. 1951–1956
    b. 1956–1961
    c. 1961–1966
    d. 1966–1971

13. Twelfth five-year plan period is between
    a. 1997–2002
    b. 2002–2007
    c. 2007–2012
    d. 2012–2017

II. Short Answer Questions (Answer in one or two sentences)

1. List two short term goals of Bhore committee.
2. List two recommendations of Mudaliar committee.
3. State two major observations of Mudaliar committee.
4. State two strategies adopted to promote "Small Family Norm" in National Population Policy of India.
5. State four "National Health Policy Goals" to be achieved by 2015.
6. State two key features of National Health Policy 1983.
7. List four national health goals of 12th five-year plan.
8. State four national health goals in 12th five-year plan related to communicable disease.

III. Write short notes on:

1. Mudaliar committee
2. Bhore committee
3. Bajaj committee
4. Chadha committee
5. Mukerjee committee
6. Shrivastav committee
7. Jungalwalla committee
8. Krishnan committee
9. Kartar Singh committee
10. National Institution for Transforming India (NITI Aayog)
11. Planning Commission of India
12. Five-year plans in India
13. National Population Policy 2000
14. National Health Policy 1983
15. National Health Policy (NHP) 2002
16. Strategies adopted to promote "Small Family Norm" in National Population Policy
17. Central Council for Health and Family Welfare

IV. Essay or Long answer questions:

1. Describe in detail about the major health problems in India.
2. What is health planning? Describe the steps involved in health planning.
3. What is NITI Aayog? What are the differences between "NITI Aayog" and "Planning Commission of India"?
4. Describe National Health Policies.
5. Describe salient features of all (from first to twelfth) five-year plans.

ANSWERS

I.   **1.** b   **2.** a   **3.** c   **4.** c   **5.** a   **6.** d   **7.** d   **8.** d

   9. d   **10.** d   **11.** d   **12.** a   **13.** d

Delivery of Community Health Services

Unit Outline

- Planning, Budgeting and Material Management: Subcenters, Primary Health Centers and Community Health Centers
  - Integrated Planning and Budgeting in India
  - Budgeting
  - Supplies and Equipment
  - Material Management
- Rural Health Services in India: Organization, Staffing and Functions
  - Levels of Health Care System in India
  - Administration at the Village Level (Panchayat)
- Urban Health Services: Organization, Staffing and Functions
  - How do you Define an *"Urban Area"*
  - Urban Administration and their Population Coverage
  - Townships
  - Cantonment Boards (Military Residential Areas)
  - Slums
  - District Family Welfare Services: Organization
  - Urban Health Posts
  - Maternal and Child Health Center
- Components of Health Services
  - Environmental Sanitation
  - Health Education
- Vital Statistics
  - Source of Vital Statistics In India
- Maternal and Child Health (MCH) Care
  - Objectives of MCH
  - Trends in MCH
  - Causes of Maternal Mortality in India
  - Preventive and Social Measures to Reduce Maternal Mortality Rates
  - Antenatal Care
  - Intranatal Care
  - Postnatal Care

- Medical Termination of Pregnancy
  - Legal Framework of MTP Act
- Female Foeticide Act
  - Important Features
- Child Adoption Act
  - Laws Related to Adoption
- Family Welfare
- School Health Services
  - Definition
  - Milestones in School Health Services in India
  - Need for School Health Services
  - Factors to Consider before Initiating School Health Services
  - Objectives of School Health Services
  - Components of School Health Services
- Occupational Health
  - Occupational Hazards
  - Occupational Health Team
  - Health Promotion of Workers
- Defence Services
- Institutional Services
- Systems of Medicine and Health Care
  - Allopathy
  - Ayush
  - Ayurveda
  - Yoga
  - Naturopathy
  - Unani
  - Siddha
  - Homeopathy
- Referral System

Learning Objectives

At the end of this unit the learners will be able to:

- Identify the structure of bottom up approach used in community health services for planning and budgeting
- Demonstrate skills in planning and budgeting for sub-center, primary health center and community health center
- Describe the principles for procuring supplies and equipment for health facility
- Describe the organization, staffing and functions of rural health services provided by government at various levels
- Describe the organization, staffing and functions of urban health services provided by government at various levels
- Describe various components of health services in India
- Describe the systems of medicine and health care
- Explain the process of referral system in health services

K E Y   T E R M S

- National rural health mission
- Subcenter
- ANM/Multipurpose health workers
- Sarpanch
- Primary health center (PHC)
- Community health centers (CHCs)
- Panchayat samiti
- Zilla parishad
- Family planning
- Contraception
- Safe abortion
- Slums
- Audio-visual aids
- Civil registration system
- Sample registration system
- Health surveys
- AYUSH
- Referral System

PLANNING, BUDGETING AND MATERIAL MANAGEMENT: SUBCENTERS, PRIMARY HEALTH CENTERS AND COMMUNITY HEALTH CENTERS

INTEGRATED PLANNING AND BUDGETING IN INDIA

Bottom-up Approach in Planning

Under **"National Rural Health Mission" (NRHM)** planning and budgeting follows a **"Bottom-up approach."** In bottom-up approach, the planning process begins at block level. (Fig. 1). This approach considers and receives the input from the concerned committees and units at the block level and prepares and submits **"block health action plan" (BHAP)** to **districts.** At district level, **BHAPs** compiled and "integrated district health action plan district health action plans (DHAP)" is prepared and sent to state. At the state level, all DHAPs compiled to form the **"state program implementation plan" (SPIP).** A thorough review of SPIPs helps in estimating the fund requirements for forthcoming year activities under NRHM.

People/Committees Responsible for Planning at Each Level

Various committees and people responsible for planning at each level are as follows:

- **At village level:** Village health, sanitation and nutrition committees (VHSNC) will be responsible for village health plan.
- **Gram panchayat level:** At this level gram panchayat pradhan, auxiliary nurse midwife (ANM), multipurpose worker (MPW) and VHSNC prepares the health action plan.
- **Primary health center (PHC) level:** The planning committee at this level facilitate planning inputs from panchayat representatives and the community.
- **Block health action plan:** At this level the "Block" or "community health center (CHC), the planning and monitoring committee takes up the planning work. This committee is formulated by block panchayat adhyaksh, block medical officer (BMO), NGO/CBO representative and head of CHC, rogi kalyan samitis (RKS) or hospital management societies (HMS).

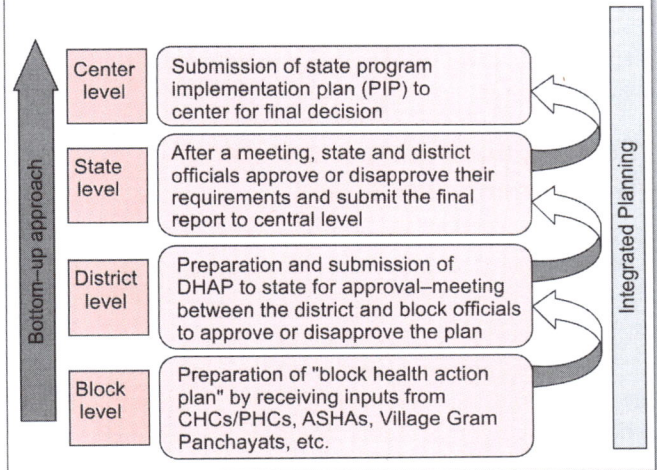

Figure 1: Planning and budgeting
Abbreviations: CHCs, community health centers; PHCs, primary health centers; ASHAs, accredited social health activists

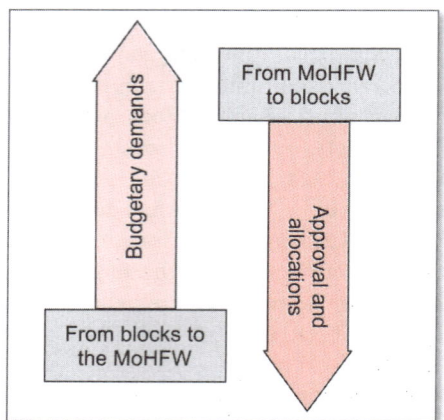

Figure 2: Two-way process of budget planning

Abbreviations: MoHFW, ministry of health and family welfare

○ **District health action plan:** Collects the resource requirements from various sub-district level units. This helps in planning and working on the infrastructure, human resource (HR), procurement, running various schemes, etc.

The Ministry of Health and Family Welfare (MoHFW), as the apex body receives the budget from all the participating states and makes a thorough review after analyzing. After this it approves the arrangement for disbursements.

Budget planning occurs as two-way process (Fig. 2):

○ "Budgetary demands" running from blocks to the MoHFW, government of India.

○ "Budgetary approvals/allocations" running from MoHFW, government of India to blocks.

National rural health mission functions with the main aim of providing health care facilities to the remotest areas of the state. Hence, planning and budgeting of SPIP should meet the basic necessity of providing a functional first referral unit (FRU) in each Block comprising of 120,000 population in plain areas and 80,000 population in hilly, tribal and remote areas of the state.

Planning, Budgeting and Material Management: Subcenters

In plain areas for every 5,000 population a subcenter is established and in hilly and tribal areas for every 3000 population a subcenter function to serve the health needs of people (Table 3).

Government health subcenters are categorized into two based on certain factors like catchment area, health-seeking behavior, case load, and availability of PHC/CHC/FRU/hospitals, etc. in the surrounding areas.

Type A: Type A subcenter is the one that provides all the recommended services but does not have the facilities needed for conducting deliveries.

The labor room facilities and ANM quarters will not be found under type A subcenters. All other facilities are similar to type B centers.

Type B subcenter: Type B subcenter is the one that provides all the recommended services including facilities for conducting deliveries.

Planning for a Health Subcenter

While planning to establish a health subcenter you need to think about money or funds and its sources (government or some other funding agencies), material (land, building, equipment, drugs and supplies, etc.) and manpower (staffing) needed to carry out the tasks at the venue.

Money/Funds

Money is the most important factor without which it is hard to initiate or complete any work. Indian government funds to start subcenters run by the government. In addition, Government of India also recommends the state governments to find availability of land or building through other funding agencies/programs to run subcenters.

The MoHFW, Government of India provides financial support and assistance to all the subcenters since 2002 in following ways:

○ Provision of building or rent for hired building

○ Salary to ANMs and LHVs

○ Contingencies

○ Drugs and equipment kits

○ Voluntary worker (paid from contingency fund by ANM)

○ State government provides the salary to the male health worker.

The subcenters run by private agencies/medical colleges are fully funded by the private owners.

Criteria to Find a Suitable Location to Start a Subcenter

○ To ensure easy access to people by choosing central place

○ To ensure safety to staff and patients

○ It should be within 3 km distance from beneficiaries residence

○ Members of the village panchayat should be involved while planning and deciding on the location of the subcenter.

Building

A subcenter that functions as an immediate care unit at village level should function in its own building. In case of nonavailability of own building a suitable building at central location should be taken on rent.

Earthquake proof: Building should be disaster proof specifically from earthquake. Low lying area should be avoided to prevent flooding.

Firefighting facilities: Equipment necessary for firefighting should be available and all staff must be trained to use those.

The building should be environment-friendly with facilities like rainwater harvesting and solar energy.

Name and signboard: The name of the center should have a name board written in the local language at the gate and on the building.

Building layout and components: The following criteria to be considered while making a layout of the building.

○ There should be a compound wall or fence with a gate to provide safety.

○ There need to be a residential quarters provided for ANM within the compound. The size of the quarters will be based on the availability of land and type of subcenters. The separate entrance is given to the residential quarters

○ If such facilities are unavailable, a house should be rented within the village for the ANM. Health worker (male) may also be accommodated by expanding the building, if there is a need.

○ The reception/entrance should be well illuminated.

○ There need to be a provision for ramp with rails to help the physically challenged and elderly people so that wheel chains trolley and stretcher can be used freely.

Building layout for type B subcenter should have the following facilities:

○ Four to five rooms that are assigned names with purposes—
  □ Waiting room
  □ A labor room with a labor table and a care corner for newborn
  □ A room (ward) with two to four beds
  □ A room for storing items
  □ A room for clinic/office
  □ One toilet each in labor room, ward room and in waiting area (essential).

Residential Accommodation for Staff (ANM/Multipurpose Health Workers)

Residential accommodation should be essentially provided for a minimum of two staffs and desirably for three staffs in **type B (MCH) subcenters**.

○ Type A subcenter with ANM residence should be of 85 square meters.

○ Type B subcenter should have an additional area of 65 square metres on ground floor and 125 square metres on first floor.

○ Each health worker should have 2 rooms, kitchen, bathroom and water closet (WC).

○ Residential accommodation for one ANM in the main subcenter area should measure:

Two rooms each measures—3.3 m × 2.7 m

Kitchen—1.8 m × 2.5 m

Water closet—1.2 m × 9.0 m

Bathroom—1.5 m × 1.2 m

Equipment at Subcenter

Subcenter has to have all the required equipment and supplies to provide quality services. This may include but not limited to:

○ Equipment and supplies needed for conducting safe deliveries at subcenter (for type B subcenters) and home deliveries (for both Type A and Type B)

○ Equipment needed for conducting immunization, contraceptive services like instruments needed for insertion of intrauterine devices

○ Kit needed for providing first aid and emergency services

○ Facilities for testing water quality and blood smear collection

○ Services for repair and maintenance of the all equipment

○ Facilities for sterilizing the items

○ Registers and records to maintain the activities.

Supply of Drugs

All the drugs should be available as per the guidelines

Furniture

Adequate furniture that is solid, strong and easy to maintain should be provided to the subcenter.

Other Support Services

Lab facilities: Testing blood for hemoglobin and glucose levels, urine testing for sugar and albumin levels should be available.

Electricity: Uninterrupted supply of electricity—when electric power shuts down there need to be a generator or solar energy for immediate help.

Water: Continuous and safe water supply for drinking and storage facility should be available in meet the emergency.

Toilet: Toilets should be provided in labor room, ward room and waiting room.

Communication: There needs to be a telephone to provide information and seek advice.

Referral system: Assure a good referral system that save lives. Referral system functions as: subcenter → primary health center → community health centers.

Table 1: Staffing in health subcenter

Type of subcenter	ANM/Health worker (Female)	Health worker (Male)	Staff nurse (or ANM, if staff nurse is not available)	Safai karamchari (cleaner)
Type A	1 (essential)	1 (desirable)	—	1
Type B	2 (essential)	1 (essential)	1 (desirable)	1

Disposal of waste: Waste disposal guidelines given by government of India should be followed.

Continuous monitoring and quality assurance: Quality of services provided by the subcenter is monitored through review meeting and onsite visits by health supervisors and by the medical officer of primary health center.

Staffing or Manpower in Subcenter (Table 1)

As per the prescribed norms, required number of qualified staff should be appointed in subcenter to carry out the activities. Staffing pattern differs in type A and type B subcenters since type A does not take up delivery conduction.

Material Management at Subcenter using Untied Fund

As part of the National Rural Health Mission (NRHM), ₹10,000 is provided as a untied fund to meet any urgent and again discrete activities that need relatively small amount of money.

This fund shall be kept in a joint bank account of the ANM and the sarpanch. The village health committee approves the amount to be spent and it is administered by the ANM.

This untied fund may be used for the maintenance of the following activities:

○ Purchase of curtains to provide privacy
○ Plumbing and repair works, replacement of new bulbs, any other minor repairs needs to be done
○ Cleaning
○ Referring emergency cases to higher order referral centers
○ Transporting samples during epidemics
○ Purchase of required consumables (bandages, cotton, etc.)
○ Purchase of cleaning agents like bleaching powder and disinfectants
○ Supplies for environmental sanitation
○ Payment/reward to accredited social health activist (ASHA) for certain identified activities.

Planning for Primary Health Center

Primary health centers and its subcenters (discussed earlier) are real boon to provide health services in rural parts of India. Currently every PHC covers the population of 30,000 in plain

Table 2: Population norms at community health facilities

Center	Plain area	Hilly/tribal/difficult area
Subcenter (SC)	5000	3000
Primary health center (PHC)	30,000	20,000
Community health center (CHC)	1,20,000	80,000

Source: MHFW (2005), Population norms (Census 2001), http://www mohfw. nic.in

areas and 20,000 in hilly and tribal areas (Table 2). Under each PHC there are 6 subcenters functioning. Primary health centers are categorized into "Type A" and "Type B" based on their delivery case load.

Type A PHC: PHC with delivery load of less than 20 in a month.

Type B PHC: PHC with delivery load of 20 or more deliveries in a month.

Objectives of PHCs

○ To provide comprehensive primary health care to the community
○ To provide standard quality care to the community
○ To provide sensitive service that meets the needs of the community.

Infrastructure

The PHC should have its own building with clean surroundings.

Location of PHC

○ PHC should be located in central area for easy access.
○ The area should have electricity, excellent communication system and water supply.
○ Primary health center should be started in places where there are no other primary health center/SC to avoid duplication of services and to save manpower money.
○ The area should be away from filthy areas like garbage collection, cattle shed, etc.
○ Primary health center shall have proper boundary wall and gate.
○ The area should have well ventilation and lighting facilities

○ The plinth area would differ from 375 to 450 sq. meters based on the inclusion of operation theater facility.

Building

○ The building should be disaster proof. It should be able to survive during earthquake, flood and have fire protective measures

○ Fire extinguishers, sand buckets should be readily available all the time to meet fire-emergencies

○ PHCs should have disaster management plan

○ All staff should be trained to prevent and manage disaster by conducting mock drills.

Name and Signboard

○ The center should have a prominent name board written in the local language at the gate and on the building. There should be pictorial signboard that provides direction to all the departments and public utilities like rest rooms and drinking water, etc.

○ The services, charges/fee and the timings of the center should be displayed in regional language

○ Education and information material to be displayed at important locations. Educating material shall be displayed at main places like waiting area, examination room, etc.

○ Patient's rights and responsibilities to be displayed in local language.

Entrance

The entrance should have a ramp facilitating easy access for elderly and physically challenged patients with a provision to wheel chairs, stretchers, etc.

Waiting Area

○ Seating arrangements for patients to wait for their turns should be available as per patient load

○ Drinking water should be available

○ Toilet facilities should available for males and female separately

○ Available services should be displayed on the board.

Outpatient Department (OPD)

○ Consultation/examination room should be provided with privacy.

○ The rooms should well-lit and ventilated.

○ There need to be a room for immunization and counseling, etc.

Wards or Inpatient Area

○ There should be 4–6 inpatient beds with a provision for keeping male and female patients separately

○ Drinking water facilities should be present

○ Toilets should be available for male and female separately

○ Cleanliness to be maintained and should be regularly monitored.

Operation Theater (Optional)

○ Procedures like vasectomy, tubectomy, hydrocelectomy are carried out.

○ The OT should be well-connected to the wards.

○ It should have a patient preparation area and post-operative area

○ Primary health care should have standard procedure for autoclaving and one staff should be trained

○ Operation theater should have power back up like generator or any other

○ Operation theater should be fumigated at regular intervals.

Labor Room

○ Labor room measures 3.8 m × 4.2 m

○ The labor room should be with good ventilation and lighting facilities

○ Hand washing facilities should be available and be carried out in labor room and OT at regular intervals

○ Fumigation should be carried out as per the schedule

○ Separate areas for septic and aseptic deliveries

○ Drinking water facilities, hot water facilities with attached toilet should be available

○ There need to be separate areas for discard of dirt, baby wash, toilet, sterilization, etc.

○ Standard treatment protocols should be available along with policies and procedures for common problems, which occur during labor and delivery and care of newborns

○ One corner of the labor room area measuring 20 × 30 sq ft is assigned with radiant warmer for newborn care

○ Oxygen, suction apparatus with baby resuscitation kit should readily available to manage newborn care and emergencies.

General Store

○ A separate area with adequate racks should be available for storing sterile and common linen and other materials/drugs/consumable, etc.

- There need to be separate storage shelves for AYUSH drugs
- Store area should be well-ventilated and free of rodents and pests
- Dispensing cum store area measures 3 m × 3 m. This is designed based on the medicine system in practice.

Minor OT/Dressing Room/Injection Room

It should be located near to the OPD and equipped with all the emergency drugs and instruments.

Laboratory

- Measures 3.8 m × 2.7 m
- It should have space with workbenches and area for collection and screening
- A marble/stone tabletop for platform and washbasins enhance easy wash.

Referral Transport Facility

It is desirable that the PHC has ambulance facilities for referral and transport of patients to functional FRUs in case any emergencies during pregnancy and childbirth.

Waste disposal pit—Waste disposal pit should be arranged as per the guidelines given by the pollution control board of India.

Cold chain room should be available in the size of 3 m × 4 m

Logistics room measures 3 m × 4 m

Generator room measures 3 m × 4 m

Office room measures 3.5 m × 3.0 m

Dirty utility room for dirty linen and used items should be available separately.

Staff Accommodation

Staff quarters with water supply and electricity should be available for the staff working in PHC. In case of non-availability of house, rent allowance may be paid provided the staff should stay near PHC so that they are available for work whenever called.

Equipment and Furniture

The necessary equipment should be available in adequate quantity and in working condition. Periodic stock taking and assessment of functioning state of all the equipment must be done. A list of suggested equipment and furniture and diagnostic kits should be available.

Quality Assurance in PHC

To ensure quality the following measures should be taken:

- Record maintenance

- Medical audit
- Death audit
- Patient satisfaction surveys to be conducted in outpatient and inpatient departments
- Evaluation of complaints and suggestions received from patients and relatives.

Maintenance of Primary Health Center

Under NRHM every PHC gets ₹25,000/-per year as untied grant for local health action and ₹50,000/- as annual grant for improving and maintenance of physical infrastructure.

Primary health care untied fund shall be maintained in the bank account of the concerned rogi kalyan samitti [Hospital Management Committee, (HMC)].

Untied fund is used by ANM for:

- Any repairs, replacement of torn curtains
- Plumbing work
- Purchase or repair of patient examination table, delivery cot, hemoglobin meter, copper-T insertion kit, infantometer, plastic sheets, dressing scissors, stethoscopes, buckets, stool, etc.
- Cleaning the center
- Referring and transporting emergencies
- Purchase of consumables like bandages
- Purchase of supplies for environmental sanitation
- Payment/reward to ASHA.

Planning for Community Health Centers

Community health centers are the main health facilities which serve as "FRUs" to manage the cases referred from lower level health facilities.

Objectives of CHCs

- To function as FRU and accept referrals from subcenter, PHC, etc.
- To provide expert secondary level care to the community
- To assure quality care to the community
- To be sensitive to the client's needs/expectations of the community.

Physical Infrastructure of CHC
Location of the Center

- The CHC should be located at the center of the block headquarter to improve access to the patients
- Community health center should be located in a clean surroundings with good natural light and ventilation

❑ The area have all weather road communication, water supply, communication and electric facilities

❑ Low lying area should be avoided to prevent flooding.

Building

The building should be disaster proof (like earthquake and flood proof) and equipped with fire protection measures. CHC should have a compound and gate.

Name and Signboard

The community health center should have a prominent name board written in the local language at the gate and on the building.

Signage

❑ There should be a pictorial sign board that provides direction to all the departments and public utilities like rest rooms and drinking water, etc.

❑ The services, charges/fee and the timings of the center should be displayed in regional language

❑ Education and information material to be displayed at important locations. Educating material shall be displayed at main places like waiting area, examination room, etc.

❑ Patient's rights and responsibilities to be displayed in local language

❑ Safety, hazards and caution signs should be displayed at appropriate places, e.g. radiation hazards in X-ray room

❑ Fluorescent fire-exit signages should be kept at needed locations.

Cubicles for Consultation and Examination

All clinics should have provision for doctor's chair, table, patient's stool, follower's seat, wash basin and examination couch with equipment for examination.

Emergency

A separate emergency area near the entrance of hospital with at least 4 rooms (for doctor-1, minor OT-1, plaster/dressing-1, and observation room-1) should be available to manage casualties and emergencies.

Nonambulant and Friendly Environment for Elderly

Provide ramp with wheelchair, stretcher, hand-railing, proper lightning, etc. to make the environment nonambulant friendly.

Registration cum inquiry counters should guide people.

❑ Pharmacy for drug dispensing and storage with adequate drugs and other supplies.

❑ Clean public utilities should be available separately for males and females.

❑ Suggestion boxes should be available to get feedback.

Outpatient department should have functional flow order and clearly defined areas to run those functions like enquiry, registration, waiting, clinic, dressing room/injection room, billing, lab/X-ray, pharmacy and exit.

Treatment Room

This should have minor OT, injection, dressing and observation room.

Nurses' Station

❑ Nurses' station should be centrally located, spacious with facilities such as medicine.

❑ Cupboard, sinks, dressing tables, color coded bins and provision for Hub cutters and needle destroyers.

❑ Nurses' rest room should be available.

Newborn Corner

Within the labor room, area measuring 20–30 sq ft is identified as newborn corner.

Facilities should be kept ready to provide care at birth, provision of warmth, for resuscitation of sick babies, IV fluids, to weigh and measure babies, etc.

Central Sterilization Supply Department

The central sterilization supply department (CSSD) department should be well established to assure quality.

❑ **Laundry:** There should be storage for dirty linen and clean linen.

❑ **Water supply:** Around 10,000 liters of potable water should be supplied to meet all the requirements except fire fighting.

Administrative Zone

Provision of separate rooms for office and stores should be available.

Residential Zone

There should be residential accommodation available:

❑ For Doctors: Minimum 8 quarters

❑ For staff nurses/paramedical staff: Minimum 8 quarters

❑ For ward boys: Minimum 2 quarters

❑ For driver: Minimum 1 quarter

○ If residential quarters are not available within the campus the staff should be paid rent allowance and advised to stay near the community health center.

BUDGETING

Funds Allocation and Budgeting under National Rural Health Mission (NRHM) for SCs, PHCs and CHCs.

Government of India allocates the following funds under NRHM:

○ 10% funds to state level
○ 20% funds to district level
○ At least 70% funds to block level and below.

So, 70% of the total funds are assigned to manage community SCs, PHCs and CHCs.

SUPPLIES AND EQUIPMENT

Ordering and procurement of supplies and equipment for SCs, PHC and CHCs is a skill. Overstocking and understocking, both are not good to health care facility.

Factors Considered while Estimating the Needed Supplies and Equipment

○ The quantity of stock normally used
○ Number of patients to be treated
○ Season and its demands
○ Usual frequency of order placements
○ The storage capacity of health facility
○ Limited quantity of extra stocks of some items to be kept to meet challenges like epidemics and natural disasters.

Quantification Methods

It functions as a tool to:

○ Prepare budget estimates
○ Adjusting quantities to match a fixed budget
○ Monitor the use of supplies and equipment by staff
○ Quantification methods help to avoid overstocking and understocking and calculate the needed supplies
○ **Consumption method:** In this method the previous consumption or the actual use is considered to calculate the quantities that will be required in future. Mostly the consumption method is preferred for estimating requirements.
○ **Morbidity data method:** Morbidity means the disease. This method considers the prevalence and incidence of disease, the existing health problems and their treatments to estimate the future needs.

Calculate the consumption for a time period

Recorded consumption = Opening stock balance + Stock received – Closing stock balance

For example,

Opening stock of 4" bandages = 200

Stock received in 2017 = 1000

Closing balance = 200 bandages

So, recorded consumption = 200 bandages + 1000 bandages – 200 bandages = 1000 bandages

Real consumption = Recorded consumption × wastage = 1000 – 0 = 1000

In the above example if the stock lasted for 10 months (bandages were in stock for 10 months), then:

Stock out: Adjusted real consumption $\times \dfrac{\text{Period in calculation}}{\text{Period in stock}}$

$$\dfrac{1000 \times 12}{10} = 1200$$

Stock Levels (Table 3)

○ The **stock level** is defined as the quantity of an item that is available for use in a given period of time. The **reserve stock** is defined as the lowest level of stock for each item, and at any cost the quantities should not fall below this level.
○ **Reserve stocks** refers to the extra supplies to ensure that there are no stock outs.
○ The **lead-time** refers to the length of time between placing an order and receiving the items. It is also known as the **delivery time**.
○ The **minimum stock level or re-order level** refers to the stock level that alerts us to place an order to avoid running short of supplies.
○ The **maximum stock level** refers to the maximum numbers or quantity of any item we should have in stock at any time.

Minimum stock level = Reserve stock + Stock used during lead time

Maximum level = Reserve stock level + Order quantity for one supply period

Calculating the Order Quantity

For example,

Table 3: Lead time and reserve stock

Lead time	1 month	2 months	3 months	6 months	12 months
Reserve stock	2 weeks	1 month	1.5 months	2 months	3 months

Annual requirement: 480 × 5 mL disposable syringes

Time between orders: 6 months

Balance: 120 × 5 mL disposable syringes

Lead time: 2 months

Average monthly consumption (AMC) =

$$\frac{\text{Total quantities issued in the time period}}{\text{No. of months in the time period}}$$

$$AMC = \frac{480}{12} = 40$$

Reserve stock   = 1 month if lead time is 2 months

= 1 × 40 = 40

Minimum stock level = Reserve level + Stock used during lead time

= 40 + (2 × 40) = 120

Order quantity   = Time between orders × AMC

= 6 × 40 = 240

Maximum stock level = Reserve level + Order quantity

Maximum stock level = 40 + 240 = 280

Quotation

The person who places order should get at least three quotations.

Include costs of any import duties, preshipment inspection, customs clearance, freight and insurance, transport, handling and storage. Seek advice on these costs from the supplier.

As a general rule:

○ Add 20–30% to the cost of the item(s)—as freight and insurance costs.

○ Add 5–7% to cover maintenance and running costs for items of capital equipment

○ If the total cost exceeds the budget, look for "not so essential" items and try to remove it.

Principles for Procuring Supplies and Equipment (Fig. 3)

○ Supplies are always based on the identified needs. Use VEN model, i.e. "vital", "essential", and "not so essential"

○ Appropriateness of the supplies or items for the chosen setting (SC/PHC/CHC), the climate (hot or cold) and its suitability and acceptability

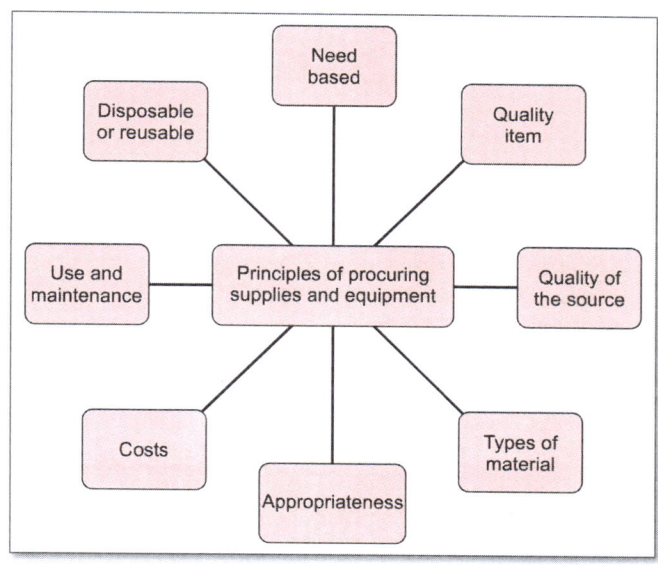

Figure 3: Principles of procuring supplies and equipment

○ Item or supplies should be culturally acceptable

○ Must be of high quality related to safety and performance

○ Quality always costs; do not hesitate to buy quality item that lasts longer than the cheaper ones

○ Pay attention on additional costs too: tax, installation, transportation, insurance and staff training

○ Check whether operational costs have been included in the budget to care the item throughout its lifespan like consumables and accessories, maintenance and servicing, spare parts, electricity or other fuel, etc.

○ Select appropriate source to order the supplies and equipment—a licensed, reputable and reliable source

○ Good maintenance facilities should be available for which all the users should be trained to use, report and maintain

○ Caring and maintenance of an item depends upon the type of material with which the item is made. Iron rusts, glass breaks, aluminium bends use maintenance standards relevant to the type of material used

○ Some of the supplies and equipment, like gloves and syringes are manufactured as disposable or reusable ones. One must select the appropriate one to procure.

MATERIAL MANAGEMENT

The basic principle of material management is the same for a SC or a PHC or a CHC. Only the number of items to be taken care varies based on their capacity to render services. For example, the population coverage of each of this health care facility varies accordingly the number of equipment and supplies varies to meet the service demands.

The provision of untied fund to subcenter, PHC, etc. help them carry out any repair or maintenance work (This has been discussed under health subcenter and primary health centers)

Management at Store

o Store should be locked

o Great care to hygiene and cleanliness

o Monitor the temperature of the store room. It should be maintained below 25°–30°C, not too hot- or cold

o Well lit and ventilated

o No exposure to direct sunlight in the store. Place curtains to avoid direct sunlight.

o The store room should have adequate space and cupboards to store medical supplies.

o Arrange the items in a logical way so that it would help you in finding items quickly and easily.

o The supplies should have a place in open shelves or in cupboards to prevent moisture and pests.

o Organize the stock into different sections like, drugs, cotton and dressings, instruments, stationery items, equipment, spare parts, laboratory supplies, disinfectants, etc.

o Provide label to each section of the store. Everything has its place and everything in its place.

o Arrange items of large supplies and dressing materials, alphabetically.

o Supplies should be divided into (1) regular use and (2) reserve stock.

o Regular use stock should be placed in the front portion of the shelves.

o Reserve stock, for example, instrument reserve stock such as artery forceps, episiotomy scissors, needle holders should be placed at the back of the shelves.

o The opened units/boxes should not be kept in the store room.

o Rotate stock, based on the expiry date using the shortest life first out (SLFO) and first in first out (FIFO) rules. Place the items with latest expiry date at the back and earliest at the front. Use the FIFO rule for items without an expiry date and mark these with the date of receipt.

o Mark a red star on the labels of expired items of the current year.

o Dispose the expired and damaged items as per approved internal policies and procedures.

o As part of stock control measure: (1) Keeping accurate and reliable records of stock, i.e. received and issued, (2) Periodic stock taking means checking stocks regularly and (3) inventory check once a year.

Routine Check on Items

o Keep items and instruments clean and dry. Check for damage or defects and report promptly.

o Switching off and unplugging the electrical items when they are not in use.

o Storing items as per design and instruction in the pack, e.g. Scissors kept closed; diagnostic sets properly kept in their case following the pattern designed.

o Checking and oiling wheels, e.g. wheels on trolleys.

o Checking screws and tightening loose screws.

o Replacing any lost/worn/cracked/broken parts, e.g. thermometer, stethoscope earpieces and diaphragms

o Keep away the batteries of any item when not in use to prevent corrosion (e.g. laryngoscope, torch light, etc.)

o Assess the sharpness of the scissors

o Open stethoscope earpieces and clean the dirt or aural wax

o Inspecting cots for any cracks, splits and rusts.

RURAL HEALTH SERVICES IN INDIA: ORGANIZATION, STAFFING AND FUNCTIONS

LEVELS OF HEALTH CARE SYSTEM IN INDIA

India's health care delivery system is organized under various levels: Central level, state level, district level and community level.

Central level: Organization, Staffing and Functions

Organization

Union ministry of health and family welfare functions at the central level in the health care system of India. The Ministry consists of three departments: (1) Department of health and family welfare, (2) Department of ayurveda, yoga-naturopathy, unani, sidha and homeopathy (AYUSH) and (3) Department of health research (Flowchart 1). Each of these departments is headed by respective secretaries to Government of India.

The official components or organs of health system at national level include:

Flowchart 1: Organization of health care system at central level

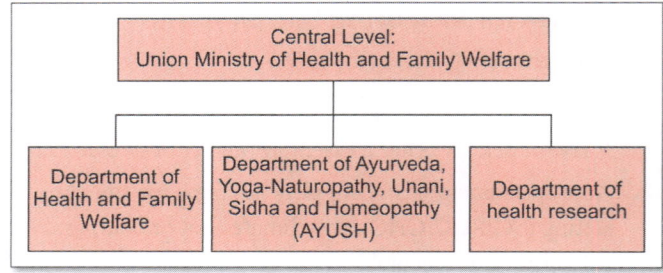

Ministry of Health and Family Welfare

The constitution of India in seventh schedule and under Article 246 describes the functions of Union Ministry of Health under (1) Union list and (2) Concurrent list.

Functions in the Union List

❍ International health relations and administration of port quarantine

❍ Administration of central institutes like All India Institute of Hygiene and Public Health, Kolkata and National Institute for the Control of Communicable Diseases, Delhi

❍ Promotion of research

❍ Regulations and development related to medical, dental and paramedical courses

❍ Establishment and maintenance of drug standards

❍ Census, collection and publication of other data

❍ Immigration and emigration

❍ Regulation of labor

❍ Coordinating with states and with other ministries to promote health.

Functions in the Concurrent List

Both union and state governments are responsible to carry out the functions of the concurrent list. The functions are:

❍ Prevention and extension of communicable disease from one unit to another

❍ Prevention of food adulteration

❍ Control of drugs and poisons

❍ Maintenance of vital statistics

❍ Labor welfare

❍ Ports other than major

❍ Economic and social planning

❍ Population control and family planning.

Directorate General of Health Services

The department of health and family welfare is supported by a technical wing, the Directorate General of Health Services, headed by Director General of Health Services (DGHS). The Director General of Health Services has a additional secretary to assist him. In addition, there are Deputy Directors and large group of administrative staff working in the Directorate of health services.

Functions

The general function may include planning, coordinating, programming, assessment of all health related issues and conduction of surveys. Specific functions are:

❍ Coordination and maintenance of international health relations

❍ Control of drug standards

❍ Responsible for running medical store depots at Mumbai, Kolkata, Chennai, Karnal, Gauhati and Hyderabad

❍ Responsible for administration of national institutes which run postgraduate training

❍ Medical education

❍ Responsible for medical research through Indian council for medical research (ICMR)

❍ Planning and coordinating various health programs

❍ Responsible for preparing various health educational material through "Central Health Education Bureau."

❍ Central Bureau of Health Intelligence is responsible for collection and dissemination of all health-related information and statistics

❍ Maintains "National Medical Library" to disseminate information.

Central Council for Health and Family Welfare

The Central Council for Health and Family Welfare was discussed under previous unit.

Functions

❍ Policy formulation regarding health-related issues

❍ To make legislations relating to medical and public health

❍ To recommend for grants to states and make periodical review on the usage of grants.

State Level: Organization, Staffing and Functions (Flowchart 2)

State Health Ministry

The states have **State ministry of health and a directorate of health**. A minister of health and family welfare and a deputy minister of health and family welfare is head of the department of health and family welfare. The **health secretariat** is the official organ of state health ministry headed by the **Health Secretary**. This secretary is the person chosen from the cader of Indian administrative Services. The organizational patterns at the states follow the style of the central. Deputy secretaries, under secretaries and a big group of administrative staff, assist the health secretary functions at the state level.

State Health Directorate

The director of health services is the appointed head of the "state health directorate" who functions as a chief technical advisor to the state for all matters related to medicine and public health. Realizing the importance of "family planning"

Flowchart 2: Organization structure of health care system at state level

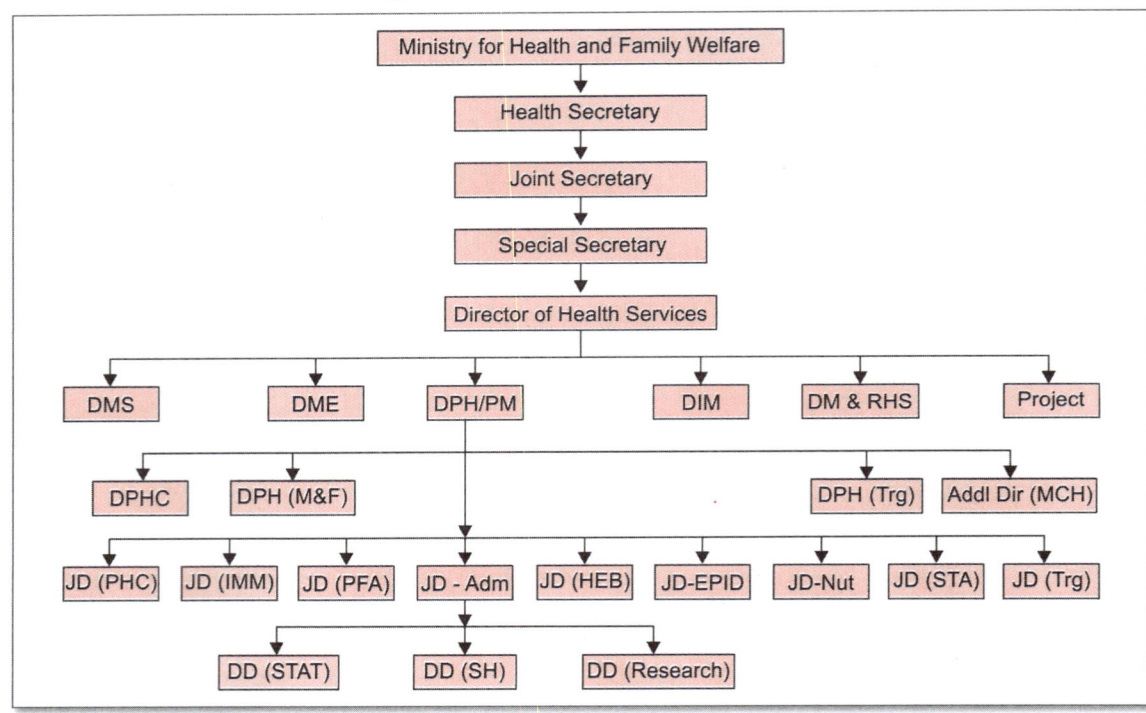

Abbreviations: DMS- Director of Medical Services; DME- Director of Medical Education; DPH and PM- Director of Public Health and Preventive Medicine; DIM- Director of Indigenous Medicine; DM and RH- Director of Medical and Rural Health Services; DPHC- Director of Primary Health Center; JD- Joint Director; DD- Deputy Director EPID- Epidemiology; Nut-Nutrition; Trg-Training; STA-Statistics.

the designation of director of health services has been changed to "Director of Health and Family Welfare." In some states, the "Director of State Health Services" is re-designated to "Director of Health and Family Welfare". Some of the states have appointed "Director of Medical Education" separately in order to meet the work demands of increasing number of medical and paramedical institutions.

The "Director of Health and Family Welfare" is assisted by **"Deputy Directors"** *and* **"Assistant Directors."** The deputy and assistant directors work under two divisions like regional and functional. The regional directors are *"generalists"* responsible for inspecting all the branches of public health under their control irrespective of their specialty. The functional directors are **specialists**, responsible for concentrating their allotted area of specialization like mother and child health, family planning, nutrition, tuberculosis, leprosy, health education, etc.

Regional Level

In some states like Bihar, Madhya Pradesh, Uttar Pradesh, Andhra Pradesh, Karnataka and others, zonal or regional or divisional setups have been created between the state directorate of health services and district health administration.

Zonal or regional or divisional setups are established in between state and district health administration in few states like Uttar Pradesh, Bihar, Andhra Pradesh and Karnataka etc.

Regional or zonal setup covers three to five districts and acts under State e of Health Services.

District Level (Flowcharts 3 and 4)

In India, Districts are the principal unit of administration. Districts function under **collectors**. The size and population of the districts vary. District comprises of six areas of administration. The districts are divided into two or more **subdivisions** and each functions under **assistant collector** or **sub-collector**. These subdivisions are further divided into Tahsils or Taluks and functions under Tahsildar. The concept of organizing the rural areas of the district in to "community development blocks" emerged after the inception of community development program in India in 1952. The community development block comprised of 100 villages that equaled 80,000 to 120,000 population. The block development officer is the incharge of the block.

A three tier structure of rural self-government functions at the rural areas known as **"Panchayati Raj."** This functions as the link between villages and districts. The three-tier structure includes:

Flowchart 3: District level—administration areas

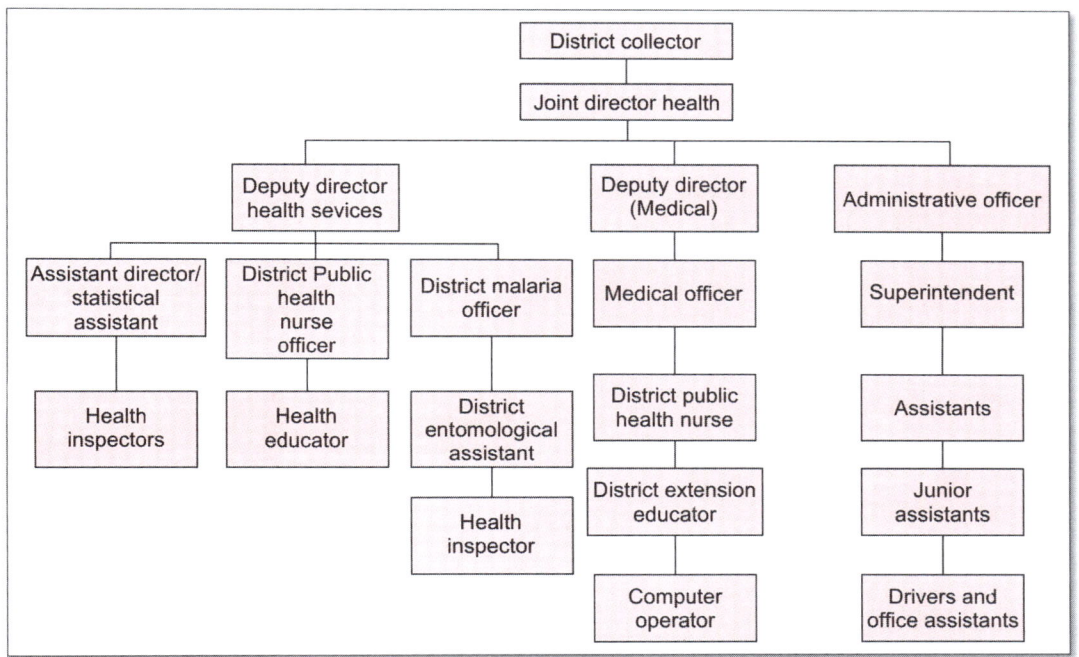

Flowchart 4: Organization structure—district level

1. Panchayat—Functions at village level

2. Panchayat samiti—Functions at the block level

3. Zilla parishad—Functions at the district level

The above three institutions are recognized as public welfare agencies that works for public development activities. This three-tiered local self-government encourages people's participation and gives the feel of democracy at qrars root level.

The panchayat raj agency that functions at the district level is **zilla parishad** or **zilla panchayat**. The member-size of zilla parishad vary from 40 to 70. Zilla parishad includes all heads of the panchayat samitis in the district, MPs and MLAs of the district, two people with experience in administration, public life or rural development, representatives from SC, ST and women. The collector is the member and has no voting

authority. It performs as supervisor and coordinator but the functions and powers may differ from state to state.

The health facility at district level functions next to state/regional structure. This also links the peripheral level structures such as PHC/subcenter with the state. The family planning officer and maternal and child health officers work at the district level are under the control of zilla parishad.

District Hospital

The district health system is the secondary level of health care whose services are curative, preventive and promotive in nature. The district hospitals cater to the population of urban and the rural areas of the district. District hospitals aims at providing quality, comprehensive secondary health care to the population of the district. The district hospitals receives the referred patients from lower and horizontal level heath facilities and provide specialist care. District hospital's inpatient bed strength varies based on the size of the population it serves. Further, for prescribing the norms the hospitals are graded based upon the number of inpatient beds:

Grade I: District hospitals norms for 500 beds

Grade II: District hospital norms for 400 beds

Grade III: District hospitals norms for 300 beds

Grade IV: District hospitals norms for 200 beds

Grade V: District hospitals norms for 100 beds. The district officer also known as the chief medical and health officer (CM and HO) or district medical and health officer (DM and HO) is the overall control. DMO/CMO is the overall responsible person for the health and family welfare programs of the district. There are deputy CMOs who assist the CMOs.

Sub-district (Subdivisional) Hospitals

Sub-district (Subdivisional) hospitals function below the district and above the block level (CHC) hospitals. These sub-divisional hospitals act as "first referral units" for the tehsil/taluk/block population. These hospitals provide specialist services and they receive referrals from CHCs, PHCs and SCs. They provide obstetrics and newborn emergency care. They serve as a link between district hospitals and SC, PHC and CHC. Subdivisional hospitals have 31–100 beds or more and caters to about 5–6 lakhs population.

Functions

Sub-district Hospital Functions

- ○ It provides effective, affordable health care services.
- ○ It serves both urban and rural population.
- ○ It is a referral center for CHCs, PHCs and SCs.
- ○ It is responsible to provide education and training for primary health care staff.

The district officer also known as the chief medical and health officer (CM and HO) or district medical and health officer (DM and HO) is the overall control. DMO/CMO is the overall responsible person for the health and family welfare programs of the district. There are deputy CMOs who assist the CMOs.

Community Level

Community Health Center

The administrative organ at the block level is "panchayat samiti". The block covers 100 villages and a population of 80,000–1,20,000. The heads (President or sarpanch) of all villages in the block, MLAs, MPs lives in the block, representatives from various denominations like women, SC/ST and cooperative societies form the panchayat samiti

at block level. The block development officer (BDO) serves as the ex-officio secretary of the panchayat samiti. The community development programs at the block level are executed with technical advice from BDO and funds received from the government.

Organization

Effective referral system is the most essential part of PHC. Considering this fact one CHC for every 80,000–120,000 population (Table 2) was proposed. Community health center should afford providing the basic services in the areas of general medicine, pediatrics, surgery, obstetrics and gynecology.

State governments take the responsibility of establishing and maintaining the CHCs. CHCs are designed to function as "**block level health administrative unit**". They also serve as a gatekeeper for referrals flowing to higher level health facilities.

Community health centers have (Table 4) four medical specialists (surgeon-1, Physician-1, gynecologist-1 and pediatrician-1), along with paramedical and other staff. It has 30 inpatient beds, 1 operation theater, 1 X-ray lab, a labor room for delivery and all laboratory facilities. CHCs functions as FRUs. Each CHC meets the specialist care needs of 4 PHCs and provides facilities for obstetric care and other consultations.

Table 4: Staffing at community health center

Staffing community health center	Existing	Proposed by IPHS
Medical officer*	4	7
Nurse mid-wife (staff nurse)	7	9
Dresser	1	1
Pharmacist/Compounder	1	1
Laboratory technician	1	1
Radiographer	1	1
Ward boys	2	2
Dhobi		
Sweepers	3	3
Mali	1	1
Chowkidar	1	
Aya	1	
Peon	1	
OPD Attendant		5
Stat assistant/Data entry operator	5	
OT attendant		
Registration clerk		
Ophthalmic assistant	1	
*, surgeon, obstetrician, physician, pediatrician, anesthetist, public health program manager, eye surgeon.		
Note: Sr No. 11, and 14–17——total 5, flexibility rests with State for recruitment		

Abbreviations: IPHS, Indian Public Health Standards

At present the eligible PHCs are upgraded to CHCs.

Supervisory cadre staff of PHC or district level with 7 years of experience is appointed as **"Community Health Officer"** in CHCs. But in states which have not accepted CHO appoint a second medical officer. The specialists at CHC can refer patient to subdivisional hospital, district hospital or if necessary, directly to state level hospitals and teaching hospitals.

Functions of CHC

- Provides in-and outpatient services in general fields of allopathy and AYUSH services.
- Emergency and routine care cases in medicine
- Maternal health
- Newborn care and child health
- Family planning
- Eye specialist services (at one for every 5 CHCs)
- Laboratory services
- National health programs
- Other services like school health, immunization, adolescents' health, etc.
- Referrals

Primary Health Center (PHC)

Organization

Primary health center is the health facility functioning at the block level between the SC and the CHC. As per recommended norms, there should be one PHC for every 30,000 population in plain areas. PHCs in hilly, tribal and backward areas covers the population of 20,000. PHCs at block level has 6 beds. There is also a plan to upgrade the PHCs at block level into 30 bedded community health centers. There are 25,020 PHCs established in India as of March, 2014.

Functions of PHC

The functions of PHCs in India meet all the **"eight essential elements"** of primary health care, as stated in Alma-Ata declaration of 1978:

- Medical care
- Maternal and child health (MCH) and family planning (FP)
- Provision of safe water supply and basic sanitation
- Prevention and control of locally endemic diseases
- Collection and reporting of vital statistics
- Health education
- National health programs as relevant
- Referral services

- Training of primary care workers (health guides, health workers, local dais and health assistants)
- Provision of basic laboratory services

Apart from the above it was also proposed for:

- Provision of surgical facilities at PHC for selected surgical procedures like vasectomy, tubectomy (female sterilization) medical termination of pregnancy (MTP) and some minor surgical procedures
- Reorientation of medical education (ROME) through attaching three PHCs to each medical colleges with the aim of reorienting the medical education to meet the needs of the community and country.

Staffing Pattern

A total of minimum 15 staff work at PHC to provide services to the public (Table 5).

Subcenter Level

Organization

Subcenters are the peripheral outpost of rural areas in Indian health care delivery system. Health sub-centers located in villages are the interface with the community at the grassroot level. They function at the most peripheral level and acts as the first contact point between the primary health care system and the community. Each subcenter covers the population of 5,000 in plain areas and 3,000 in hilly, tribal, and backward areas. Subcenters stores basic drugs to treat minor ailments and take care for the important health needs of men, women and children.

Table 5: Staffing at primary health center

Staff	Existing	Recommended
Medical officer	1	3 (At least 1 female)
AYUSH Practitioner	Nil	1 (AYUSH or any ISM prevalent locally)
Accounts manager	1	Nil
Pharmacist	1	2
Staff nurse Nurse–Midwife	1	5
Health worker (F)	1	1
Health educator	1	1
Health assistants (one male and one female)	2	2
Clerks	2	2
Laboratory technician	1	2
Driver	1	Optional (can be outsourced)
Class-IV workers	4	4
Total	15	24/25

Table 6: Staffing at subcenter

Staff for subcenter	Existing	IPHS proposed
Health worker (Female)/ANM	1	2
Health worker (Male)	1	1
Voluntary worker (Helper-optional)	1	1

Staffing of Subcenter

Subcenter is staffed with one female health worker who is known as ANM and one male health worker known as multipurpose worker (male). The health assistant (female) commonly known as lady health visitor (LHV) and one health assistant (male) who are placed at the PHC level are accountable for supervision of all the subcenters (generally six subcenters) that function under the PHC (Table 6).

Functions of Subcenter

Subcenters provide primary health care services at village level. The functions may include:

Maternal health care

- Early registration of all pregnancies within first trimester (before 12th week of pregnancy)
- Advise minimum 4 antenatal visits including registration
- General examination that includes height, weight, BP, anemia, abdominal examination, breast examination, etc.
- Supplementation of folic acid from first trimester and Iron and folic acid from 12 weeks onwards.
- Tetanus toxoid immunization
- Check blood HB and treat anemia
- Counseling on birth preparedness and diet, avoidance of tobacco, need for rest and sleep
- Screening for any high-risk pregnancy
- Timely referral in case of any need.

Intranatal care

- Promotion of institutional deliveries and skilled attendance at home deliveries
- Timely referral in case of any high-risk cases or complications
- Advice on diet, hygiene and contraceptive measures to be adopted.

Postnatal care

- Initiation of early breastfeeding within 30 minutes (1/2 hour) of birth.
- Ensure at least 2 postnatal home visits during early postpartum period.

- Plan postnatal visits on 2, 3 and 42nd day to assess and provide advice for those delivered at subcenter and home.

Child health care

- Provision of essential newborn care as per the standards Advise and promote exclusive breastfeeding for 6 months
- Immunization and vitamin A prophylaxis
- Prevention and control of diseases like diarrhea, malnutrition, respiratory infections, fever and anemia.

Family planning and contraception

- Education, motivation and counseling to adopt appropriate family planning methods.
- Provision of contraceptives such as condoms, oral pills, emergency contraceptives, intrauterine device (IUD) insertions (In places where ANM is trained on IUD insertion).
- Follow-up services for eligible couples who are adopting terminal/spacing methods of family planning.

Safe abortion services

- Counseling and referral services for mothers who need safe abortion services [medical termination of pregnancy (MTP)]
- Follow-up and referral in case of any complications.

Adolescent health care

- Education, counseling on prevention of anemia and avoidance of tobacco
- Timely referral for any health problems.

School health services

- Screening for any deficits and referral, treatment of minor ailments, immunization, deworming, prevention and management of vitamin A and nutritional deficiency anemia and referral
- Provision of school health services staff team.

Control of endemics

- Early detection and control and reporting of endemic diseases such as malaria, kala-azar, etc.
- Japanese encephalitis, filariasis, dengue, etc.
- Assistance in control of epidemics
- Curative services for minor diseases and referrals
- Disease surveillance and reporting
- Provision of safe drinking water and sanitation measures that include use of toilets and proper disposal of garbage.

Works for National Health Program Implementation

Works for all national health programs like *National AIDS Control Program (NACP), National Vector Borne Disease Control Program (NVBDCP), National Leprosy Eradication Program (NLEP), Revised National Tuberculosis Control Program (RNTCP), National Program for Control of Blindness (NPCB) etc.*

Antenatal Visits

1st visit: Within 12 weeks

2nd visit: Between 14 and 26 weeks

3rd visit: Between 28 and 34 weeks

4th visit: Between 36 weeks and term

ADMINISTRATION AT THE VILLAGE LEVEL (PANCHAYAT)

The panchayati raj at the village level includes:

○ Gram sabha

○ Gram panchayat

○ Nyaya panchayat

○ **Gram sabha:** The gram sabha means the adult-assembly where all the adults of the village participate. This gram sabha meets at least twice a year to accept taxation, elect the members of the sabha and plan for village annual programs.

○ **Gram panchayat:** It is the most important executive organ of the "**gram sabha**". The member strength of gram panchayat may vary from 15–30 and it covers the population of 5000 to 15000 and above. The elected president (Sarphanch/Sabhapatilayat/Mukhiya), vice president and secretary hold office for 3–4 years. All planning and development activities at village level are taken care by **gram panchayat. Secretary post** of the panchayat is powerful and he covers the full range of activities of civic administration that includes but not limited to sanitation and public health.

○ **Nyaya panchayat:** It is an informal and old form of adjudication. This consisted of 4–5 respected senior members of the society who is known for integrity to hear cases informally and provide judgment.

Health Care Services at Village Level

The Government of India launched rural health scheme in 1977 with the aim of placing people's health in people's hands considering the recommendations from Shrivasthav committee. Following this India became the signatory of Alma-Ata declaration (1978) and committed to achieve health for all by 2000 AD through "**Primary health care**

Flowchart 5: Health care services at village level

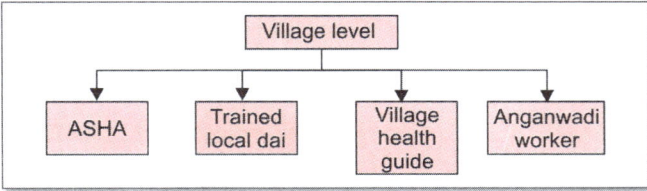

approach." This primary health care approach focuses on providing universal comprehensive health care at a cost, which is affordable by people.

The most important of primary health care is taking health care to farthest reaches to all remote rural areas and assure that every person has access to it. The basic idea was to make universal coverage and assure equitable distribution of health services. To operate this approach at village level India has introduced some schemes. They are as follows (Flowchart 5):

○ Village health guides scheme

○ Training of local *dais*

○ Integrated child development service (ICDS) scheme

○ Accredited social health activist (ASHA) scheme

Who are These Workers?

○ The above schemes encourage community participation in health care.

○ The above workers are volunteers from the same community and work at village level.

○ They are trained people who serve as the first contacts between the villagers and the government health facilities.

○ They should be willing to spend some time for the community health work.

○ Government provides honorarium for these workers.

Village Health Guide

Village health guide (VHG) scheme was introduced on October 2, 1977 under rural health scheme with aim of encouraging people's participation. This scheme was not launched in states like Kerala, Tamil Nadu, Karnataka, Arunachal Pradesh and Jammu and Kashmir, which had other equal systems in place.

Criteria to Select VHGs

○ Preferably woman and should be permanent resident of the community

○ Should be acceptable to all sections of the community

○ Should be able to read and write with minimum formal education of up to VI standard.

○ Should be able to spare at least 2–3 hours every day for community health work.

VHG-Training

After the selection, the VHGs are provided with short training in primary health care facilities (subcenter or PHC) for 200 hours spread over a period of 3 months with a stipend of Rs. 200/month. After training, they receive a working manual, kit of simple medicines both modern and traditional medicine system. The manual plays the role of the guide.

Duties of VHGs

- Treating minor ailments
- *Refer* in time if required
- First aid
- Mother and child health
- Family planning
- Health education and sanitation
  - Honorarium to VHG is ₹50 per month (revised time to time)
  - VHG also receives medicines of worth of ₹600 per year
  - No VHG to be trained from the same village, before three years, as it involves expenditure
  - There should be one VHG per village or 1000 rural population (The VHG scheme has now been discontinued by the GOI)
  - The community health work is now delivered by ASHA, AWW and trained *dai*.

Local Dais

Many women lost their lives because of nonavailability of trained health care professional or people to conduct their deliveries in the community. Dais training program was launched under rural health scheme to train all categories of traditional birth attendants (dais) in basic concepts of maternal and child health and sterilization. The training is for 30 working days.

Each dai is paid ₹300 stipend during the training period. Training given at PHC/SC/MCH center for 2 days in a week, and the remaining 4 days she accompanies the female health worker (HWF) to villages.

She is required to conduct at least 2 deliveries under the supervision of HWF, ANM or HAF during the training. At the time of training it is to emphasize on asepsis while carrying delivery at home to reduce material mortality. After completion of training each *dai* is provided with a delivery kit and a certificate. She is also expected to spread message on small family norms. The national target is to train one local *dai* from each village.

Anganwadi Worker

Under the ICDS scheme one *anganwadi* worker (AWW) is placed for a population of 400–800. There are 100 AWW function in each ICDS project. Recent data reveals that there are 6,719 ICDS blocks function in India. The AWW is a part-time worker selected from the community where she is to serve. She is provided 4 months of training in different aspects of health, nutrition and child development. She receives an honorarium of ₹1,500 per month. Her job responsibilities may include:

- Health check up
- Growth chart monitoring
- Immunization
- Supplementary nutrition
- Health education
- Nonformal pre-school education
- Referral services

Beneficiaries

- Nursing mother
- Pregnant women
- Women in reproductive age (15–45 years)
- Children below the age of 6 years
- Adolescent girls

Accredited Social Health Activist

National rural health mission (NRHM) was launched on 5th April 2005 for the period of 7 years (2005–2012), later extended for another 5 years (2012–2017). Though this program is in operation in all the states, special attention is given to 18 states. ASHA cadre is created under NRHM.

Guidelines to Select ASHA

- Must be a woman (married/widow/divorced) resident of the village
- Preferred age group 25–45 years
- Should have had the formal education up to VIII standard
- Should have good communication skills
- Should have leadership qualities
- One ASHA for every 1,000 population and it is relaxed for hilly and tribal areas (One ASHA per habitation).

Training and Incentive to ASHA

- ASHA undergoes training and receives a drug-kit. She is also given in-service periodic training.
- Performance-based incentives given to ASHA for promoting universal immunization, referrals and escort

services for reproductive and child health (RCH), and other health programs and construction of household toilets.

○ ASHA works in liaison with women's committees (self-help groups or women's health committees), village health, nutrition and sanitation committee (VHNSC) of the gram panchayat, ANMs and AWW.

Roles and Responsibilities of ASHA

○ ASHA functions as the first point of contact to meet the demands of weaker sections specifically women and children, who find it hard to access health services.

○ ASHA, the health activist functions to create awareness on health and motivates community to involve in local health planning.

○ She involves herself in teaching healthy practices and promotes health.

○ She also provides a minimum package of curative care and makes timely referrals.

○ ASHA provides information on nutrition, hygiene, basic sanitation, healthy living, effective utilization of available health services, etc.

○ ASHA counsel women on preparation for delivery, importance of safe delivery, breastfeeding and complementary feeding, immunization, contraception, prevention infections (reproductive tract infection/sexually transmitted infections—RTIs/STIs) and care of the young child.

○ ASHA will mobilize the people and help to access health services like immunization, antenatal check-up (ANC), postnatal check-up, supplementary nutrition, sanitation at the *anganwadi*/SC/PHCs.

○ She will acts as a depot older to community for essentials and supplies like oral rehydration therapy (ORS), iron folic acid tablet (IFA), chloroquine, disposable delivery kits (DDK), oral pills and condoms, etc.

○ ASHA needs adequate institutional support to function. Women's committees, self-help groups, village health and sanitation committee and the peripheral health workers like ANMs, *anganwadi* workers, and the trainers of ASHA should support ASHA. In addition, periodic in-service training is the big source of support to ASHA.

URBAN HEALTH SERVICES: ORGANIZATION, STAFFING AND FUNCTIONS

Lord Ripon was the first one to introduce the democratic local self-government system for municipal governance in India in the year 1882. Government of India Act, 1935, placed

Flowchart 6: Administrative structure of India

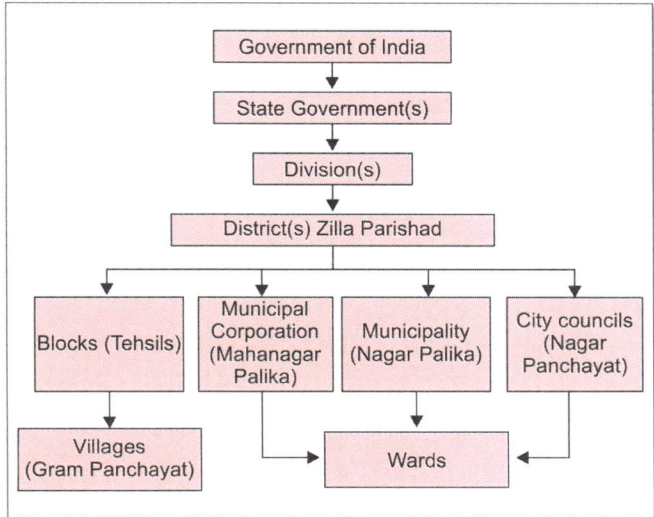

local government under the purview of the state government by giving specific powers (Flowchart 6).

In 1992, the 74th Constitutional Amendment Act highly recognized the local governments and provided greater responsibilities and authorities. Further, the local government was considered as a third tier government.

HOW DO YOU DEFINE AN *"URBAN AREA"*

Census, 2011 defines urban as:

○ Places that are administered by municipality/corporation/cantonment board or notified town area committee (and)

○ All the other places that meet the following conditions: A minimum population of 5000, population density-400 people/sqkm and at least 75% of the male are involved in nonagricultural job/work.

As mentioned previously the "Municipalities Act" or "Nagar Palika Act" introduced in 1992 through 74th Amendment Act. Municipality functions as a three-tier system like Panchayati Raj system of rural areas.

URBAN ADMINISTRATION AND THEIR POPULATION COVERAGE

○ Municipal corporation—for a larger urban area

○ Municipal council—for a smaller urban area

○ Nagar panchayat—for a rural area in transition to become urban

Corporation (Nagar Nigam/Mahanagar Palika)

It covers more than 200,000 populations. Corporation is the apex body of the urban governance. The cities and state capitals hold comparatively higher populations like 100,000 and above for the corporation to administer. Municipal corporations usually formed as per the statute of the state legislature but the only exception is Delhi, where, the power lies with the parliament.

The corporation governs cities with mayor the political head and deputy mayor the subsequent political authority. Corporation is divided as small units called *wards*, which are headed by the councilors. The city's residents directly elect the *councilors*. The councilors elect a mayor and a deputy mayor who lead and direct over about 10 standing committees.

The corporation functions of big metropolitan area has and many larger and smaller suburbs under its jurisdictions. The **municipalities** govern the **larger suburbs** and the **panchayats** (town councils) govern the **smaller ones**.

Mayor and deputy mayor: They are elected political executives. The mayor heads the municipal corporation, but for the most time his role is ceremonial. As executive power are vested in him he can appoint executive head, the municipal commissioner.

- Mayor is the elected political executive. Mayor is the head person of the corporation.
- He is the proud owner of the "first citizen" of the city.
- He is responsible for conducting meetings.
- The mayor gets report from the commissioner regularly and he has the access to records or reports of the corporation.
- Mayor acts as the line of communication between the municipal commissioner and the state government.

Municipal commissioner: The municipal commissioner is the Indian Administrative Service (IAS) officer who holds the executive power and authority, appointed by the state government.

Functions of the Corporation

- Birth and death registration and issue of certificates
- Health services
- Collection and maintenance of vital statistics
- Land survey and regulation of land and construction
- Urban planning and town planning
- Activities of social and economic development
- Maintenance and laying of roads and bridges
- Activities on improvement of slums
- Water supply for domestic, industrial and commercial purposes
- Public health, sanitation, conservancy and solid waste management
- Fire services

- The removal of hurdles or obstruction in public places
- Property assessment and taxation
- Collection of taxes
- The regulation and maintenance of places for the disposal of dead; maintenance and establishment of burial grounds, crematoriums grounds and electric crematoriums.

Municipalities (Nagar Palika/Municipal council/Nagaratchi)

Municipalities are usually set up for the population of 100,000 and above but earlier, the municipal set up was provided to the areas with the population of >20,000. Further, the municipal bodies that were set for lesser population were allowed to continue and retain the name 'Municipality" even if the population fall below one lakh. The small city or town is further divided into "wards" (subdivision/district of the municipality/town etc.) as per the size of the population. One or more members elected from each ward. The ward members elect a president to conduct meetings and other coordinating activities.

Functions of Municipality

- Hospitals
- Registration of births and deaths
- Laying and maintenance of roads
- Water supply
- Sanitation
- Street lighting
- Solid waste management
- Conduction of fire brigade
- Drainage maintenance
- Collection of tax
- Receiving grants from state government

Nagar Panchayat for a Rural Area in Transition to Become Urban

Nagar panchayat is set up for a very small urban area or the rural area that is fast transitioning to urban area. To give the nagar panchayat status to a place certain factors are considered:

Population density, the revenue by local government, higher percentage (75%) of employment in non-agricultural activities and the economic importance of the area. The members are directly elected by the people; each ward elects one member. The member of the State Legislative Assembly (MLA) representing that area is the ex-officio member of nagar panchayat.

Every nagar panchayat has a president and a vice-president who are elected by all the elected members. The president presides over its meetings.

TOWNSHIPS

Township covers 5000–10000 population. Townships emerge due to the establishment of colonies, or specific worksites provided under the government. Township is one of the areas administered by municipality or municipal corporation. A town administrator appointed by the Municipality and assisted by engineers and technicians takes care of roads, lights, water etc. in township.

CANTONMENT BOARDS (MILITARY RESIDENTIAL AREAS)

Cantonment boards were set up to administer established military station. Usually when there is a military personnel station at a place, the civilian population moves in to provide supporting facilities like market and provision, etc. In such situations, the cantonment boards are set up. Cantonment boards are formed for every cantonment residency, which take care of all the facilities and civic amenities in concerned locations. India has 63 cantonment boards.

About 30% of population of India lives in urban areas. There is a humongous growth in urban migration specifically in the last decade. This has raised the population growth in urban slums. Consequently, the living conditions of the cities the deteriorated to a large extent. Department of family welfare and externally aided projects (like India population project-VIII) provide the family welfare services to the urban population in selected cities.

After the 74th constitutional amendments, the local bodies are insisted to play an efficient role in planning, monitoring and coordinating urban health care activities at local level.

SLUMS

Slums are the communities characterized by insecure residential status, poor structural quality of housing, overcrowding, and inadequate access to safe water, sanitation, and other infrastructure (United Nations Human Settlements Program, 2003). The slum population meets every day challenges and bigger health problems because of poor housing, overcrowding, unhygienic surroundings, poor sanitation, lack of safe drinking water and environmental pollution. Urban slum is the place for all vulnerable populations such as homeless, rag pickers, street children, rickshaw pullers, construction and brick and lime kiln workers, sex workers and other temporary migrants.

Dispensaries

Dispensaries are fourth order medical facilities providing normally outdoor treatment with the help of one physician and one pharmacist. The dispensaries in slum areas provide medical facilities to the growing urban population. The dispensaries are opened in areas of the towns where predominantly poor and economically weaker sections of the society live. The dispensaries provide medical facilities for slum dwellers near to their home.

Staffing patterns of dispensaries include one MO, two pharmacists and 2–3 ANMs.

Slum Health Programs by Mobile Dispensaries

Slum population also gets services by mobile units attached to UPHC/UHP. Mobile unit in the slum consists of: School health team (medical officer, pharmacist and a health worker) provided with a van to reach the slum areas to provide health services. One urban health post or urban primary health center covers two schools. On daily basis a mobile van visits one zone. Mobile units continue to provide services in slum areas using available van/vehicle and staff.

DISTRICT FAMILY WELFARE SERVICES: ORGANIZATION (FLOWCHART 7)

Followings are the main functions of family welfare services:

- Information, education and communication (IEC) activities to create health awareness
- Prevention of disease and health promotion
- First aid
- Treatment of minor illnesses
- Referrals for treating major illnesses
- There are shelters functioning for homeless/migrants/mobile population.

URBAN HEALTH POSTS

Based upon the recommendations given by the Krishnan Committee (1983), India introduced four types of urban health posts (UHP) in 10 States and Union Territories. This health facility mainly aimed at helping the slum dwellers to have access to health services. These health posts should be located in slum areas or within the vicinity.

India population project-V aimed to strengthen and expand the health care services with a special concentration on family welfare and maternal and child health services. These health posts are either attached to hospital/maternity homes/dispensaries or function individually. Health posts

Flowchart 7: District family welfare

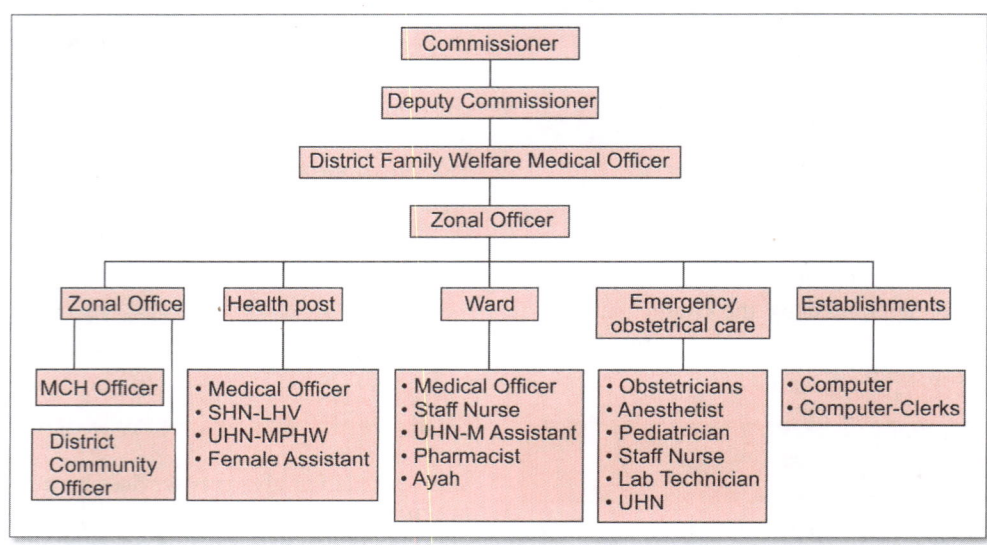

Table 7: Urban health post

Category	Population covered	Staffing pattern
Type A	<5000	ANM-1
Type B	5,000–10,000	ANM-1, multiple worker—Male-1
Type C	10,000–20,000	ANM (2), multiple worker—Male (2)
Type D	25,000–50,000	Lady MO (1), PHN (1), ANM (3–4), multiple worker—male (3–4), Class-IV Women (1)

and dispensaries provide preventive, promotive and outreach services for maternal child health/family planning services. Depending upon the population coverage the urban health posts are categorized as A, B, C and D (Table 7).

Core Functions of Urban Health Post

- To provide outreach
- Primary health care
- MCH and family welfare services.

Other Functions

- Conducting baseline survey in the community
- Early registration and care of antenatal mothers
- Distributing iron-folic acid to mothers
- Antenatal care, deliveries, postnatal and newborn care
- Maintaining eligible couple register
- Motivating people to adopt small family norms and providing services on contraception

- Out reach services
- Growth monitoring for under-five age group
- Immunization
- Administering vitamin A prophylaxis
- De-worming of children
- Issue oral rehydration solution (ORS) packets to children with diarrhea
- Health education
- Detection and treatment of leprosy, tuberculosis and malaria
- Notification of certain infectious diseases
- Maintenance of records, statistics and reports
- IEC activities
- Referral system

Special Clinics

Special clinics in urban areas concentrate on providing specialized care for urban population. The specialists of the concerned field conduct these clinics. Some of them to mention here are:

- Dental clinics conducted in morning and evening hours
- Geriatric clinics conducted to help the old people
- De-addiction center
- Diagnostic centers
- Rehabilitation clinics for destitute and mentally ill
- Dialysis clinics to help the patients with kidney failure
- Shelter for the homeless
- Lifestyle clinics—mainly conducted in school and colleges to inculcate healthy lifestyle among school and college students.

Table 8: Staffing in CGHS dispensary

Designation	Nos
CMO incharge	1
Other doctors	11
Nurses and midwives	3
Laboratory staff	2
Clerks	2
Pharmacists	6
Storekeeper	1
Others (Attendants, dressers, peons, sweepers and chowkidars)	12
Total	38

Dispensaries-ESI (Employee State Insurance Scheme)

There are dispensaries run under ESI scheme to help employees mentioned as mentioned in the beneficiaries' regulations of ESI.

Dispensaries

Under Central Government Health Scheme (CGHS), dispensaries provide comprehensive health care to all retired and serving central government employees, current and ex-members of Parliament, sitting and retired judges of the Supreme Court of India, VIPs, freedom fighters, and their dependent family members. CGHS started its first dispensary in New Delhi in 1954. Now there are 319 CGHS dispensaries functioning in 24 locations in India. The population coverage approximates to 43 lakhs. They have appointed staff members to provide following services (Table 8).

Functions of Dispensaries

- Outpatient and emergency services
- Free supply of necessary drugs
- Laboratory services
- Home visits of seriously ill
- Family welfare and RCH services to the beneficiaries as well as general population
- Specialist consultation and treatment in government and recognized private hospitals through referrals.

Staffing at ESI Dispensary

Norms for opening of ESI dispensaries/hospitals (Table 9):

An ESI dispensary will be opened in an area as per the following norms:

- 2 doctor type, if the number of insured persons is 3,000–5,000

Table 9: Staffing norms for ESI dispensaries

Designation ESI	2 Dr. Type Dy. (3,000–5,000 IP)	3 Dr. Type Dy. (5,000–10,000 IP)	5 Dr. Type Dy. (10,000 and above IPs)
Doctors	2	3	5
Assistants	2	2	2
Junior assistants	1	1	3
LHV/ANM/SN	2	2	
Lab technician	1 per 25–30 tests/day		
Dresser	1	2	2
Record sorter	3	2	2
Class IV workers		5	5

- 3 doctor type, if the number of insured persons is 5,000–10000
- 5 doctor type, if the number of insured persons is 10,000 and above number of IPs

MATERNAL AND CHILD HEALTH CENTER

Maternal and child health (MCH) centers are the health care facility specifically designed to provide care for the mother and child. National rural health mission has identified matching health facilities to offer MCH care at various levels.

The all time continuous health services provided by trained personnel level-I care. Provision of emergency obstetric care refers to level-II care. In this context, all the PHCs function as Level I centers for MCH care.

Functions of MCH Centers

Community health centers referred to Level II MCH centers provide:

- Reproductive and child health (RCH) services that include antenatal and postnatal care, emergency obstetric care, safe abortion services, sterilization services including temporary methods, adolescent clinics, RTI/STI management, etc.
- Newborn stabilization units of these centers would help in providing excellent care.
- Round the clock delivery services
- Referrals and follow-up.

Level I MCH center-staffing: 2 more VHNs and sanitary worker.

Level-II MCH center-staffing: 2 additional doctors (preferably specialists), 3 more staff nurses, pharmacist, junior assistant, hospital workers, sanitary workers.

COMPONENTS OF HEALTH SERVICES

ENVIRONMENTAL SANITATION

Sanitation means **hygiene**. Keeping the environment clean and adopting hygienic practices can prevent us from many diseases that occur due to unhygienic practices and environment. Health promotion measures prevent harmful contact that can cause hazards to human beings. Poor living conditions, using polluted water for drinking and cooking, improper waste disposal are some of the activities that invite infection to man. Safe disposal of the solid waste is one of the practices that promote our health.

Types of Sanitation Based on Situations

o   Provision of toilet at household level helps in preventing the unsafe disposal of human feces. Safe disposal of human feces at the level of individual houses refers to **basic sanitation**.

o   Once the waste is collected it is treated in a place where it is dumped is known as **on-site sanitation**.

o   The hygienic practices adopted during the process of storage, preservation, cooking, serving and eating all refers to food hygiene or **food sanitation**.

o   Paying careful attention to the house and its surroundings for cleanliness refers to **housing sanitation**.

The chains of human activities that occur in the environment turn it as an unsafe atmosphere to live. Some of the major activities those cause unsafe living atmosphere are improper treatment or management of solid waste, wastewater and industrial waste. In addition, it also includes the practice of poor implementation of pollution and noise control measures. Controlling all these factors through proper management of wastewater from all sources, such pollution control measures refer to **environmental sanitation**.

HEALTH EDUCATION

Definitions

Health education is any combination of learning experiences designed to help individuals and communities to improve their health, by increasing their knowledge or influencing their attitudes.

Health education like general education is concerned with the change in knowledge, feelings and behavior of people. In its most usual 'form it concentrates on developing such health practices as are believed to bring about the best possible state of well-being'

—**WHO**

Health education is a process that informs, motivates and helps people to adopt and maintain healthy practices and lifestyles, advocates environmental changes as needed to facilitate this goal, and conducts professional training and research to the same end.

—**National Conference USA,1977**

Health education is "any combination of learning experiences designed to facilitate voluntary actions conducive to health". —**Green and Kreuter, 2005**

Health education is an attempt to close the gap between what is known about optimum health practice and that which is actually practiced. —**Griffiths, William 1972**

Health education is the principle by which individuals and groups of people learn to behave in a manner conducive to the promotion, maintenance, or restoration of health. The ultimate aim of health education is positive behavioral modification.

Lawrence Green defined it as "a combination of learning experiences designed to facilitate voluntary actions conducive to health."

Approaches to Health Education

There are four main approaches to health education. They are:

1. **Legal or regulatory approach:** Legal approach forces to control the "human behavior" that may cause harmful consequences to self and the public by using the law and order. This legal approach is considered as pragmatic strategy with quick results. For example: Air pollution and noise pollution. Under the regulations of air pollution and noise pollution act, any person violating the rules is liable to be prosecuted.

The childhood marriages are prevented in India through enforcement of "The Child Marriage Restraint Act, 1929."

The legal approach has many limitations: (1) This is not an appropriate measure for all problems. For example, the government cannot force people to have cholesterol free diet or balanced diet because there are many issues connected to it. (2) This may not change the behavior of people.

However, it is very much appropriate to manage emergencies and epidemics.

2. **Administrative or service approach:** This approach intends to provide all the health facilities to the people at their doorsteps. India attempted to use this approach through provision of basic health services at doorsteps in the year 1960, but it was a failure since it was not planned considering the felt needs of the people.

3. **Educational approach:** Health education has the ability to protect, promote and maintain people's health. It can

prevent many communicable and noncommunicable diseases and thereby reduce morbidity and mortality rates. Health education aims at bringing about desired change in people's behavior, attitude and practices. However, we may not be able to see these changes within a short time. It may take weeks, months, or years because every individual has his/her own belief and value system and functions accordingly.

4. **Primary health care approach:** Primary health care approach delivers health services using the principles of primary health care through community participation and an efficient intersectoral coordination. In this approach, the health care providers play a key role in providing necessary guidance to the community in finding the problems/needs and making an action plan to solve the problems. In a long run the community will be empowered to make brilliant workable plans against the problems discovered.

Scope of Health Education

The scope of health education stretches to all areas beyond our usual calculations or plans. Some of the broad fields or areas of health education are stated under content of health education.

Focused Areas for Health Education (Fig. 4)

○ Human biology
○ Nutrition
○ Hygiene
○ Family health care
○ Control of communicable and noncommunicable diseases

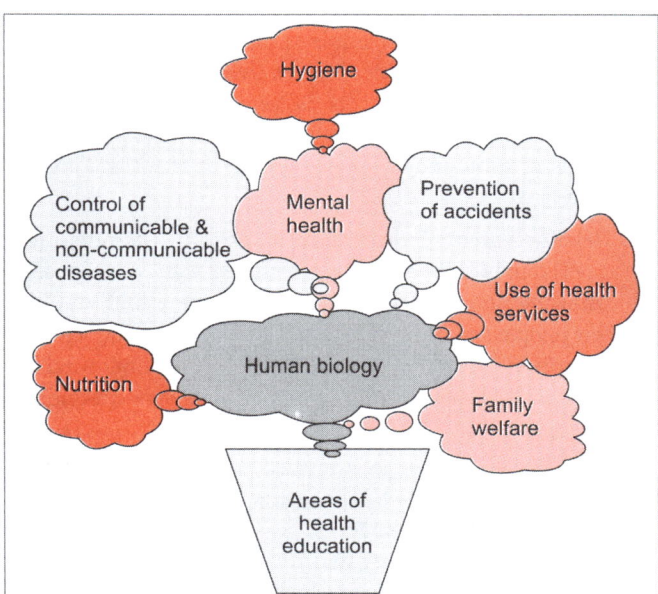

Figure 4: Focused areas for health education

○ Mental health
○ Prevention of accidents
○ Use of health services

1. **Human biology:**
   ❑ Children need to have understanding on biology prior to learning about health, hence biology sessions begin from the kindergarten itself
   ❑ As beginners they are taught different parts of the human body and their functions
   ❑ Importance of good health and practices to keep physically fit
   ❑ Importance of exercise, adequate sleep and rest
   ❑ Consequences of poor habits

2. **Nutrition:**
   ❑ Nutrition is the very basic need to survive. All age groups must know about nutrients and their daily-recommended allowances.
   ❑ Teach on balanced diet
   ❑ Nutrient value of foodstuff
   ❑ Meaning of malnutrition and ways to prevent children from it
   ❑ Signs and symptoms of deficiency disorders and prevention
   ❑ Cooking demonstration
   ❑ Specific diets for people with diseases (Diabetes, hypertension, etc.)

3. **Hygiene:** Hygienic practices of people help in keeping away the communicable diseases. Person as an individual should know how to keep himself and his surroundings clean. Hygienic practices taught should include: (1) personal hygiene and (2) environmental hygiene.

   Personal hygiene: Bathing, brushing, clothing, washing hands after defecation, urination; personal care like nail, feet and hair care, etc. Adequate precautions while coughing, sneezing; one should avoid public spitting, defecating and voiding in places. Inculcating good habits in childhood help the children to grow as a responsible citizen.

   Environmental hygiene: It has two aspects:

   i. *Domestic hygiene:* This includes clean house, cross ventilation, good lighting and fresh air, proper waste disposal systems, avoidance of pests, insects, etc.

   ii. *Community hygiene:* Proper garbage disposal, adequate sewage and drainage facilities

4. **Family health care:** Family is the first institution, which a person comes across in life. Family gives identity, love, affection, and facilities needed to live. Family teaches the religion, language, behavior, habits, etc. One person's ill health may affect the entire family. Health education

tries to strengthen the health of the family as a single unit rather than an individual. It promotes self-reliance specifically in the areas of child bearing, self-care and adoption of healthy life style practices.

5. **Disease prevention and control:** Treatment alone cannot cure a disease. Creating awareness about the disease like cause, spread, prevention and management will not only help in curing the disease but also help in caring the others. Provision of basic knowledge may help in promoting health, preventing the diseases and reducing the complications. There are many national health programs run in India to eradicate some diseases like malaria, filarial, leprosy, tuberculosis, etc. Recent malaria eradication showed the importance of placing health education other antimalarial measures.

6. **Mental health services:** Mental illnesses are slow killers because most often, the mentally ill brought to medical attention very late. People are not aware much about mental illnesses like other chronic diseases. There are specific situations where mental health need to be cautiously observed and supported: Postnatal mother, child at entry into school for the first time, Student at entry to secondary school and college, single mother, man who lost his affectionate wife, young lady who lost her husband recently, etc. Health care professional need to take a lead role in educating the people who are in need.

7. **Prevention of accidents:** Accidents are the most common "People-killer" in the world. Accidents can occur at home, road and in work-site.

   Teaching road safety rules and prevention of accidents at home, in the work site will help to great extent to reduce disability and mortalities caused by accidents.

   For example, provision of mouth guards while playing contact sports will help you greatly.

8. **Use of health services:** In most communities, people are not aware of health services available in the community and the approaches to use such services. It is the role of health care professionals to inform the people about various health services and preventive programs available in the community and the way to use those services. Community should be educated and encouraged to participate in the health programs.

Principles of Health Education

○ **Credibility:** Interest refers to the extent to which the receiver perceives the message as trustworthy. The message should be scientific; facts based and should be congruent with local culture and goals. The health educator must win the confidence of the people before he delivers the message. This would help them accept and adopt the message.

○ **Interest:** If the health education topic is of interest to the people, they will listen to it.

   Health educator should identify the "felt needs" of the people and then prepare a program that they can actively participate in to make it successful.

○ **Participation:** Success of any program depends upon people's participation. Community health nurses should encourage people to participate in the program. The Alma-Ata declaration stated that the peoples have right and duty to participate in the planning and implementation of their health care.

   Encouraging teaching methods like group discussion, panel discussions, etc. would enhance the chances of people's participation.

○ **Motivation:** Motivation is "the fundamental desire to learn." Motives are primary (hunger, sex, survival) and secondary (love, praise, rewards and punishment). In motivation incentives takes role of changing the learning behavior. For example, instruction to obese woman:

   "If you do not reduce your weight you will get cardiac problems." It is a **negative reinforcement**; probably she may not listen to the educator.

   "You will look more beautiful if you reduce your weight."—**Positive statement**. She may listen to it and act accordingly.

○ **Comprehension:** Health educator must always assess the level of literacy understating of the audience and use the words accordingly. Simplified message always reach the audience well and gets a good feedback. Avoid using high-level jargon. Convey the message in such a way so that the participants understand it. Avoid technical and medical terms.

   A community health nurse says, "Please, add 'vitamin A-rich foods" into your under-fives diet." The mother may not know what foods are rich in Vitamin A. Therefore, the CHN should name the vitamin A-rich foods recommended for preventing or treating Vitamin A deficiency disorders.

○ **Reinforcement:** Reinforcement refers to the repetition needed in health education. Health education is repeated until the desired behavioral changes are achieved. Only few people can learn new things in a short period. Hence, repetition is a strategy to make people remember used for easy understanding and remembering of new messages.

○ **Known to unknown:** People tend to show interest in listening when the educator starts with what the audience know and get into what he wants them to know. Health education always functions as: Concrete to abstract, simple to complex, easy to difficult, known to unknown.

   Before the start of health education session, the community health nurse should find out the existing knowledge of people on the topic. This provides the foundation to build further knowledge. For example, a community health nurse planned to teach on "Prevention of childhood obesity" to urban mothers will be better appreciated if she starts the program with "Do all the children of same age look alike in size"? If not why so?. Then start building from big size and taking the session into—obesity, causes, prevention and management.

○ **Setting an example:** The health educator automatically becomes a role model to an individual or public while providing education. Hence, he or she should follow what he/she preaches.

For example, a health educator provides education on ill effects of tobacco should not be seen smoking because if he does so, he sends the opposite message and again, the seriousness of the situation will be lost.

○ **Learning by doing:** Lessons are always by doing and not by saying. Learning is an action-oriented task not simple recitation. Action oriented learning methods (demonstration) better registers in people's mind. The Chinese proverb appropriately states this principle: "If I hear, I forget; if I see, I remember; if I do, I know".

○ **Community leaders:** Getting into a community itself is a big task when you are a stranger to the place. It is easy to approach or educate the community through the respected people of the locality like the village president or headman, village administrative officer, panchayati members, school teachers, politician, etc. The word of mouth from the leaders or the important people is *the most basic* requirement to make a rapport with the community. Community leaders can be used to reach the community. Leaders also can be involved to educate the people. The leader will have an idea about the needs of the community.

○ **Good health relations:** The health educator should have good pleasing manners and admirable qualities to build professional relations with the people. The health educator should be kind and empathetic. He or she must be a task-focused person with a smile that extends invitation to take the message what he has for them.

○ **Feedback:** Feedback refers to the receiver's indication that the message has been understood (decoded) in the way that the sender intended (encoded). It helps to find out if any modifications are sought to make the program more effective.

Audio-visual Aids used in Health Education

No health education is successful without audio-visual aids. Audio-visual aids are appreciated for their smart appeal to more than one sense and prevention of monotony. Advancing technology greatly supports the field of education and teaching methodologies by introducing many new teaching aids.

Audio-visual aids are classified into:

○ **Auditory aids:** Auditory aids works on the principles of sound, electricity and magnetism.

It helps in reproducing the spoken words. Examples include:

- Megaphones
- Microphones
- Gramophone records and discs
- Tape recorder
- Radios
- Sound amplifiers

○ **Visual aids:** Visual aids function on the principle of projection. It is of 2 types: (1) projected aids and (2) nonprojected aids

- **Projected aids:** This requires projection from a source to the screen. Examples include:
  - Film strips
  - Slides
  - Transparencies

- **Non-projected aids:** This does not require any projection:
  - Blackboard
  - Pictures, cartoons, photographs
  - Flip charts, flashcards
  - Flannel boards
  - Printed materials—leaflets, pamphlets, folders, booklets, brochures
  - Models, specimens

○ **Combined audio-visual aids:** This helps to see and hear. The examples include:

- Televisions
- Tape and slide combinations
- Video cassette players and records
- Motion pictures or cinemas
- Multimedia computers.

Approaches in Health Communication

There are three approaches used for communicating health messages. They are:

1. Individual approach
2. Group approach
3. Mass approach

Individual Approach

Individual approach refers to one to one basis of health education. The community health nurses have many opportunities to provide health education to individuals. Woman at home seeks individual health education on various health issues from community health nurses during the home visits. Apart from thus, community health nurses provide health education to antenatal, postnatal, sick men, women and adolescents at home, special clinic, health centers, worksites and schools, etc. The teaching program is planned or incidental.

Advantages

- One to one discussion makes individual more comfortable
- The individual feels free to ask questions and clear doubts.

Disadvantages

Only a single individual receives education during the session.

Group Approach

Chalk and Talk (Lectures)

It is a planned oral presentation of facts, organized thoughts, and ideas by a qualified person on a specific topic or phenomenon.

Advantages

- This method is used for a group of 30 or less.
- Duration of talk lasts for 15–20 minutes
- Should be based on topics of current interest
- The ability of the speaker to write and draw legibly is the biggest plus point.

Disadvantages

- It is a one-way communication and the learners are passive
- It does not stimulate problem solving among audience
- Message taken away depends upon comprehending ability of the individual.

Symposium

Symposium is a meeting in which experts on a particular subject give series of speeches.

- Each speaker presents on a specific aspect of the given topic
- Symposium does not include any discussion among speakers
- At the end, the audience may ask questions
- The chairman presents the summary at the end of the session

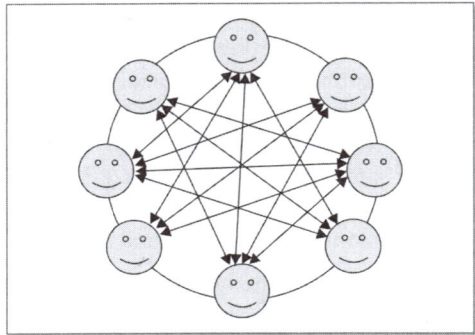

Figure 5: A good group discussion

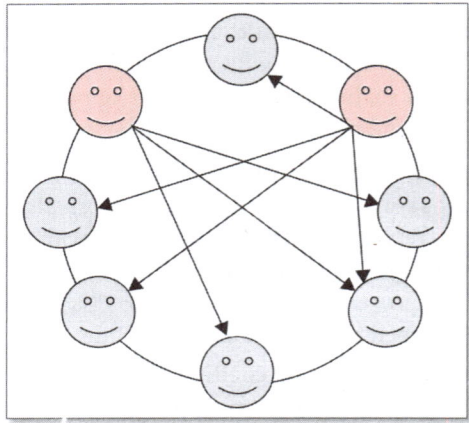

Figure 6: Dominated group

Group Discussion (Figs 5 and 6)

In group discussion a group of individuals with similar interest gather formally or informally to bring up ideas, solve problems or give comments. People in group discussion interact face-to-face.

- Group consists of 6–12 members
- Participants sit in a circle for discussion
- The leader of the group opens the topic of discussion. The leader controls any side conversations, and encourages everyone's participation
- The leader presents the summary at the end
- The member assigned as "recorder" prepares the report on issues discussed and agreements reached.

Panel Discussion

A panel of 4–8 members who are qualified to talk about the specific issue or topic present information and discuss personal views in front of a large group of audience. This may help audience to clarify and evaluate their positions regarding specific issues being discussed.

- Chairman opens the session, introduces the speakers and keeps the discussion going
- No specific agenda or order to deliver the speeches

- After exploring the main aspects of the topic or subject audience are allowed to ask questions
- At the end, the chairman sums up the different views presented.

Workshop

Workshops are teaching and learning arrangements, usually in small groups, that are structured to produce active participation in learning. Workshops conducted traditionally, provided the participants with some opportunity to practice skills and receive feedback. Conversely, current usage is so loose that any learning event that aspires to engage the learners actively may be called a workshop.

- Workshop has series of meetings that highlights the individual practicing a work with the help of resource persons.
- In workshop series the participants are divided into small groups and each with a selected chairman and a recorder.
- Group works in democratic way under the guidance of the resource person.
- The individuals work, solve a part of the problem with the help of resource person.
- The group discussion takes place at the end, and the group walks with a plan of action for the problem.

Conferences or Seminars

- Program ranges from half day to one week
- Held on a regional, state or national level
- They usually have a theme.

Role Playing/Sociodrama

- Situation is dramatized to make communication more effective
- It is followed by a discussion on the problem
- Puppet shows is a type of sociodrama
- Useful for children's health education.

Demonstrations

- Step-by-step procedures performed in front of the audience using set principles
- Following which the audience perform the procedure themselves with expert help
- Best method for transfer of skills.

Mass Approach

Mass media are the most effective means of communication to reach people as well as the remote residents. The audience

or the beneficiaries of this kind of mass health education do not belong to one particular group or geographical region. Initially, only printed materials like newspaper, pamphlets, books and periodicals took the important place in mass approach. Later, radio and television came to play a role.

Various Mass Media

Television

Nowadays television is the most powerful among mass media.

The followings are the advantages and disadvantages of television.

- **Advantages**
  - Large number of people can be reached
  - People of all socioeconomic status have access to health education.
- **Disadvantage**
  - One way communication
  - It is simply one of the aids in teaching since it cannot cover all aspects of learning.

Radio

Radio is the oldest form of mass media that uses audio technology. Radio has been used extensively to disseminate information on health, nutrition and agricultural education, etc. Because of its commercial nature and appeal to mass audiences, it has been most specifically used for pleasure and entertainment than for education.

The followings are the advantages and disadvantages of radio

- **Advantages**
  - Helps the students to keep their knowledge updated
  - Easy reach to all people
  - Portable
  - Serves as major source of information to public.
- **Disadvantages**
  - Radio-jockeys are required to get public attention
  - Repetition of information is not possible
  - One-way communication
  - Scheduled programs, those stick on to specific.

Only a few schools have their own system of broadcasting to educate students.

Print material

These are the oldest and widely used forms of educational resources. Examples include books, pamphlets, magazines and newspapers. Printed materials are frequently combined with other forms of media to form multimedia packages, which may be either locally or commercially produced.

Followings are the advantages of print material.

- Advantages
  - Medium of communication and instruction
  - Produced in multiple copies
  - Easily portable
  - Revision and updating of information is easy and fast
  - Familiar to teachers and students.

Types of Printed Material

Books, picture book, textbooks, workbooks, paperback books, reference books, newspaper and magazines, etc.

Posters: "A poster or placard is usually pictorial or decorative. It utilizing an emotional appeal to convey a message aimed at reinforcing an attitude or urging a course of action".

It aims at conveying the specific message, teaching a particular thing, giving a general idea, etc. Posters exert a great influence on the observer.

The followings are the advantages and limitations of poster

- Advantages
  - Captures attention
  - Motivates the audience
  - Presents a single idea
  - Strong lasting impression
  - Satisfy the viewer emotionally and esthetically.
- Limitations
  - Poster conveys only a single theme.
  - If the message on the poster is not attractive and accurate than it makes the poster illegible.
  - It is time consuming to produce quality posters.

Museums

A museum is a building displaying a collection of historical relics, antiques, curiosities, works of arts, works of science, literature and other artifacts of general interest.

Museums can be useful both for public education and specific class room instructions.

VITAL STATISTICS

Vital statistics include indicators such as birth rate, death rate, natural growth rate, life expectancy at birth, mortality and fertility rates. The most common way of collecting information on these events is through civil registration, an administrative system used by governments to record **vital** events which occur in their populations.

Our country keeps a continuous check on demographic changes through registration of vital events. If registration of vital events is complete and accurate, it serves as a reliable source of health information. Dependable vital statistics related to births and deaths are vital to assess the health of the population, conduct epidemiological research, health planning and for evaluating any program. Civil registration is the best suited source of statistics on vital events (i.e. births and deaths). The office of the "registrar-general and census commissioner", functions under the ministry of home affairs is the national authority for civil registration in India.

SOURCE OF VITAL STATISTICS IN INDIA

- Population census: Ancient literature reveals that the population count was practiced between 600 and 800 BC in India. India initiated its first census in 1881, and continued it once every 10 years.
- The last census of India was undertaken in 2011 and it was the 15th census of India.

Civil Registration System

- The task of "civil registration system" is recording of vital events, i.e. live births, stillbirths and deaths.
- Present registration of births and deaths is being done under Act, 1969.
- "Registration records" are very useful legal documents
- It is a source of statistics.

Sample Registration System (SRS)

- It is one of the largest demographic household sample survey in the world.
- This was initiated in 1969–70 with the purpose of complete registration from CRS.
- Provides reliable annual estimates of birth, death and infant mortality rates at the State and National levels.
- This system provides estimates and rates separately for rural and urban areas.
- Some of the other rates which could be elicited from this are: child mortality rate (CMR), total fertility rate (TFR), sex ratio at birth and 0–4 age, rate of institutional deliveries, medical attention before death, etc.
- From the year 2008, it also provides under 5 mortality rate.

Demographic Sample Surveys (NSSO)

National sample surgery office (NSSO) established in 1950 in India conducts regular socio-economic surveys (household expenditure, employment and unemployment, health and medical services, etc.)

- "National sample survey organization" currently known as "National Sample Survey Office," functions under the ministry of statistics, Government of India.

Health Surveys

National Family Health Survey (NFHS): It is a large-level, multiple surveys conducted in a representative sample of households throughout India." International Institute for Population Sciences", Mumbai, provides coordination and technical guidance for the survey. The multiple survey rounds were funded by USAID, DFID, the Bill and Melinda Gates Foundation, UNICEF, UNFPA, and MOHFW, GOI.

Specific Goals of NFHS

- To provide essential data on health and family welfare needed by the Ministry of Health and Family Welfare and other agencies for policy and program purposes
- To provide information on important emerging health and family welfare issues

Four rounds of the survey have been conducted so far:

- NFHS-1 (1992–93)
- NFHS-2 (1998–99)
- NFHS-3 (2005–06)
- NFHS-4 (2014–15)

Reproductive and child health survey (DLHS-RCH): The largest ever demographic and health surveys carried out in India, with a sample size of about seven lakh households covering all districts of the country. The main purpose of RCH is to provide district level estimates on health indicators that would assist in policy making, decentralized planning and evaluation.

Survey provides information on—maternal and child health, reproductive health, practice of family planning, performance of National Rural Health Mission (NRHM) and accessibility and utilization of health facilities.

Health facility adequacy and performance

- Three rounds of the survey have been conducted since
- RCH-1 (1998–99)
- RCH-2 (2002–04)
- DLHS-3 (2007–08)
- DLHS-4 (2011–12)

Annual Health Survey

The annual health survey (AHS) is a comprehensive, representative dataset on core vital indicators like IMR, MMR and TFR along with their co-variates of the districts to provide special attention on needy districts.

Concurrent Evaluation of NRHM

Concurrent evaluation assesses the extent of reach of NRHM activities to the rural communities and provide information for policy making and program planning.

Multiple Indicator Cluster Survey

The multiple indicator cluster survey (MICS) enable all the countries to elicit statistically sound and internationally comparable data on certain indicators in the areas of health, education, etc. MICS is extensively used in policy making and program interventions.

Longitudinal Aging Study in India

The longitudinal aging study in India (LASI) mainly focuses on the issues related to elderly population of India on health, economic, and social well-being. IIPS Mumbai, Harvard School of Public Health and RAND Corporation extend the technical support to LASI.

Vital Statistics Indicators

Birth Rate

Birth rate is the most basic and the simplest indicator of fertility.

Crude birth rate is defined as, "the number of live births occurring during the year, per 1,000 population, estimated at midyear."

Birth rate is not considered as a satisfactory measure of fertility because the total population is not open to fertility.

$$\text{Birth rate} = \frac{\text{Number of live births during the year}}{\text{Estimated midyear population}} \times 1000$$

Subtracting the crude death rate from the crude birth rate would give the rate of natural increase, which is equal to the rate of population change in the absence of migration. But it cannot provide true idea about the fertility of a population.

General Fertility Rate

The general fertility rate (GFR) is defined as the total number of live births per 1,000 women of reproductive age (ages 15 to 49 years) in a population per year.

$$\text{GFR} = \frac{\text{Number of live births in an area during the year}}{\substack{\text{Midyear female population age 15–49 years} \\ \text{in the same area in same year}}} \times 1000$$

This is the most suitable way to measure "fertility in a population" than crude birth rate because the GFR accounts for the female population ages 15–49 years in the denominator, rather than considering the whole population.

General Marital Fertility Rate

General marital fertility rate (GMFR) is defined as the number of live births for 1000 married women in the reproductive age group (15–49) in a given year.

$$\text{GMFR} = \frac{\text{Number of live births in a year}}{\substack{\text{Midyear married female population} \\ \text{in the age group 15–49 years}}} \times 1000$$

Age-Specific Fertility Rate

The age-specific fertility rate (ASFR) is defined as the annual number of births to women of a specified age per 1,000 women in that age group. ASFR is the sensitive indicator of family planning.

$$\text{ASFR} = \frac{\text{Number of live births in particular age group}}{\substack{\text{Midyear female population of} \\ \text{the same age group}}} \times 1000$$

Age-Specific Marital Fertility Rate

Age-specific marital fertility rate (ASFR) is defined as the number of live births in a year to 1000 married women in any specified age group.

$$\text{ASMFR} = \frac{\text{Number of live births in particular age group}}{\substack{\text{Midyear married female population} \\ \text{of the same age group}}} \times 1000$$

Total Fertility Rate

Total fertility rate (TFR) is defined as the number of children that would be born to a woman if she were to live to the end of her childbearing years and bear children in accordance with current age-specific fertility rates.

Total fertility rate is the sum of the age-specific birth rates (5-year age groups between 15 and 49) for females of a specified geographic area during a specified time period multiplied by 5.

The TFR is calculated as: $\text{TFR} = \sum \text{ASFR}_a$ (for single year age groups)

or

$\text{TFR} = 5 \sum \text{ASFR}_a$ (for 5-year age groups)

Where:

ASFR$_a$ = age-specific fertility rate for women in age group *a* (expressed as a rate per woman).

Net Reproduction Rate

Net reproduction rate (NRR) is defined as the number of daughters a newborn girl will bear during her life time assuming fixed age specific fertility and mortality rates.

NRR of India is 1.171 (2015)

Crude Marriage Rate

The crude marriage rate is defined as the annual number of marriages per 1,000 population. Principles and recommendations for a vital statistics system-revision 2 (UN) define marriage as "the act, ceremony or process by which the legal relationship of husband and wife is constituted. The legality of the union may be established by civil, religious or other means as recognized by the laws of each country."

$$\text{Crude marriage rate} = \frac{\text{Number of marriages in the year}}{\text{Midyear population}} \times 1000$$

According to demographers this is very unsatisfactory rate since the denominator comprised primarily of population that is not eligible to marry.

Other method that is very sensitive for calculating marriage rates.

General Marriage Rate

General marriage rate

$$= \frac{\text{Number of marriages within 1 year}}{\substack{\text{Number of unmarried} \\ \text{persons age 15–49 years}}} \times 1000$$

Pregnancy Rate

Pregnancy rate is defined as the total number of pregnancies including live births, induced abortions and fetal deaths per 1,000 women aged 15–44 years for a specified geographical area during a specified time period.

Pregnancy rate

$$= \frac{\substack{\text{Number of resident pregnancies} \\ \text{(live births + induced abortions + fetal deaths)}}}{\text{Number of women aged 15–44 years}} \times 1000$$

Pregnancy ratio

$$= \frac{\text{(live births + induced abortions + fetal deaths)}}{\text{Number of women in reproductive age (15–44 years)}}$$

Abortion Ratio

It is defined as the number of abortions of all types in a year to number of live births over the same period.

$$\text{Abortion ratio} = \frac{\text{Number of all types of abortion}}{\text{Number of live births}}$$

World abortion ratio = 32:100 live births. This means for every 100 live births in the world there are 32 abortions.

Abortion refers to the termination of pregnancy from whatever cause before the fetus is capable of extra uterine life.

—**WHO**

Child Woman Ratio

It is defined as the number of children of 0-4 years to 1000 women of child bearing age (5–44 years). This is not an accurate measure of fertility, it is more like a measure of population structure.

Child/woman ratio

$$= \frac{\text{Living children aged 0–4 years}}{\text{Women of child bearing age (15–44 years)}}$$

Any birth or deaths that have occurred in government hospitals or private hospitals or nursing homes or medical institutions should be reported within 21 days by the head of the institutions to the registrars (births and deaths) of the area.

○ In case birth or death that has occurred at home, it becomes the responsibility of the head of the family or any other family member to report within 21 days to the sub registrars (births and deaths).

○ Birth or death can be registered only at the place where it took place

○ According to registration of births and deaths (RBD)Act, 1969 Fees and penalties imposed for delayed registration are to be paid to the concerned registrar of births and deaths.

Barriers to Registration of Vital Events

There are various factors functioning as the barriers to registration of vital events. They may include—1 political factors, administrative factors, economic factors, legislative factors and neglect of cultural and community realities.

MATERNAL AND CHILD HEALTH (MCH) CARE

World Health Organization defined maternal and child health services as "promoting, preventing, therapeutic or rehabilitation facility or care for the mother and child."

The MCH or maternal and child health is not a new entity to health care professionals. However, it is definitely a significant area of importance since this package include two vulnerable groups the mother and children, whose health has major contribution in determining the health status of a country. The women of reproductive age group (15–44 years) and under five children constitute major (32.4%) portion of our India's population. MCH services concentrate on preventive, curatives and social aspects of mother and child care.

OBJECTIVES OF MCH

○ Reduce morbidity and mortality among mothers and children

○ Promote reproductive health

○ Promote physical and psychological development of child within the family

Lifelong health is the overall aim of MCH services.

The MCH services focus on many subareas to provide complete care to mothers and children (Fig. 7).

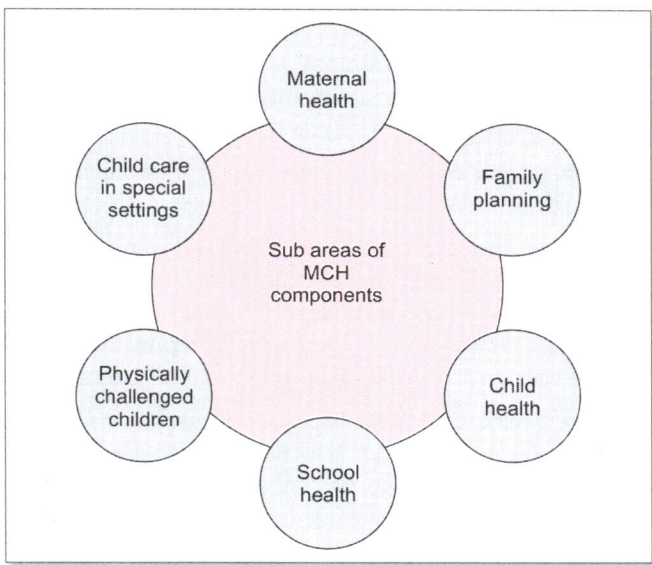

Figure 7: Sub areas of MCH components

TRENDS IN MCH

Maternal mortality rate in India just before our independence was estimated at 20/1000 live births. Further, 30% of all babies born, died before their 1st birthday. After independence, Indian government included MCH programs and emphasized its importance in all "five-year plans."

The recently stated trends in MCH care are—Integration of care, Risk approach, Manpower changes, Primary health care.

Integration of care: Integrated approach in MCH care had replaced the conventional care, in which mother needs to attend various health facilities to get care for mother and child. In this approach all members of health team (from obstetrician to local dai) work as a team. The obstetric and pediatric unit should have good coordination by including community physicians and community workers to provide quality MCH care.

Risk approach: The main purpose of this approach is to identify the "high-risk" mothers and children and provide appropriate specialized care using available resources. The others (normal mother and child) receive routine care.

Risk approach is the major strategy to match the available resources with the type of care required. This tackles the problem of scarce resources and provides care to all.

Manpower changes: There are many changes adopted to assure quality services to the mothers and children. The recent one is the phasing out of ANMs and health visitors work in peripheral health care facilities. The second strategy is to add the following categories to enhance the quality of MCH care:

Professionals-specialist doctors and other practitioners

Field workers: Multipurpose health workers, health guides, *dais, bal sevikas,* anganwadi workers extension workers, ASHA etc.

Voluntary workers such as members from women health organization.

Earlier, the dais' "delivery practices" were criticized calling it as a menace. However, country like India where 70% population live in rural areas definitely needs person like dai who can help them greatly. Hence, the government initiated "dai training" to assist rural women in a skilled manner.

Primary health care: This approach ensures that essential health care is available to all. The elements of primary health care—(MCH, family planning, control of infection, nutrition, health education, etc.) have higher level positive impact on MCH.

CAUSES OF MATERNAL MORTALITY IN INDIA

- Medical causes
  - Obstetrical causes
  - Nonobstetrical causes and
- Social factors that influence maternal mortality (Table 10)

PREVENTIVE AND SOCIAL MEASURES TO REDUCE MATERNAL MORTALITY RATES

As stated in the table there are many causes and social factors influencing maternal mortality:

- Promote early registration of pregnancy

Table 10: Causes of maternal mortality in India

Medical causes- ◻ Obstetrical	○ Toxemias of pregnancy ○ Hemorrhage ○ Infection ○ Obstructed labor ○ Unsafe abortion
◻ Non- obstetrical	○ Anemia ○ Associated diseases—cardiac, renal, metabolic, etc. ○ Malignancy ○ Accidents
○ Social factors	○ Age at child birth, parity, Too close pregnancies ○ Family size, malnutrition, poverty, illiteracy, ignorance and prejudices ○ Lack of maternal services, delivery by untrained dai, poor communication and transportal facilities, societal customs, etc.

- Four antenatal visits
- Supplementation of diet and anemia correction
- Preventing hemorrhage and infection in puerperium
- Prevent complications (PIH, uterine rupture, etc.) and treat medical conditions
- Antimalaria and tetanus prophylaxis
- Clean delivery practices by training dais
- Advise institutional deliveries for women with high risks
- Promote family planning
- Safe abortion services
- Identify all maternal deaths and its causes.

ANTENATAL CARE

Antenatal care refers to the comprehensive health supervision provided to pregnant woman before delivery. Antenatal care defined as planned examination, observation and guidance given to the pregnant woman from conception till the time of labor.

Objectives

- Promote, protect and maintain the health of the mother and growing fetus
- Identify and provide special attention to the high-risk cases
- Prevent complications
- Reduce maternal mortality rates
- Provide health education on various topics (child care, nutrition, hygiene, environmental sanitation, etc.)
- Sensitize mother on need for family planning and advice on safe abortion and MTP
- Attend the under-fives who are attending OPD along with the mother

Principle elements of antenatal care:

- Early registration of all pregnancies ideally in the first trimester before 12th week of pregnancy. If a woman comes late she should be registered and care given to her according to gestational age. Collect proper history and keep record on tobacco use for all antenatal mothers
- There should be minimum 4 antenatal check ups and complete package of services should be provided.
- Antenatal visits:
  - 1st visit: Within 12 weeks—preferably, as soon as pregnancy is suspected
  - 2nd visit: Between 14 and 26 weeks
  - 3rd visit: Between 28 and 34 weeks
  - 4th visit: Between 36 weeks and term

- At least 1 ANC—preferably the 3rd visit—the antenatal should be examined by a doctor.
- Provision of iron and folic acid tablets and injection for tetanus toxoid, etc.
- Laboratory investigations like hemoglobin, urine albumin and sugar, RPR test for syphilis and blood grouping and Rh typing
- Nutrition and health counseling
- Identification and management of high-risk pregnancies
- Timely referral to higher-level care.
- Chemoprophylaxis for malaria in high malaria endemic areas.

INTRANATAL CARE

The main idea of intranatal care is to prevent complications that may arise during the process of delivery. Septicemia is one of the complications that may endanger the life of mother and the baby. The health centers and hospitals should be well equipped to prevent sepsis in the delivery rooms and in newborn care units. The home deliveries to be done under trained birth attendant/*dai* taking all necessary precautions to prevent sepsis there by save the lives of mother and baby.

POSTNATAL CARE

Care of the mother and the newborn after delivery is known as postnatal or postpartum care. Care focuses on mother and newborn. The obstetrician and pediatrician play an important role in caring the mother and newborn.

Objectives

- To prevent complications that may occur during postnatal period
- To help in rapid restoration of optimum health of the mother
- To assess of breastfeeding adequacy
- To educate on family planning services
- To educate mother and family on related health topics

Complications of Postpartum Period

- *Puerperal sepsis:* This refers to the genital tract infection that occurs within 3 weeks of delivery. The signs and symptoms may include rise of temperature, pulse, foul smelling lochia and lower abdominal pain and tenderness.
- *Thrombophlebitis:* This is the infection of the leg veins more often linked with the varicose veins.
- *Secondary hemorrhage:* This refers to the vaginal bleeding that occurs any time after 6 hours of delivery to the end of the puerperium (6 weeks).

- *Others*
  - Urinary tract infection
  - Mastitis

Restoration of Mother's Health

Mother's optimum health is restored by postnatal assessment (includes physical and psychosocial assessment) psychological support wherever necessary, breastfeeding, anemia prevention, adequate nutrition and postnatal exercises, family planning and health education.

MEDICAL TERMINATION OF PREGNANCY

The aims of medical termination of pregnancy (MTP) act

- To improve the maternal health and prevent unsafe abortions and thereby high incidence of maternal mortality and morbidity
- To legalize abortion services
- To promotes access to safe abortion services wherver applicable
- To protect medical practitioners who otherwise would be penalized under the Indian penal code (Sections 315–316)

LEGAL FRAMEWORK OF MTP ACT (FIG. 8)

The MTP Act highlights the approved conditions and suitable candidates, places and qualifications required from the medical practitioner to terminate pregnancies.

What is a Legal Abortion?

Abortions are termed legal only when it fulfills the following conditions:

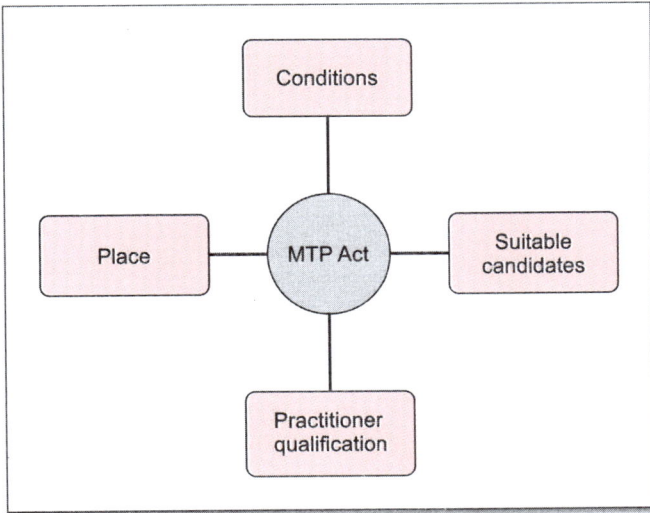

Figure 8: Legal framework of MTP act

- Termination is done by an approved medical practitioner.
- For conditions approved and gestation as prescribed by the Act.
- At an approved place, abiding all rules and regulations.

Following are the permitted conditions to do MTP:

- *Medical:* Continuation of pregnancy constitutes risk to the life or grave injury to the physical or mental health of woman.
- *Eugenic:* Substantial risk of child being born with serious handicaps (mental or physical abnormalities).
- *Humanitarian:* Pregnancy caused by rape (presumed grave injury to mental health).
- Contraceptive failure in married couple (presumed grave injury to mental health)
- *Socioeconomic:* When the environment could lead to injury to the mother.

Who Can Perform MTP?

A registered medical practitioner (RMP):

- Who has a recognized medical qualification as defined in clause (h) of section 2 of Indian Medical Council Act, 1956
- Whose name has been registered in a State Medical Register and
- Who has such experience or training in gynecology and obstetrics as prescribed by rules made under the Act.

Eligibility of the medical practitioner to terminate pregnancies that did not cross 12 weeks gestation:

- A practitioner who has assisted a registered medical practitioner in performing 25 cases of MTP of which at least 5 were performed independently in a hospital established or maintained or a training institute approved for this purpose by the government.

Eligibility of the medical practitioner to terminate pregnancies up to 20 weeks:

- A practitioner who holds a postgraduate degree or diploma in obstetrics and gynecology
- A practitioner who has completed 6 months house job in obstetrics and gynecology
- A practitioner who has at least 1 year experience in practice of obstetrics and gynecology at a hospital which has all facilities
- A practitioner registered in state medical register immediately before commencement of the Act, experience in practice of obstetrics and gynecology for a period not less than 3 years.

Permitted Guidelines to Terminate Pregnancy

- Registered medical practitioner shall not be guilty of offence under law
- Only up to 20 weeks of gestation
- After obtaining the consent of the woman
- Get consent from the guardian if the woman is below 18 years or is mentally ill
- With the opinion of a registered medical practitioner, formed in good faith, under certain circumstances
- Opinion of two RMPs required for termination of pregnancy between 12 and 20 weeks.

Place for Conducting MTP

- A hospital established or maintained by Government (or)
- A place approved by a district-level committee constituted by the government
- It should be done in strict confidence.

FEMALE FOETICIDE ACT

The government of India had passed "**Preconception and Prenatal Diagnostic Techniques (PCPNDT) Act**" in 1994.

This Act was introduced to stop female feticides and as a measure to stop the trend of declining sex ratio in India. The Act put a full stop to prenatal sex determination. In 2003, the PNDT Act was amended and renamed as the **preconception and prenatal diagnostic techniques (Prohibition of Sex Selection) Act, 1994.**

IMPORTANT FEATURES

Main provisions in the Act are:

- Prohibition of sex selection, before or after conception.
- No laboratory or center or clinic will conduct any test including ultrasonography for the purpose of determining the sex of the fetus.
- No person, including the one who is conducting the procedure as per the law, will communicate the sex of the fetus to the pregnant woman or her relatives by words, signs or any other method.
- Any person advertises for prenatal and preconception sex determination facilities in any form—notice, circular, label, in electronic or print and any other can be imprisoned for up to three years and penalized with ₹10,000.
- Prenatal diagnostic techniques, like ultrasound and amniocentesis are allowed only to detect:
  - Genetic abnormalities
  - Metabolic disorders
  - Chromosomal abnormalities

- ❑ Certain congenital malformations
- ❑ Hemoglobinopathies
- ❑ Sex-linked disorders.

CHILD ADOPTION ACT

Adoption is a legal procedure through which a child is placed with a married couple or a single female who agree to raise the child as own child assuming all responsibilities.

The Adoptions and Maintenance Act of 1956 provides guidelines on the legal process of **adopting** children by **Hindu** adult, and with the legal obligations of a **Hindu** to provide "maintenance" to various family members including their wife or wives, parents, and in-laws. It extends to the whole of India except the State of Jammu and Kashmir.

LAWS RELATED TO ADOPTION

- ○ **Hindu Adoption and Maintenance Act of 1956:** It is applicable to Hindus, Jain, Sikhs or Buddhists
- ○ **Guardian and Wards Act of 1890:** It is applicable to foreign citizens, NRIs and Indian nationals who are Muslims, Christians or Jews)
- ○ **Juvenile Justice Act of 2000:** A part of it deals with adoption of children by non-Hindu parents

Adoption is valid only when the following criteria are met:

- ○ The person adopting is **legally capable of taking** in adoption.
- ○ The person giving in adoption is **legally capable of giving** in adoption.
- ○ The person adopted is **legally capable of being taken in for adoption**.
- ○ The adoption is said to be complete only when after the ceremony called *Datta Homan* (oblation to the fire) has been performed. However, this is not essential in all cases to accept the validity of adoption.

Who can adopt?

- ○ An Indian
- ○ Non-resident Indian
- ○ A foreign citizen
- ○ A single female (unmarried, widowed or divorced) or a married couple.

Who is Entitled to Give the Child for Adoption

- ○ Father or mother or guardian of the child has the capacity to give the child for adoption
- ○ The father alone, if mother has completely and finally renounced the world or has ceased to be a Hindu, or has been declared by a court of competent judges to be of unsound mind.
- ○ The mother may give the child in adoption, if the father is dead or has completely and finally renounced the world or has ceased to be a Hindu, or has been declared by a court of competent judge to be of unsound mind.
- ○ Where both the father and mother are dead (or) have completely and finally renounced the world (or) have abandoned the child (or) have been declared by a court of competent jurisdiction to be of unsound mind (or) where the parentage of the child is unknown—the guardian of the child may give the child in adoption with the previous permission of the court.

Eligibility Criteria to be an Adoptive Parent

- ○ Medically fit and financially able to care for a child
- ○ Must be at least 21 years old
- ○ No legal upper age limit for parents
- ○ Adoption of the older children, age of the parents may be relaxed
- ○ Adopted child with special needs, the age limit may be relaxed
- ○ If the adoption is of a son, the adoptive father or mother by whom the adoption is made must not have a son living at the time of adoption
- ○ If the adoption is of a daughter, the adoptive father or mother by whom the adoption is made must not have a daughter living at the time of adoption.
- ○ Hindu Adoption and Maintenance Act of 1956: An adoptive parent is allowed to ask for a child, as per her preferences (age, gender, skin color, religion, specific features and health condition). A single parent or married couples are not permitted to adopt more than one child of the same sex.

FAMILY WELFARE

After independence, India took many steps to improve the health, education and economic status of our country by introducing various plans and policies and targets during the five year plans. One of the most important steps was "National Planning Program" introduced in the year 1951 with the objective of "reducing the birth rate to the extent necessary to stabilize the population at a level consistent with the requirement of the National economy." Family Welfare Program, considered priority area, was a fully sponsored program by the central government. Initially (I and II five year plan period), the government used a clinical approach. In 1961, "Extension and Education Approach" had replaced clinical approach disseminating small family norm through slogans. Though there was a continuous reduction in birth rates the program received a set-back in 1977–78 due to the rigidity shown by field functionaries in enforcement of targets.

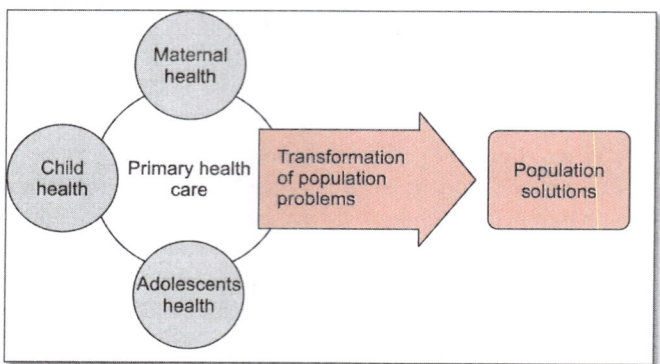

Figure 9: Family health care

Consequent to this, the Government of India made it clear that no one should compel or force people to undergo family planning procedures. The delivery of the program became an integral part of "Family Welfare" using mass education and motivation. The name of the program changed to **"Family Welfare"** from Family Planning. The Family Welfare Program during VII five year plan (1985–90) gave importance to "voluntary approach" with a specific interest on promoting spacing methods. This approach continues to exist even today through self-motivation and community participation.

In 1997, India moved from "National Family Welfare Program" into "Reproductive and Child Health Strategy" expecting a complete change during the ninth five-year plan (1997–2002).

This strategy took great effort in integrating maternal, child and adolescent health into primary health care paving the big way for healthy nation and population control (Fig. 9).

Many programs in India like family planning, maternal and child health, universal immunization, diarrheal control, acute respiratory tract infection control, nutritional deficiency control had the same objectives. During ninth five-year plan period all the mentioned programs were brought under one umbrella that is the "Reproductive and Child Health (RCH) Program" in the year 1997 providing better service packages and wider coverage.

SCHOOL HEALTH SERVICES

DEFINITION

School is one of the social institutions where the students learn many things that help him grow into a person with intellectual abilities, positive attitude, matured behavior and a responsible citizen. Initially, the school health services focused on attending children through periodical medical examinations. Recent years the provision of "comprehensive health care services" to promote the health and well-being of children had gained higher popularity.

The school health policy and program study (SHPPS) describes **school health services** as a coordinated system that ensures a continuum of care from school to home to community health care provider and back (Allenworth et al., 1997).

School health nursing: Specialized practice of professional nursing that advances the well-being, academic success, and lifelong achievement of students.

The **school health program** is defined as "the school procedures that contribute to the maintenance and improvement of the health of pupils and school personnel including health services healthful living and health education".

MILESTONES IN SCHOOL HEALTH SERVICES IN INDIA

1909: Medical examination conducted for the first time for schoolchildren in Baroda city.

1946: Bhore committee report had revealed the non existence and underdeveloped state of school health services.

1953: Secondary education committee suggested on medical examination and school feeding program.

1960: Government of India had appointed a committee under the chairmanship of Smt. Renuka Ray to assess the status of schools and to recommend strategies to improve.

1961: The above committee submitted report with its recommendations.

Five-year plans: Following the committee's recommendations many state governments came forward to implement feeding programs and other services.

With all the efforts school health services are still in infancy level only.

1977: Centrally Sponsored National School Health Scheme was started.

1981: A task force was established by Ministry of Health and Family Welfare to study the progress of School Health program functioning in various states of the country.

1989: Central Health Education Bureau, Directorate General of Health Services, had launched an intensive school health education project.

NEED FOR SCHOOL HEALTH SERVICES

Followings are the needs for school health services

○ Constitute a vital and substantial segment of population.

○ Constitute the vulnerable section of the population by virtue of growth and development during this period.

○ They are prone to get exposed to various stressful situations.

- They belong to different socioeconomic and cultural backgrounds which affect their health and nutrition status.
- They are prone to get specific health problems.

FACTORS TO CONSIDER BEFORE INITIATING SCHOOL HEALTH SERVICES

- Existing health problems/needs of the local community from where school children enrolled.
- Culture of the community.
- Available resources to tackle the problems in terms of money, material, manpower and time. Government schools are funded by the state or the central government. Apart, self-financing schools initiate their own funding resources.
- Parents/Community participation.
- Health problems vary from place to place. Hence, Government of India's comprehensive survey picked up five main area to concentrate in school health services but it not be limited to this (Fig. 10).

OBJECTIVES OF SCHOOL HEALTH SERVICES

- To promote positive health
- To maintain and protect health
- To prevent diseases
- To promote early diagnosis, treatment and follow-up
- To refer cases when needed
- To create health awareness among children
- To provide safe and healthful environment.

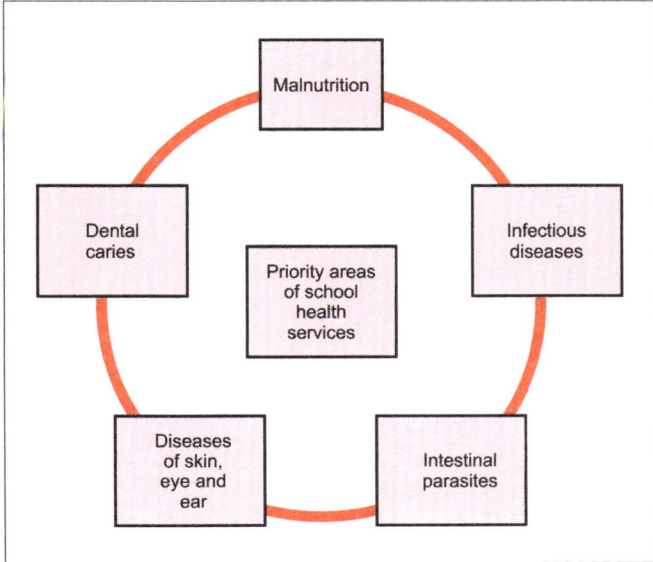

Figure 10: School health services

COMPONENTS OF SCHOOL HEALTH SERVICES

Physical Infrastructure of the School

Schools are the institutions where students spend more time next to their homes. Schools should not only function as the nurturing units of the young brains but also the providers of conducive environment where pupils learn while living full heartedly. Schools should be a model for "sanitation and healthful living" to community. *Minimum standards for sanitation and environment in India:*

Location: Centrally located with road facilities and away from cinema hall, railways, factories, etc.

Protection: To be free from hazards and it should be properly fenced.

Site: Should be on high land and not subject to inundation.

Land area required: Primary schools-5 acres with an additional 1 acre of land for every increase in numbers of 100 Higher elementary schools-10 acres.

Structure: Nursery and secondary schools should it single storied, exterior walls should be 10" thickness, heat resistant *Class rooms*: Should be attached to varandhas. **Per capita space**-10 sq ft per student and no class should exceed 40 students. **Furniture** should suit to the age group. Desirable is single desk and chair. **Desks**-minus type, Chairs should have backrests and desk work facilities. **Doors and windows** should be 2–6' from floor level, windows and doors should constitute 25% of the floor space. Windows should be placed on different walls for cross ventilation. **Color:** Inside wall, color should be white.

Lighting: Sufficient natural lighting from left to right. **Water:** Safe potable continuous water supply.

Eating facilities: Separate place to eat, no vendors allowed other than permitted.

Lavatory: Privies and urinals should be provided as-1 urinal per 60 students 1 latrine per 100 students (Girls and boys separately).

Disposal of wastewater and refuse: School should have a wastewater drainage system. Most often schools in rural areas drain wastewater into a soak pit or school garden or nearby agricultural field. The refuse comprised of dust, paper, dirt, peelings of fruit, vegetable-remains should be disposed off in a dustbin.

Health Assessment

For Students

- Regular and periodical medical examinations of schoolchildren is essential to find any deviation from normal structure and functioning of the body.

- Complete physical and medical examination required. It is done at the time of entry and thereafter every 4 years.
- Initial appraisal at entry to school includes history taking, physical and medical examination.
- Physical examination includes observation of child from head to toe, measuring age appropriate anthropometric measurements (height, weight, arm and chest circumference).
- Testing of vision, hearing and speech.
- Assessing vital signs—pulse, respiratory rate and temperature, BP and pain assessment.
- A routine examination of blood, urine and stool.
- Tuberculin testing to identify tuberculosis in clinic.

For School Staff

Routine health examinations are done for all teaching and nonteaching staff of the school since they form the part of the environment where child is exposed to.

Daily Inspection by the Teacher

- Daily inspection by teachers on her own class students help to a great extend in detecting the health problems.
- The symptoms that may alert teacher to bring the child to medical attention: Fever, rashes, flushed face, acute cold, cough, sneezing, watery eyes and nose, sore throat, headaches, sleepiness, headache, body ache, lack of interest to play, diarrhea, vomiting, skin conditions, frequent urination, pediculosis, etc. For making good observation, teachers should have adequate training.

First Aid and Emergency Care

Generally, all teachers must have first aid training to take of any injuries or emergencies that may happen in students, specifically where there is no school health nurse appointed.

There need to be a "first aid-post" available in all schools as per the guidelines of St John ambulance association of India.

Commonly found emergencies are injuries and emergencies. Medical emergencies like gastroenteritis, epileptic fits and fainting are most common ones.

Health Promotion, Health Maintenance and Disease Prevention

Personal Hygiene

Personal hygiene is taught to the students.

Nutritional Services

Nutritional disorders are widely prevalent among children. A child who is not physically well may not be active to perform the daily activities. A specific attention need to paid on the nutrition of the children. To combat malnutrition, school health committee appointed in 1961 recommended at least one nourishing meal should be by the school. School meal should meet 1/3 of calorie requirement and half of daily protein requirement.

UNICEF extends help in developing school gardens by providing seeds, manure, water supply equipment, etc. It is important to concentrate on use of specific nutrients in order to prevent diseases like dental caries, endemic goiter, night blindness, etc.

Promotion of Mental Health

School is the place, which nourishes the child to grow into an individual with his own cognitive skills. Teachers should observe all the children to identify any abnormal behaviors and seek medical attention through parents. Teacher must never discriminate students as: rich and poor; clever and dull; and no difference should be shown based on creed, color and caste. There need to be health psychologists and counselors available in the school.

Health Education

Health education should be an ongoing activity in school. Based on the need and priority health education should be planned using individual, group or mass approach.

The topics dealt are closely related to their personal hygiene, environmental hygiene and family life.

Dental Health

Children always report with dental problems like caries, gum defects, etc. School health program should have provision for dental check-up at least once a year. The dentists in schools perform dental examinations. Apart a dental hygienists are appointed in schools.

Eye Health Services

Basic eye health services like treatment of eye infections, squint and amblyopia and early detection of refraction errors, administration of vitamin A to high risk children.

Treatment Services

- Treatment and follow-up
- Specialized health services

School Health Records

- Record maintenance is the vital part of school health services.
- It is essential to maintain complete, accurate and continuous records of school children.

○ Such health records help as a tool to monitor and retrospectively evaluate the health of the students. They are used for identification of personal data, results of physical and medical examination and delivery of services and the progress.

Rehabilitative Services

Rehabilitative services are very essential for all people who are born with some kind of disability. The child or a person may be born with the disabilities. In other cases they may have acquired disability or handicap through road accident/infection, some serious diseases, burns, injury, etc. The children of special disabilities like autism, blindness, deafness should get training in special institutions for rehabilitation.

OCCUPATIONAL HEALTH

Occupational health explains the dynamic equilibrium that should exist between the worker and his occupational environment. Occupational health is defined as "The highest degree of physical, mental and social well-being of workers in all occupations." (The Joint International Labor Organization Committee, 1950).

Occupational health deals with all aspects of health and safety in the workplace and has a strong focus on primary prevention of hazards. **(Harrington and Gill, 1992)**.

OCCUPATIONAL HAZARDS

An industrial worker is exposed to 5 types of hazards (Table 11) based upon the type of the occupation.

Table 11: Types of occupational hazard

○ **Physical hazards**	**Heat:** Heat syncope, heat cramps, heat exhaustion, heat stroke, heat burns etc. **Cold:** Frost bite, Reynaud's disease, chilblains, trench foot, gangrene, etc. **Light:** Due to inadequate light: Headache, eye strain, eye fatigue. Due to excessive light: Glaring, visual fatigue, blurring of vision, accidents. **Noise:** Deafness, fatigue, irritability, interference with speech and communication. **Vibration:** Numbness, white fingers, injuries. **Radiation:** Leukemia, aplastic anemia, cancer, congenital defects, sterility

Contd...

○ **Chemical hazards**	**Irritants:** Dermatitis, eczema, ulcerations, cancer **Inhalants:** Dust-pneumoconiosis, fumes—mental fume fever **Gases-**asphyxia
○ **Biological hazards**	**From animal:** Zoonotic diseases like—anthrax, bovine TB, rabies **From soil:** Tetanus, gas gangrene
○ **Mechanical hazards**	Mainly accidents
○ **Psychosocial hazards**	Anxiety, hostility, depression, sickness, absenteeism

OCCUPATIONAL HEALTH TEAM

Occupational health team includes professional members from various disciplines (Box 1).

Box 1: Occupational health team

- Occupational health physician
- Occupational health nurse
- Occupational health epidemiologist
- Occupational hygienist
- Industrial toxicologist
- Industrial psychologist
- Ergonomist
- Occupational therapist
- Physiotherapist
- Health educator
- Safety engineer

HEALTH PROMOTION OF WORKERS

Nutrition

○ Malnutrition is the major problem among workers.

○ There need to be a canteen if the number of employees exceeds 250

○ Provide diet and snacks at reasonable rates

○ If worker brings his own food, there need to place to store food safely, before eaten.

○ Dining room.

Communicable Disease Control

○ Early diagnosis and treatment

○ Isolate the cases from working environment

○ Protective measures

○ Regular medical checkup

○ Immunization against specific diseases—TB, typhoid, hepatitis, etc.

○ Anthrax, undulant fever, Q fever diseases have occupational origin.

Environmental Sanitation

- Avoid common glass tumbler to drink water and install drinking water fountains
- Food hygiene and education to food handlers
- Sufficient number of toilets and urinals separately for males and females
- One sanitary convenience for 25 employees till 100; thereafter one for every 50
- General cleanliness to be maintained
- Sufficient floor space-minimum 500 cu ft per worker
- Adequate lighting
- Protection from, dust, fumes and toxic hazards
- Housing facilities near to work area desirable.

Mental Health

- Mental health facilitates good physical health. We cannot separate mind and body
- Promotion of health and happiness
- Detection of any signs of emotional stress
- Identify the cause and treat promptly
- Rehabilitation of the ill.

Measures for Women and Children

There are many measures to protect women and children. Some of them are:

- Maternity leave for 12 weeks with cash benefit under ESI Act
- Ante/Intra/Postnatal services
- Provision of crèches for children
- Prohibition of employing women and children in certain dangerous occupation
- Prohibition of night work between 6 pm and 7 am
- Prohibition of work-underground
- No child below 14 shall be employed.

Health education: Health education is encouraged in all levels of planning to promote employees health and to protect them from occupational hazards and other communicable and noncommunicable diseases. Health education should cover all the areas specifically wherever lifestyle and behavior plays a major role in causing the diseases.

Family planning: Employees are encouraged to adopt "small family norm" and lead physically and economically healthy family.

Measures to Prevent Occupational Diseases

The various measures to prevent occupational diseases are classified into—Medical, Engineering and Legislative measures.

Medical Measures

Pre-placement Examination

This refers to the medical examination carried out prior to placement in order to place right man in right job. This includes thorough medical, family, occupational history and physical examination. Preplacement examination of the employee will function as yardstick to make future comparisons.

Periodical Examination

- Periodical examination will help in diagnosing the disease since occupational diseases take very slow process of development.
- Usually, the workers are examined once in a year, again it also depends upon the kind of occupational exposure. Like lead, toxic dyes needs monthly examinations.

Medical and Health Care Services

In India, Employee State Insurance (ESI) Scheme provides medical services to the employee and his family. Prompt first aid and vaccination services rendered to protect the worker and the family.

Notification: There are 22 diseases recognized internationally to avail workmen's compensation. This is for the purpose ensuring preventive and protective measures of workers and to identify the causes in case of occurrence.

Visit to Working Environment

- Physician takes all the efforts to visit the work environment periodically. He assesses for adequate lighting, ventilation, noise levels, etc.
- He also studies on various aspects like fatigue, night work, shift work, etc.
- These reports will help in improving the work environment.

Records: The compilation and frequent review of records of workers will help in further planning and goal setting.

Health Education and Counseling

- A thorough induction session before starting his service
- Worker is aware of the risks related to his job, the personal protective measures and how to use those
- The worker adopts hand-hygiene practices
- The worker learns to adjusts between work, home and community.

Engineering Measures

- Design of building
- Good housekeeping

- General ventilation
- Mechanization
- Substitution
- Dusts
- Enclosure
- Isolation
- Local exhaust ventilation
- Protective devices
- Research
- Statistical monitoring
- Environmental monitoring

Legislative Measures

There are laws that regulate and assure health services to workers. It may include:

- The Factories Act, 1948
- The Employees State Insurance Act, 1948
- Mine and Mineral Act, (Development and Regulation) Act, 1957
- Noise Pollution (Regulation and Control) Rules, 2000
- The Child Labor (Prohibition and Regulation) Act, 1986
- The Air (Prevention and Control of Pollution) Act, 1981
- Maternity Benefit Act (1961)
- Minimum Wages Act (1948)

DEFENCE SERVICES

People who are in defence services (Army/Navy/Air Force/Indian Coast Guard/Special Frontier Force) get all the medical facilities free of cost from defence hospitals. The family and dependents also get all kinds medical services from defence hospitals.

Ex Service Men Contributory Health Scheme (ECHS)

Retired (Ex) defence personnel get a range of medical facilities. Ex-servicemen and their families can avail in-patient and outpatient treatment at military hospitals at any time. Non-pensioner ex-servicemen are provided financial assistance to meet medical expenses.

India had introduced ECHS on 1st April 2003. ECHS is a publicly funded medicare scheme, specifically to provide health services to ex-servicemen and pensioners and their eligible dependents.

Outpatient services: ECHS provide outpatient services through 227 polyclinics all over India.

In-patient hospitalization and treatment: ECHS provide in-patient services at all these 227 locations through Military Hospitals and out-sourced civil hospitals and diagnostic centers.

This medical facility is meant for Ex-servicemen, who have served in Army/Navy/Air Force/Indian Coast Guard/Special Frontier Force.

Since March 31, 2007 there is also a provision for getting 75–90% financial assistance from the Kendriya Sainik Board for the cost of treatment incurred for those military personnel who are unable to avail medical treatment at military hospitals.

INSTITUTIONAL SERVICES

"Institutional health services" means the health services provided in or through health care facilities and includes the entities in or through which such services are provided. (Oregon, 2007). Institutions are residential facilities that assume total care responsibilities of the individuals who are admitted. Most often, it gives comprehensive care that may include room and board.

Institutions should have genuine license to run such facilities. Hospital or institutional residential care is suggested when age or illness of an individual reduces his/her ability to cope with the activities of daily living, thus making it impossible to live at home.

Institutional care is provided through big organizations with the help of a professional team from various discipline. The team may include doctors, nurses, therapists, nutritionists and many more. Institutional care facilities, e.g. nursing home care, old age home, hospice centers, rehabilitation homes for alcoholics and drug addicts, etc. Institutional care is particularly intended for those who need constant care and assistance with daily activities. Institutional care is the most common form of long-term care.

SYSTEMS OF MEDICINE AND HEALTH CARE

ALLOPATHY

The Concise Medical Dictionary defines allopathic medicine as "the orthodox system of medicine, in which the use of drugs is directed to producing effects in the body that will directly oppose and so alleviate the symptoms of a disease."

Dictionary of Public Health defines allopathy as "the prevailing form of conventional or orthodox medical practice, based as far as feasible on formally arrived at diagnostic categories of conditions that are treated on the basis of best available evidence for efficacy of therapeutic measures.

CFS Hahnemann coined the term 'allopathy' in 1842 to designate its contrast to homeopathy, a system of medicine that he founded during 19th century. Other names that have been used for "Allopathy" are: Traditional western medicine, regular medicine, mainstream medicine, orthodox medicine, modern medicine and conventional medicine. In general, this approach views the body as a machine. This was the reason earlier allopaths were addressed as mechanics.

The practitioners and the technologies that accompany this system do extremely well in treating acute illness and injuries. The imaging systems of modern medicine discover the hidden problems in the body in its early stages itself. Surgical procedures, the real boon help in repairing or removal of the diseased area or damaged organs. Pharmacological drugs and therapies cure serious infections. Allopathy helps in realigning the fractured bones. Allopathy is a method of treating diseases with remedies that produce effects different from those caused by the disease itself.

People of the recent decades most often opt for "Allopathy" and considered as the main system of practice in the hospitals." As per the law, patients have rights and protection. All the health care professionals who cure and care for patients—like doctors, nurses, technicians, must have qualification as per the norms and appropriate license to practice. The medical facilities must obtain license to practice and ensure quality care. There need to be continuous research and development to adopt evidence-based practice.

AYUSH

AYUSH is the term used for referring a group of systems of medicine. AYUSH stands for Ayurveda, Yoga and Naturopathy, Unani, Siddha and Homeopathy (Table 12).
AYUSH is synonymous with:

- Department of Indian Systems of Medicine and Homeopathy (ISMH)
- Allied sciences
- Traditional health care
- Indigenous system of medicine
- Alternative medicine
- Complementary and alternative medicine (CAM)

India introduced the Department of Indian Systems of Medicine and Homoeopathy (ISMH) in the year 1995 under Ministry of Health and Family Welfare (MoHFW) and

Table 12: Practice of Indian systems of medicine in India

The Ayurveda system—popular in the States of Kerala, Himachal Pradesh, Gujarat, Karnataka
The Siddha system—widely accepted in Tamil Nadu and Kerala
The Unani system—popular in Andhra Pradesh, Karnataka, Tamil Nadu, Bihar
The Homeopathy—practiced all over the country but primarily popular in Uttar Pradesh, Kerala, and West Bengal.

re-named it to "Department of Ayurveda, Yoga and Naturopathy, Unani, Siddha and Homeopathy (AYUSH)" in November, 2003.

Integration of AYUSH in National Health Care Delivery System (under "NRHM")

The main reasons for merging AYUSH under NRHM are:

- These practices are accepted by the rural community
- The medicines used under this system locally made using the available resources hence, easily available
- These medicines are safe and economic
- Unwillingness of allopathic doctors to work in rural areas
- A single system of health care is unable to solve all health needs/problems of the society.

AYURVEDA

Ayurveda, means the science of life (Ayur = Life, Veda = Science). The Ayurveda system of medicine originated from the "Atharva veda", the fourth among "vedhas" and it was practiced in India since 5000 years. We can find "Ayurveda" practiced as a system of medicine in India, Nepal, Sri Lanka, Pakistan, Tibet, China, USA and in some European countries.

Initially, the sages of India disseminated information about Ayurveda by communicating orally to the disciples. After many years, texts on Ayurveda **Charaka Samhita, Sushruta Samhita,** and the **Ashtanga Hrudaya** *published*. These texts explain about the five elements (earth, water, air, fire, space) and keeping them balanced for a healthy and happy life.

Each individual will be dominated by some elements in a way more than others. This is due to prakriti (natural constitution). The different constitutions are placed under three different doshas:

1. **Vata dosha**— the air and space elements dominate
2. **Pitta dosha**—the fire element dominates
3. **Kapha dosha**—the earth and water elements dominate

Most people have the combination of two doshas of the above stated.

Different Ayurvedic Therapies

Ayurvedic Treatment is categorized into two: (1) *Shodhana* (purificatory therapy) (2) *Shamana* (palliative therapy).

The shodhana therapy practice some procedures to remove the vitiated humors from the body. The procedures may include: vamana (emesis), virechana (purgation), vasti (enema), nasya (nasal administration).

The *shaman* procedure includes procedures that calm down the doshas or put back to normalcy. e.g. *deepana* (carminative), *pachana* (digestive), *upavasa* (fasting), etc.

Some of the ayurvedic drugs are given below:

- Saubhagya sunthi
- Ksheerbala taila
- Bal rasayan
- Ark pudhina
- Ark ajawain
- Punarnavadi mandoora
- Ayushgutti

YOGA

Yoga is in practice since 5000 years. Yoga is a healing system of practice of medicine which renders therapy through breathing exercises, physical postures, and meditation. **Yoga** is believed to cause calming effect on the nervous system and through which balances the body, mind, and spirit are maintained. This system of yoga does not use any medicine or pills to treat the disease.

It is learned through the literature the founders of yoga was the *saints* and *sages* who practiced and taught this. *Maharishi Patanjali* is popularly called "The Father of Yoga."

The practice of Yoga prevents the psychosomatic disorders and enhances ability to tolerate stressful situations.

NATUROPATHY

Naturopathy is an ancient system of medicine that is capable of preventing or curing the disease through integration of various aspects of body, mind, and spirit. Dr Benedict Lust is "the Father of naturopathy."

Naturopathy states that the improper diet, faulty lifestyle, and violation of laws are the factors those influence the accumulation of toxins in the body and giving rise to problems.

Principles of Naturopathy

- All disease, their cause, and their treatment are one
- Acute diseases are our friends, not the enemies. Chronic diseases emerge as the outcome of wrong treatment and suppression of the acute diseases.
- The bacteria is not the basic cause of disease
- Naturopathy treats patient and not the disease.

Therapies in Naturopathy

- Hydrotherapy
- Air therapy
- Fire therapy
- Space therapy
- Mud therapy
- Sun therapy
- Food therapy

UNANI

Unani a system of medicine originated in Greece. Hippocrates laid the foundation for "Unani system". Arabs introduced the "Unani system" in India.

Unani system of medicine is known for treating arthritis, leucoderma, jaundice, bronchial asthma in comparison to other systems of medicine.

Various Therapies in Unani System

- Diet therapy (Ilaj-bil-Ghiza)
- Climatic therapy (Ilaj-bil-Hawa)
- Regimental therapy (Ilaj-bit-Tadbir)
- Pharmacotherapy (Ilaj-bid-Dawa)—Unique, remarkable and popular system that differed from other systems.

SIDDHA

The Siddha System of Medicine is the "Traditional Tamil System of medicine." Its origin can be traced back to BC 10,000 to BC 4,000 in the ancient Tamil land. This is the foremost of all other medical systems in the world. Mythically, Siddha's origin was attributed to Lord Siva, from whom it was handed to Parvathi (Shakthi), passed on to Nandi. Nandi transmitted to the "Siddhars".

Guiding Principles of Siddha Medicine

- The individual a microcosm of the universe.
- The human body is made up of: five primordial elements (earth, water, fire, air and space)
- The three humours (vatha, pitta and kapha) and seven physical constituents.
- The food basic building material of the human body gets processed into humours, tissues and wastes.
- The equilibrium of humors is "health" disequilibrium leads to a diseased state.

Materia Medica

Drugs in Siddha is classified into three groups: *Thaavaram* (herbal product), *Thaathu* (inorganic substances), and *Jangamam* (animal products).

Diagnostic Methods

This is unique made on the basis of the clinical knowledge of the physician. The pulse, skin, tongue, complexion, speech, eye, stools and urine are examined. This approach is known as "Eight types of examination." The examination of pulse is the most important one in confirming the diagnosis.

Education

Traditionally, *Guru* (Teacher) transmitted his intellectuals to *sishya* (disciple) through verses, most often in ambiguous language and the sacred medicines and techniques were taught only to a close circle of disciples.

HOMEOPATHY

It is a method of treating diseases with remedies that produce effects similar to those caused by the disease itself. The word Homeopathy, originated from the Greek, through Latin into English, literally means "like disease". This means that the medicine given is like the disease that the person is expressing, in his totality, not like a specific disease category or medical diagnosis.

Principles of Homeopathy

Homeopathy functions on 3 main basic principles. They are (Fig. 11).

The First Principle: Let Likes Cure Likes

The concept of "like curing like" dates back to the Greek Father of Medicine, Hippocrates (460–377 BC). However, it was Dr CF Samuel Hahnemann (1755–1843), German physician who first incorporated this principle into a system of medicine. He gave the medicinal substances to the healthy volunteers called "provers" (presently experimental group) and assessed for the symptoms that appeared. Homeopathy is a branch of medicine originated in Germany in 1794, which is based on the principle of "The Law of Similars."

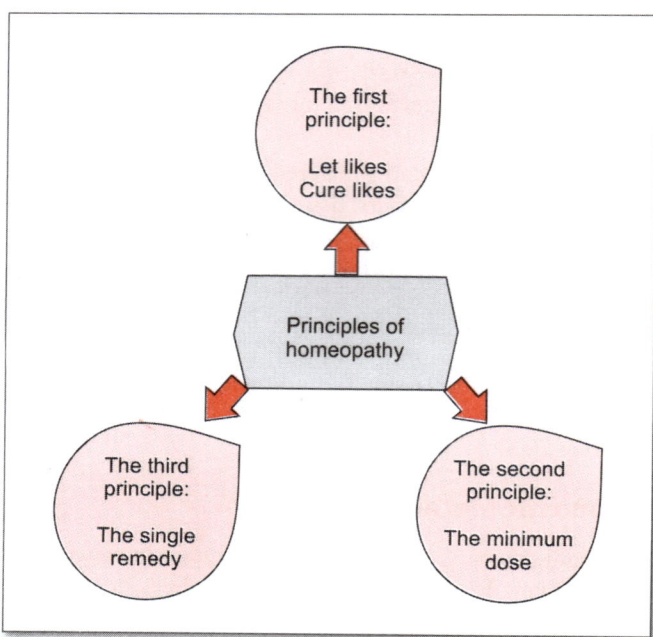

Figure 11: Principles of homeopathy

Homeopathic case-taking includes the physical, psychological and emotional aspects and complaints of the individual. After case taking the practitioner finds the matching remedy similar to the patients' problems from "drug picture"(materia medica).

That homeopathic prescription is known as the *similimum.* The similimum is given to the patient helps him get healed.

The Second Principle: The Minimum Dose

Dr Hahnemann began initially used his medicament on patient who presented with alike symptoms. He used the medicament, *Cinchona* or Peruvian bark, for treating the relapsing fever. Though the patient got cured there were side effects of the medicament. Hence, he avoided using the raw forms of medicament and started to dilute the drugs. The "minimum dose" strategy came into practice. Though the dose is minimized, has the maximum therapeutic effect with fewest side effects.

The Third Principle: The Single Remedy

Single remedy is the third principle of homeopathy. Prescribing one remedy at a time is the usual practice of homeopathy. The homeopathic remedy produces its own unique drug picture. That remedy is matched (prescribed) to the sick person having a similar picture. Then the results are observed and noted. This single remedy principle avoids the confusion of which medicament caused what side effect.

Types of Treatment

Based upon the duration of the disease it has two types –Acute and chronic. Acute treatment is prescribed for the illness of recent onset. For example, common cold. Long standing diseases are treated with chronic treatment.

Research councils: Central Council for Research in Homoeopathy (CCRH) located in New Delhi.

REFERRAL SYSTEM

A referral can be defined as a process in which a health worker at a one level of the health system, having insufficient resources (drugs, equipment, skills) to manage a clinical condition, seeks the assistance of a better or differently resourced facility at the same or higher level to assist in, or take over the management of, the client's case.

Reasons for referral (emergency/routine case)

○ To get expert opinion about the client

○ To seek additional or different services for the client

○ To admit the client for further management

○ To seek use of diagnostic and therapeutic tools

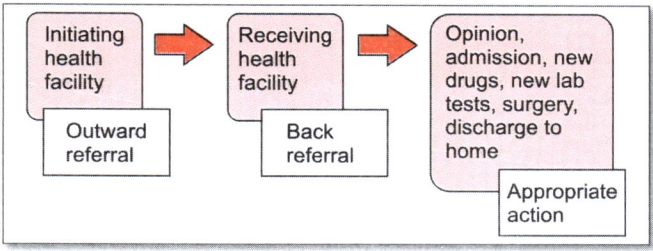

Figure 12: Process of referral

The health facility that initiates the referral process is "**the initiating facility**", and the referral that communicates the client condition and status is an **outward referral.**

The health facility that accepts the referred case is called the **receiving facility** and at the end of their involvement, they prepare a **back referral** on the lower part of the forms to let the initiating facility know what has been done. This completes the referral loop between the two facilities (Fig 12). A patient may be referred due to various reasons:

- When qualified doctors of the concerned specialty not available in health facility
- When diagnosis needs second opinion
- When needed facilities not available to manage the case
- When major complications build up and cannot manage during the process of management
- When the disease takes up unexpected routes
- When patient is unable to meet cost of the health facility
- When insured company has link with a particular health facility
- When patient demands for higher level care and change of hospital

A **referral register:** This has all inward and outward referrals in a health facility. Information of the register includes:

- Name of the client and address details, diagnosis:
- Referred to
- Time of referral
- Reason for referral
- Whether the case is closed or continuing (If returning referral is received-rehabilitation or follow-up)
- Referring doctor
- Nurses involved

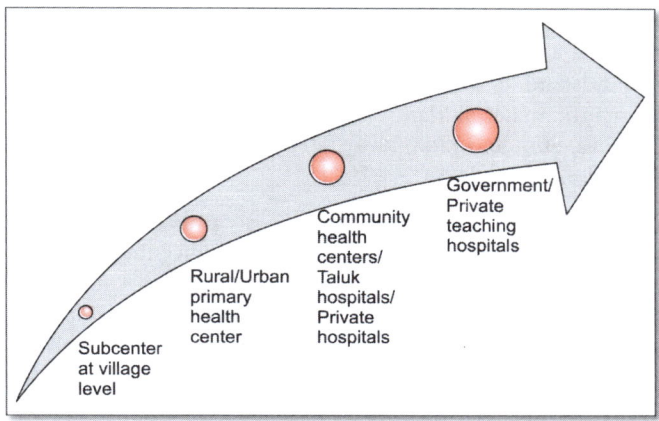

Figure 13: Referral flow in community

- Documents (Case sheet, any previous reports—lab investigations, X-rays, scan, etc.) sent along with the patient.

Village health nurses functioning at the village subcenters refers the cases on basis of emergency or the case is such that higher level opinion or management. The referred cases sometimes return back with opinion and advise to follow or the patient get treated in higher level health facility and discharged from the health facility at the end of the care (Fig. 13).

Summary

Under "**National Rural Health Mission**" planning and budgeting follows a "**Bottom-up approach**." In bottom-up approach, the planning process begins at block level. Government health subcenters are categorized into two based on certain factors like catchment area, health-seeking behavior, case load, and availability of PHC/CHC/FRu/Hospitals etc. in the surrounding areas. While planning to establish a health subcenter you need to think about money or funds and its sources (government of some other funding agencies), material (land, building, equipment, drugs and supplies, etc.) and manpower (staffing) needed to carry out the tasks at the venue.

As per the prescribed norms, required number of qualified staff should be appointed in subcenter to carry out the activities. Staffing pattern differs in type A and type B Subcenters since type A does not take up delivery conduction. As part of the National Rural Health Mission (NRHM), ₹10,000 is provided as an untied fund to meet any urgent and again discrete activities that need relatively small amount of money.

Primary covers the population of 30,000 in plain areas and 20000 in hilly and tribal areas. Under each PHC there are 6 subcenters functioning. Primary health centers are categorized into "Type A" and "Type B" based on their delivery case load. Under NRHM every PHC gets ₹25,000/per year as untied grant for local health action and ₹50,000/as annual grant for improving and maintenance of physical infrastructure. Government of India allocates the following funds under NRHM-10% funds to State level, 20% funds to district level, At least 70% funds to block level. So, 70% of the total funds are assigned to manage community health centers, primary health centers and health subcenters.

Supplies are always based on the identified needs. Use VEN model, i.e "vital", "essential", and "not so essential." Union ministry of health and family welfare functions at the central level in the health care system of India. The Ministry consists of three departments: (1) Department of Health and Family Welfare, (2) Department of Ayurveda, Yoga-Naturopathy, Unani, Sidha and Homeopathy (AYUSH) and (3) Department of Health Research. The department of Health and Family Welfare is supported by a technical wing, the Directorate General of Health Services, headed by Director General of Health Services (DGHS). The Central Council for Health and Family Welfare was discussed under previous unit. A minister of health and family welfare and a Deputy Minister of Health and family welfare head the Department of Health and Family Welfare. The *health secretariat* is the official organ of state health ministry headed by the **health secretary.** The "Director of Health and Family Welfare" is assisted by "**deputy directors**" and "**assistant directors.**"

The **health secretariat** is the official organ of state health ministry headed by the **health secretary.** The director of health services is the appointed head of the "State health Directorate" who functions as a chief technical advisor to the state for all matters related to medicine and public health. In India, districts are the principal unit of administration. Districts function under **collectors.** The size and population of the districts vary. District comprises of six areas of administration. The districts are divided into two or more **subdivisions** and each functions under *assistant collector* or **sub-collector.** These subdivisions are further divided into Tehrits or Taluks and functions under Tahsildar. The concept of organizing the rural areas of the district into "community development blocks" emerged after the inception of community development program in India in 1952. The community development block comprised of 100 villages that equaled 80,000 to 1,20,000 population.

A three tier structure of rural self-government functions at the rural areas known as *"panchayati raj."* This functions as the link between villages and districts. The three-tier structure includes:

1. Panchayat—Functions at village level

2. Panchayat samiti—Functions at the block level

3. Zilla parishad—Functions at the district level

The district health system is the **secondary level** of health care whose services are curative, preventive, and promotive in nature.

Subdistrict (Subdivisional) **hospitals** function below the district and above the block level (CHC) hospitals. These subdivisional hospitals act as "**first referral units**" for the Tehsil/Taluk/block population.

The administrative organ at the block level is "**Panchayat Samiti**". The block covers 100 villages and a population of 80,000 to 1,20,000.

As per recommended norms, there should be one **PHC** for every 30,000 population in plain areas. PHCs in hilly, tribal and backward areas covers the population of 20000. PHCs at block level has 6 beds. There is also a plan to upgrade the PHCs at block level into 30 bedded community health centers. **Sub-centers** are the peripheral outpost of rural areas in Indian health care delivery. Each subcenter covers the population of 5,000 in plain areas and 3,000 in hilly, tribal, and backward areas.

India became the signatory of Alma-Atta declaration (1978) and committed to achieve health for all by 2000 AD through **"Primary health care approach."**

To operate this approach at village level India has introduced some schemes. They are:

○ Village health guides scheme
○ Training of local dais
○ ICDS scheme
○ ASHA scheme

Village health guide scheme was introduced on 2nd October, 1977 under Rural Health Scheme with aim of encouraging people's participation. **Dais training program** was launched under rural health scheme to train all categories of traditional birth attendants (dais) in basic concepts of maternal and child health and sterilization. Under the Integrated Child Development services Scheme (ICDS) one **Anganwadi Worker (AWW)** is placed for a population of 400 to 800 population. There are 100 AWW function in each ICDS project. NRHM was launched on 5th April 2005 for the period of 7 years (2005–2012), later extended for another 5 years (2012–2017). Though this program is in operation in all the states, special attention is given to 18 states. **Accredited Social Health Activist (ASHA)** cadre is created under National Rural Health Mission (NRHM).

Corporation (Nagar Nigam/Mahanagar Palika): It covers more than 200,000 populations. Corporation is the apex body of the urban governance. **Municipalities** are usually setup for the population of 100,000 and above but earlier, the municipal setup was provided to the areas with the population of > 20,000. Nagar panchayat is set up for a very small urban area or the rural area that is fast transitioning to urban area. **Township** covers 5000–10000 population. Townships emerge due to the establishment of colonies, or specific worksites provided under the government.

Cantonment boards were set up to administer established military station: Usually when military personnel station at a place the civilian population too move in to provide supporting facilities like market and provision etc. About 30% of population of India lives in urban areas.

Slums are the communities characterized by insecure residential status, poor structural quality of housing, overcrowding, and inadequate access to safe water, sanitation, and other infrastructure (United Nations Human Settlements Program, 2003). Urban slums is the place for all vulnerable population such as homeless, rag pickers, street children, rickshaw pullers, construction and brick and lime kiln workers, sex workers, and other temporary migrants.

Dispensaries are fourth order medical facilities providing normally outdoor treatment with the help of one physician and one pharmacist. The dispensaries in slum areas provide medical facilities to the growing urban population. Based

upon the recommendations given by the Krishnan Committee (1983), India introduced four types of Urban Health Posts (UHP) in 10 States and Union Territories. This health facility mainly aimed at helping the slum dwellers to have access to health services. Depending upon the population coverage the urban health posts are categorized as A, B, C and D.

Special clinics in urban areas concentrate on providing specialized care for urban population. The specialists of the concerned field conduct these clinics. There are dispensaries run under ESI scheme to help employees mentioned as mentioned in the beneficiaries' regulations of ESI. **Maternal and child health centers** are the health care facility specifically designed to provide care for the mother and child. National rural health mission has identified matching health facilities to offer MCH care at various levels. Level I MCH center staffing: 2 more VHNs and sanitary worker. Level-II MCH center-staffing: 2 additional doctors (preferably specialists), 3 more staff nurses, pharmacist, junior assistant, hospital workers, sanitary workers.

The chains of human activities that occur in the environment turn it as an unsafe atmosphere to live. Some of the major activities those cause unsafe living atmosphere are improper treatment or management of solid waste, wastewater, and industrial waste. **Health education** is any combination of learning experiences designed to help individuals and communities improve their health, by increasing their knowledge or influencing their attitudes. There are **four main approaches** to health education. They are: Legal or regulatory approach, administrative or service approach, educational approach and primary health care approach.

Principles of health education may include: (1) Credibility, (2) Interest, (3) Participation, (4) Motivation, (5) Comprehension, (6) Reinforcement, (7) Known to Unknown, (8) Setting an Example, (9) Learning by doing, (11) Community leaders, (12) Good health relations and (13) Feedback.

Audio-visual aids are classified into: (1) Auditory aids, (2) Visual aids, (3) Combined audio-visual aids.

There are three approaches used for communicating health messages. They are: Individual approach, Group approach, Mass approach.

Vital statistics include indicators such as birth rate, death rate, natural growth rate, life expectancy at birth, mortality and fertility rates. Source of vital statistics in India includes— civil registration system (CRS), sample registration system (SRS), demographic sample surveys, health surveys.

Maternal and child health services—World Health Organization defined Maternal and child health services as "promoting, preventing, therapeutic or rehabilitation facility or care for the mother and child."

The government of India had passed "**Pre-Conception and Prenatal Diagnostic Techniques (PCPNDT) Act**" in 1994. This act prohibits of sex selection, before or after conception.

Adoption is a legal procedure through which a child is placed with a married couple or a single female who agree to raise the child as own child assuming all responsibilities. The Adoptions and Maintenance Act of 1956 provides guidelines on the legal process of **adopting** children by **Hindu** adult, and with the legal obligations of a **Hindu** to provide "maintenance" to various family members including their wife or wives, parents, and in-laws. It extends to the whole of India except the State of Jammu & Kashmir.

School health services: School one of the social institutions where the student learn many things that help him grow into a person with intellectual abilities, positive attitude, matured behavior and a responsible citizen. **Need for School health services-school children** constitute substantial segment of population, they are vulnerable and are prone to get exposed to various stressful situations and get specific health problems.

Occupational health explains the dynamic equilibrium that should exist between the worker and his occupational environment. Occupational health is defined as "The highest degree of physical, mental and social well-being of workers in all occupations." (The joint international labor organization committee, 1950).

Occupational hazards: An industrial worker is exposed to 5 types of hazards based upon the type of the occupation: Physical, biological, chemical, psycho-social and mechanical.

The various **measures to prevent** occupational diseases are classified into (1) Medical, (2) Engineering, (3) Legislative measures.

There are **laws** that regulate and assure health services to workers. Some of them are: The Factories Act, 1948, The Employees State Insurance Act, 1948, Mine and Mineral Act, (Development and Regulation) Act, 1957.

Defence health services: People who are in **defence services** (Army/Navy/Air Force/Indian Coast Guard/Special Frontier Force) get all the medical facilities free of cost from defence hospitals. The family and dependants also get all kinds medical services from defence hospitals.

Ex Service Men Contributory Health Scheme (ECHS)

Retired (Ex) defence personnel get a range of medical facilities.

"Institutional health services" means the health services provided in or through health care facilities and includes the entities in or through which such services are provided. (Oregon, 2007).

Institutions are residential facilities that assume total care responsibilities of the individuals who are admitted. Most often, it gives comprehensive care that may include room and board.

People of the recent decades most often opt for "Allopathy" and considered as the main system of practice in the hospitals."

AYUSH is the term used for referring a group of systems of medicine. AYUSH stands for Ayurveda, Yoga and Naturopathy, Unani, Siddha and Homeopathy. **Yoga** is believed to cause calming effect on the nervous **system** and through which balances the body, mind, and spirit. This system of Yoga does not use any medicine or pills to treat the disease.

Naturopathy is an ancient system of medicine that is capable of preventing or curing the disease through integration of various aspects of body, mind, and spirit. Dr Benedict Lust is "the Father of naturopathy."

The Ayurveda system—popular in the States of Kerala, Himachal Pradesh, Gujarat, Karnataka

The Siddha system—widely accepted in Tamil Nadu and Kerala.

The Unani system—popular in Andhra Pradesh, Karnataka, Tamil Nadu, Bihar.

The Homeopathy—practiced all over the country but primarily popular in Uttar Pradesh, Kerala, West Bengal.

Unani system of medicine originated in Greece. Hippocrates laid the foundation for "Unani system". Arabs introduced the "Unani system" in India. **The Siddha System** of Medicine is the "Traditional Tamil System of medicine." Its origin can be traced back to BC 10,000 to BC 4,000 in the ancient Tamil land. This is the foremost of all other medical systems in the world.

Homeopathy: It is a method of treating diseases with remedies that produce effects similar to those caused by the disease itself.

A **referral** can be defined as a process in which a health worker at a one level of the health system, having insufficient resources (drugs, equipment, skills) to manage a clinical condition, seeks the assistance of a better or differently resourced facility at the same or higher level to assist in, or take over the management of, the client's case.

The health facility that initiates the referral process is "**the initiating facility**", and the referral that communicates the client condition and status is an **outward referral.**

The health facility that accepts the referred case is called the **receiving facility** and at the end of their involvement, they prepare a **back referral** on the lower part of the forms to let the initiating facility know what has been done. This completes the referral loop between the two facilities.

Assess Yourself

I. Multiple Choice Questions (Choose the Correct Answer)

1. Which of these following approaches appropriates the planning and budgeting of "National Rural Health Mission"?
   a. Bottom-up   b. Top-down
   c. Vertical   d. Horizontal

2. Which of these following committees is responsible for planning at the village level?
   a. Block health committee
   b. Village health, sanitation and nutrition committees (VHSNC)
   c. State health ministry
   d. District health committee

3. Which of the following refers to immediate care unit of the village?
   a. Community health center   b. Primary health center
   c. Subcenter   d. All of the above

4. Which of these following appropriates the population coverage of primary health center in plain areas?
   a. 20,000   b. 30,000
   c. 40,000   d. 50,000

5. Which of these following appropriates the population coverage of primary health center in hilly and tribal areas?
   a. 10,000   b. 20,000
   c. 30,000   d. 40,000

6. Which of these following equals the population coverage of a subcenter in plain areas?
   a. 3000   b. 4000
   c. 5000   d. 6000

7. Which of these following equals the population coverage of a subcenter in plain areas?
   a. 3000   b. 4000
   c. 5000   d. 6000

8. Which of these following refers to the first referral unit (FRU)?
   a. Subcenter
   b. Primary health center
   c. Community health center
   d. Teaching hospital

9. Which of these following best describes "type B Primary health center"?
   a. Delivery load of <20 deliveries in a month
   b. Delivery load of 20 and above deliveries in a month
   c. Has lying in beds of 100
   d. Attendance of 100 outpatients per day

10. Which of the following refers to the funds allocated by Government of India under NRHM at for block level management?
    a. 40%   b. 50%
    c. 60%   d. 70%

II. Short Answer Questions

1. List the people/committees responsible for planning at each level.
2. List the factors to categorize subcenters under NRHM.
3. What is the main feature that differentiates type A subcenter from type B subcenter?
4. List the financial support and assistance provided to all the subcenters by the ministry of health and family welfare, Government of India.
5. List down the criteria to find a suitable location to start a subcenter.
6. State the staffing pattern in subcenter.
7. Enlist the objectives of primary health centers.
8. List the objectives of community health centers.
9. State the factors considered while estimating the needed supplies and equipment.
10. List two functions of subcenter.
11. List two functions of primary health centers.
12. List two functions of community health center.
13. State the three tier structure of panchayati-raj.

III. Write short notes on:

1. Integrated planning
2. Staffing and functions of subcenter
3. Functions of primary health center
4. Organization and functions of community health center
5. Health services at a slum
6. Urban health post
7. Dispensary
8. Village level health workers
9. Accredited social health activist
10. Village health guide
11. Anganwadi worker
12. AYUSH
13. Indian systems of medicine
14. Homeopathy
15. Siddha and Ayurveda system of medicine
16. Maternal health center
17. Occupational health
18. Occupational health services
19. Occupational hazards
20. Principles of health education
21. Referral system
22. Family welfare
23. Medical Termination of Pregnancy Act
24. Adoption Act
25. Female Feticide Act

26. Ex Service Men Contributory Health Scheme (ECHS)
27. Functions of the corporation
28. Functions of Municipality
29. Approaches in health education
30. Audio-visual aids

IV. Write Essays

1. Describe the process of planning, budgeting and material Management for establishing a subcenter.
2. Describe the process of planning, budgeting and material management for establishing a primary health center.
3. Describe the process of planning, budgeting and material management for establishing a community health center.

4. Describe the organization, staffing and functions of community health center (CHC).
5. Describe the organization, staffing and functions of primary health center (PHC).
6. Describe the organization, staffing and functions of subcenter (SC).
7. Describe the organization, staffing and functions of urban health services.
8. Define occupational health. List the occupational diseases and various preventive measures.
9. Explain the components of school health services.
10. Enlist different systems of medicine. Describe the existing systems of medicine in India.

ANSWERS

I. **1.** a **2.** b **3.** c **4.** b **5.** b **6.** c **7.** a **8.** c **9.** b **10.** d

Community Health Nursing Approaches, Concepts and Roles and Responsibilities of Nursing Personnel

4 Unit

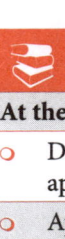

Learning Objectives

At the end of this unit the learners will be able to:

- Describe various community health nursing approaches to provide care in the community
- Apply nursing theories while providing care
- Demonstrate skills in using epidemiological approach
- Demonstrate skills in using problem solving approach
- Recognize the importance of various concepts of primary health care
- Describe various the roles and responsibilities of community health nurse in family health services, MIS, IEC and Environment and sanitation.
- Demonstrate skills in applying the roles and responsibilities of community health nurse in the areas of maternal and child health, school health and occupational health
- Demonstrate skills in providing care to minor ailments at home
- List the principles of home visit
- Explain the process of home visit
- Demonstrate skills in using community health nursing bag
- Apply the qualities of community health nurse
- Describes the job description of various categories of community health nursing personnel

KEY TERMS

- Approaches
- Nursing theories and nursing process
- Key concepts in nursing theories and models
- Nightingale's theory of environment
- Betty Neuman's systems theory
- The Roy's adaptation model
- The Orem's self-care model
- Nursing process –application
- The health promotion model (HPM)
- Epidemiological approach
- Disease and health status surveillance
- Problem solving approach
- The managerial decision-making process
- Evidence based practice (EBP) approach
- Problem solving approach
- The managerial decision-making process
- Evidence based practice (EBP) approach
- The PICO method
- Primary health care
- Comprehensive health care
- Basic health services

Contd...

KEY TERMS

- Elements of primary health care
- Equitable distribution
- Community participation
- Multisectoral coordination
- Appropriate technology
- Focus on prevention
- Family health services
- Information education communication (IEC)
- Focus on prevention
- Family health services
- Management information system (MIS)
- Good record keeping
- Training and supervision
- Community health workers
- Asha, local dais,
- Anganwadi workers
- Environmental sanitation
- Maternal health
- Treatment of minor ailments
- School health services
- Occupational health
- Organization of clinics, camps
- Waste management
- Home visit: Concept, principles, process, home visit
- CHN bag
- Qualities of community health nurse nursing
- Job description

APPROACHES

According to American Holistic Nurses Association, the holistic nursing is "all nursing practice that has healing the whole person as its goal." This model of caring focuses on the complete person, not alone the physical body is in existence and witnessed from the time of Florence Nightingale, "the mother of modern nursing." Nursing, practiced in various settings grouped under two major heads: Nursing service in the hospital, nursing service in the community. Community health nurses use various approaches to provide care in the community. Some of them are:

- Nursing theories and nursing process
- Epidemiological approach
- Evidence-based practice (EBP) approach
- Empowering people to care for themselves

NURSING THEORIES AND NURSING PROCESS

Experts look at theory as a process and a product. Theory can be a process that includes numerous activities in sequential phases that are applied into practice. The phases of theory may include: (1) analyzing concepts, (2) constructing relationships, (3) testing relationships, and (4) validating relationships.

Theory can also be a product because it provides a set of concepts and relationships that help us to describe, explain, predict, and prescribe phenomena of interest and this information is used for guiding nursing practice (Kenney, 1995, 2006). It is not possible to separate theory and nursing practice since nursing profession is a skill-oriented practice or discipline.

Application of theory and research-based practice are the pillars to the professional and autonomy in nursing practice.

> Theory is a set of systematically interrelated concepts or hypotheses that seek to explain or predict phenomena.
>
> Model is a description or analogy used as a pattern to enhance our understanding of something that is known.

Model is a hypothetical/theoretical representation of something that exists in reality. Model attempts to explain a complex reality in a systematic and organized manner.

For example, hospital organizational chart. This attempts to demonstrate the interrelationships of the various levels of the hospital's administration.

There are many theories, frameworks and models available in nursing. The theories discussed have been selected because they are appropriate to apply in community health nursing.

Scope of Theories in Community Health Nursing Practice

Community health nursing is a field with broader scope in which community health nurses practice at various levels in many branching specialties.

Influence of theories on nursing practice (Fawcett, 1992). Theories include:

- Identify standards for nursing practice
- Identify settings in which nursing practice should occur
- Identify distinctive nursing processes and technologies to be used
- Direct the delivery of nursing services
- Serve as the basis for clinical information systems including the admission database, care plan, discharge summary, etc.
- Guide the development of client classification systems
- Direct quality assurance program

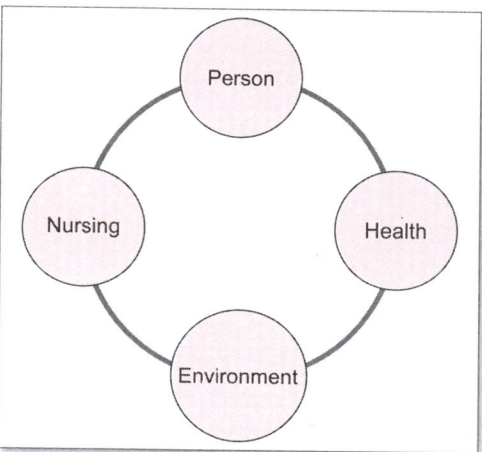

Figure 1: Key concepts of nursing theories and models

Key Concepts in Nursing Theories and Models

> There are four common concepts on which nursing theories and models are constructed. They are: Client or patient or person (individual or collective), health, environment and nursing (Fig. 1)

Each nursing model has its own specific definition of these terms, but the underlying definitions of the concepts are similar.

The concepts of nursing's metaparadigm have been linked in four propositions identified in the writings of Donaldson and Crowley (1978) and Gortner (1980). These are as follows:

- **Person and health:** Nursing is concerned with the principles and laws that govern the life-process, well-being, and optimal functioning of human beings, sick or well.

- **Person and environment:** Nursing is concerned with the patterning of human behavior in interaction with the environment in normal life events and critical life situations.

- **Health and nursing:** Nursing is concerned with the nursing action or processes by which positive changes in health status are effected.

- **Person, environment and health:** Nursing is concerned with the wholeness or health of human beings, recognizing that they are in continuous interaction with their environments (Fawcett and Malinski, 1996).

Nightingale's Theory of Environment
Major Concepts

Nightingale stated that nursing "ought to signify the proper use of fresh air, light, warmth, cleanliness, quiet, and the proper selection and administration of diet—all at the least expense of vital power to the patient."

"What nursing has to do…is to put the patient in the best condition for nature to act upon him" (Nightingale, 1859/1992 statements).

Human beings: Person/man is not defined specifically. This theory described human beings and the effect of the environment on them.

Environment: Nightingale gave big importance to the physical environment. Nightingale's writings get along with community health model in which human being's health status is determined by the environment.

Health: Nightingale (1859/1992) did not define health specifically. She stated, "We know nothing of health, the positive of which pathology is the negative, except from the observation and experience."

She strongly believed nursing should focus on healthy as well as the ill. She also had recognized health promotion as an activity in which nurses should engage.

Nightingale's (1859/1992) Statements

Health of houses: "Badly constructed houses do for the healthy what badly constructed hospitals do for the sick. Once insure that the air is stagnant and sickness is certain to follow."

Ventilation and warming: "Keep the air he breathes as pure as the external air, without chilling him."

Assumptions: Florence Nightingale believed that "pure air, pure water, efficient drainage, cleanliness and light" are five essentials to have healthful house.

She maintained that "nature alone cures" and healthy environment is essential for sick to heal.

She stressed on the importance of nurses being good observers of their patients and report the patient's state to the physician in an organized way.

She considered nursing is an art and medicine a science. Nurses should be honest in carrying out the medical plan, but not servile.

Betty Neuman's Systems Theory

This theory shows interest on how a patient/client system responds to actual or potential environmental stressors. The focus is also on the use of primary, secondary and tertiary level of nursing interventions toward the prevention for retention, attainment and maintenance of patient system wellness.

Basic Assumptions

○ Patient system is a unique combination of various factors and characters those respond accordingly.

○ There are known, unknown and universal stressors that may disturb the patient's normal stability level.

○ Each patient system is tuned with a normal set of responses to its environment refers to normal line of defence and this serves as the reference scale to identify if any deviation.

○ The line of defence tends to break when the outer layer of flexible line of defence is incapable.

○ A patient system is a dynamic entity of wellness and illness which responds accordingly.

○ The internal resistance factors specific to each patient system helps in realigning the patient to the normal state of wellness.

○ Primary prevention helps to assess the patient system to provide necessary intervention and reduce actual or potential risk factors.

○ Secondary prevention treats to reduce harmful effects.

○ Tertiary prevention helps in reconstitution of the system, refreshes the cycle toward primary prevention.

○ The patient is in dynamic, continuously in interaction with the environment and constant energy exchange.

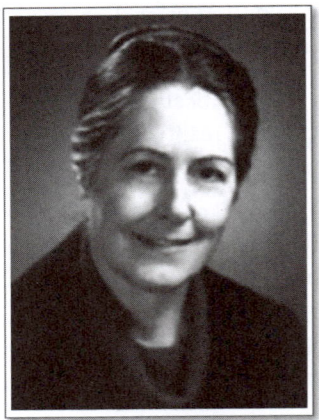

Betty Neuman

Application of Neuman's Theory at Community Level

Betty Neuman's system theory presents the concepts in concentric circles (Fig. 2). The innermost center circle represents the core, the basic amenities available for survival, and the abilities of the community to use its natural resources effectively. Three outer concentric circles called boundaries encircle the core. The innermost circle is a flexible line of resistance that means the internal defences like community's collective sense of responsibility for population control, inculcating healthy lifestyle in children, etc. The second boundary is the system's normal line of defence, like community's existing health system, law and regulations on water pollution, sanitation, road safety, etc. The third boundary is a dynamic, flexible line of defence. This functions as a buffer to prevent the stressors that try invading the system's normal line of defence. Regular maintenance of roads and bridges, disaster alert and precautions are some examples for the third boundary.

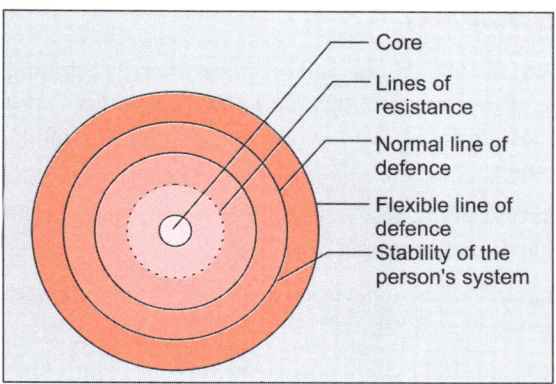

Figure 2: Betty Neuman's systems theory

This Neuman's model applied to community level (as stated in the previous paragraph) or to an individual level comparing and contrasting his or her core system and how the stressors within or out (external) affect the person's system.

Application at Individual Level

Person: Person is an open system that works together with other parts of its body while interacting with the environment. Person as a system made up of five variables, which are interrelated. They are physiological, psychological, sociocultural, developmental and spiritual. Person's protective structural mechanisms maintain stability of the system. The protective defences are flexible line of defence, normal line of defence and lines of resistance.

Health: Health is a dynamic condition equals the stability of normal line of defence. Wellness exists when all the parts or system of person works harmoniously with each other.

Environment: Environment refers to the internal, external, and created force (stressors) that interacts with a person's state of health. Environment influences a person's system positively or negatively. Hence, it is capable of altering or improving the stability of systems.

Nursing: Nursing is a unique profession that uses holistic approach by considering all factors that tend to impact person's health. The major aim is to promote optimal wellness of the individual, family and community through retention, attainment or maintenance of the stability of patient's system.

Nursing intervention modes can be primary, secondary and tertiary.

Application: When a person experiences stress, the flexible line of defence gets an "alarm" to protect the normal (solid) line of defence thereby to keep the system free from stressor reactions. On the other hand, the exposures to stressors on continuous basis will make the flexible line of defence to fail, unable to cope up with the stressors. As a result, the normal line of defence alters. Threat occurs to the wall that protects the basic structure of the individual causing instability to the person's system leading to development of illness.

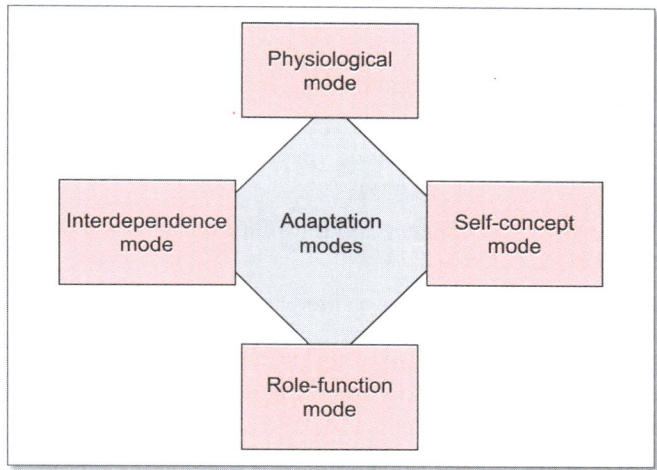

Figure 3: Adaptation modes by sister Callista Roy

Roy's Adaptation Model

Sister Callista Roy developed this model which is closely related to systems theory. The major goal of this model is to allow the client to reach his or her highest level of functioning through adaptation (Fig. 3).

Man/Person: In this model the man is considered as a dynamic entity and has both input and output. The person/client is a biopsychosocial being, affected by various stimuli and constantly displays various behaviors to adapt to the stimuli. Therefore, adaptation to stimuli is a continual process.

Inputs are stimuli arise from internal (from within) and external (physical surroundings, family, and society) environments. Output equals the behavior that the patient may demonstrate consequent to the stimuli that are affecting him or her.

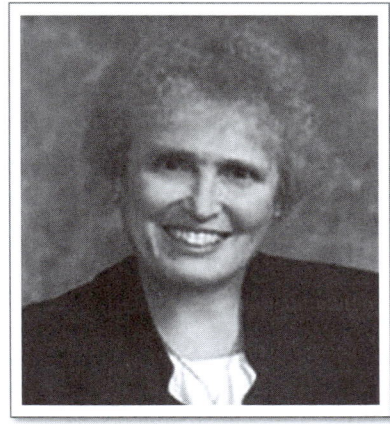

Sister Callista Roy

Generally, the output (behavior) is modified by the patient's internal attempts to adapt to the input or stimuli. Four adaptation modes identified by Roy, are:

1. The physiological mode (using internal physiological process)
2. The self-concept mode (developed throughout life by experience)
3. The role function mode (dependent on the patient's relative place in society)
4. The interdependence mode (indicating how the client relates to others).

Health: In the Roy Adaptation Model, she finds person's health along a continuum between perfect health and complete illness. Person's health is not an absolute phenomenon. It is how a person is going to adapt to stimuli. The stimuli may be an event that gave psychological trauma/stress, injury, disease or anything that disturbed the normal life that have an impact on health status. Adaptation is the person's ability to adjust, live and come out of the same.

For example, a MSc nursing student whose mother passed away on the day of her final examinations, joined the mother's funeral after writing the theory examination and ultimately joined as teacher in a nursing college. This person had the ability to adapt such a stressful situation and she would be considered by Roy's adaptation model to have a high degree of health because of the ability to adapt to the stimuli imposed.

Environment: The environment consists of all those factors that influence the patient's behavior, either internally or externally. This model categorizes environmental stimuli, into three: (1) focal, (2) contextual and (3) residual.

Nursing: The major task of the nurse is to help the patient to overcome the stimuli in all four-adaptation modes. As a first measure, the nurse assesses the patient's behavior (output) to find whether he/she is adaptive or maladaptive. The patient's behavior is the output for primary data collection.

For example, a suspected client of tuberculosis in the community—Physical debility, fever, productive cough and loss of weight, fatigue and tiredness will be the initial assessment by the community health nurse to build on the diagnosis and to send for further investigations.

Second set of assessment (input) includes knowing about what stimuli causing the problem. Testing the sputum and doing other investigations would help in finding the stimuli. She would also try to find about any other person in the family or neighborhood had predisposed the disease. She also would assess the environmental factors like crowded house, availability of the smoke outlet, dietary pattern, earning members, income, etc. These are the input. This would help the nurse formulate nursing diagnosis about the person's adaptive or maladaptive behavior and the environment. As a next step, the nurse sets the goals to plan. The focus should be on manipulation of the stimuli to promote optimal adaptation. Finally, the outcome is evaluated to assess whether the goals are attained.

Key Definitions

Adaptation: The process and outcome whereby thinking and feeling of persons, as individuals and groups, use conscious awareness and choice to create human and environmental integration.

Adaptation processes: Activity of subsystems for coping of individuals and relational persons.

Coping processes: Innate or acquired ways of responding to the changing environment.

Adaptive modes: Followings are the ways of adaptive modes:

- **Stimulus** is that provokes a response, or more generally, the point of interactions of the human system and environment.
- **Focal stimulus** is the internal or external stimulus most immediately confronting with the human adaptive system.
- **Contextual stimuli** are all other stimuli present in the situation that contribute to the effect of the focal stimulus.
- **Residual stimulus** is an environmental factor within or without the human system that have an undetermined effect on the behavior of the human adaptive system.
- **Self-concept** is the composite of beliefs and feelings that is held about oneself at a given time, formed from the internal perception and perceptions of others' reactions.
- **Role** is the functional unit of society; each role exits in relation to another.

Interdependence is the close relationships of people aimed at satisfying needs for affection, development and resources to achieve relational integrity.

Orem's Self-Care Model

Dorothea E Orem's (2001) model of nursing on self-care believes that health care is each individual's own responsibility. She described people who need nursing care as those who lack ability in self-care.

When self-care demand exceeds the patient's ability, the condition of self-care deficit arises. This situation calls for nursing intervention. The major goal of nursing intervention is to help people know their self-care demands and limitations and increase their self-care ability. Nursing meets patient's self-care needs until they are capable of performing those by themselves.

Self-care is "the practice of activities that individuals initiate and perform on their own behalf in maintaining life, health and well-being" (as cited in Cardinal Stritch University Library, 2011)

Orem's theory is made up of three related theories (Fig. 4)

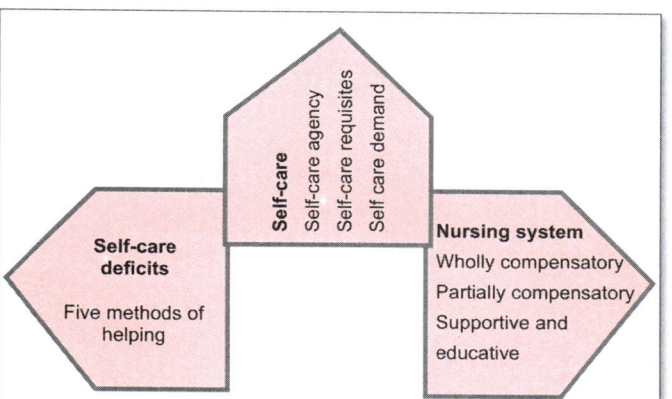

Figure 4: Orem's self-care model

1. **Theory of self-care:** This talks about the care demands of self (person) in order to stay healthy or get better from illness.

2. **Theory of self-care deficit:** When a person is unable to meet the self-care demands, or when self-care demands exceeds self-care capabilities, he or she needs assistance from nursing. Nurses can help patients meet their self-care needs by utilizing the five methods in the theory of self-care deficit.

3. **Theory of nursing systems:** The nurse must appropriately assess the level of self-care required by a patient and utilize the nursing system (as stated in the theory of nursing system) that suits the patient's ability to perform self-care.

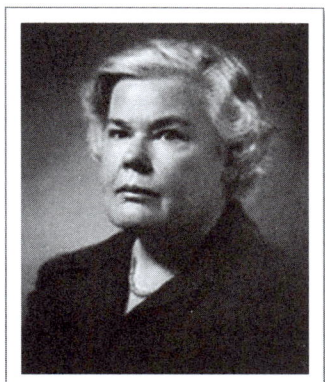

Dorothea E Orem

Components of Self-care Model

Person: The core of this model is the person who is biological, psychological, and social well-being capable of performing his self-care activities which is necessary to maintain his life and optimal functioning. Self-care is defined as the practice of activities that individuals initiate and perform on their own behalf to maintain life, health and well-being. Self-care is a requirement both for maintenance of life and for optimal functioning.

Health: In this model, health is defined as the person's ability to live fully within a particular physical, biological and social environment, achieving a higher level of functioning that distinguishes the person from lower life forms. A healthy person lives life to the fullest capable to maintain life through self-care. An unhealthy person has self-care deficit.

This deficit is identified by the individual's inability to perform one or more of the key health-care activities grouped under:

- Air, water and food
- Excretion of waste
- Activity and rest
- Solitude and social interactions
- Avoiding hazards to life and well-being
- Being normal mentally under universal self-care.

Environment: Environment is the venue or condition through which patient perform daily activities. This model considers environment as a negative factor because many environmental factors distracts the ability to provide self-care. Social interactions and physical elements that affect health are some of the examples.

Nursing: The primary goal is to help the patient conduct his self-care activities to reach the highest level of human functioning. Three distinct levels of nursing care delineated depending upon the individual's ability to perform self-care activities. When persons are less able to care for themselves, nursing care is sought.

Self-care deficit: Nursing care is categorized under three headings. They are:

1. **Wholly compensated care:** A person who is able to perform few or no self-care activities fall under this category in which the nurse must provide for most or all of the patient's self-care needs.

2. **Partially compensated care:** A person can meet some to most of their self-care needs but still have certain self-care deficits that require nursing intervention fall under this category.

3. **Supportive developmental care:** Clients who are able to meet all of their basic self-care needs require very little or no nursing interventions fall under this category. Here, the main nursing tasks include education and support.

Nursing Process—Application

Nursing process can be achieved through three steps. They are:

First step determines whether nursing care is needed by assessing the patient's health care needs and problems.

Second step assigns the appropriate nursing care-category and plans nursing care accordingly.

Provides the appropriate nursing care or actions to meet the patient's self-care needs.

Third step extends help through one or a combination of five nursing methods. This includes:

- Acting or doing for another person
- Guiding another person
- Supporting another person (physically or psychologically)
- Providing an environment that promotes personal development
- Teaching another person.

> All the three theories of the Orem's self-care model can be used in the community at various settings to promote healthy lifestyle (self-care) in general population, to provide care (partial or full compensatory) in extended care facilities, terminally ill centers, old age homes, etc.

Nola J Pender's Health Promotion Model

The health promotion model (HPM) was proposed by Nola J Pender in 1982 and revised in 1996. This was actually a complement to the other models of health protection (Flowchart 1).

Health: This model defines health as a positive dynamic state not merely the absence of disease and health promotion is aimed at increasing a patient's level of well-being.

Person: This model states that people show multidimensional nature as they interact within their environment to pursue health.

Focus of HPM Model

This model focuses on three areas. They are:

1. Individual characteristics and experiences
2. Behavior-specific cognitions and affect
3. Behavioral outcomes

Individual Characteristics and Experiences

Personal Factors

Personal factors categorized as biological, psychological and sociocultural. These factors are predictive of a given behavior and shaped by the nature of the target behavior being considered

- **Personal biological factors:** These include variable such as age, gender, body mass index, pubertal status, aerobic capacity, strength, and agility or balance.
- **Personal psychological factors:** These include variables such as self-esteem, self-motivation, personal competence, perceived health status and definition of health.
- **Personal sociocultural factors:** These include variables such as race ethnicity, acculturation, education and socioeconomic status.

Prior Behavior

It refers to the frequency of the similar behavior in the past and direct and indirect effects on the likelihood of engaging in health-promoting behaviors.

Flowchart 1: Health promotion model, Nola J Pender (1982; revised 1996)

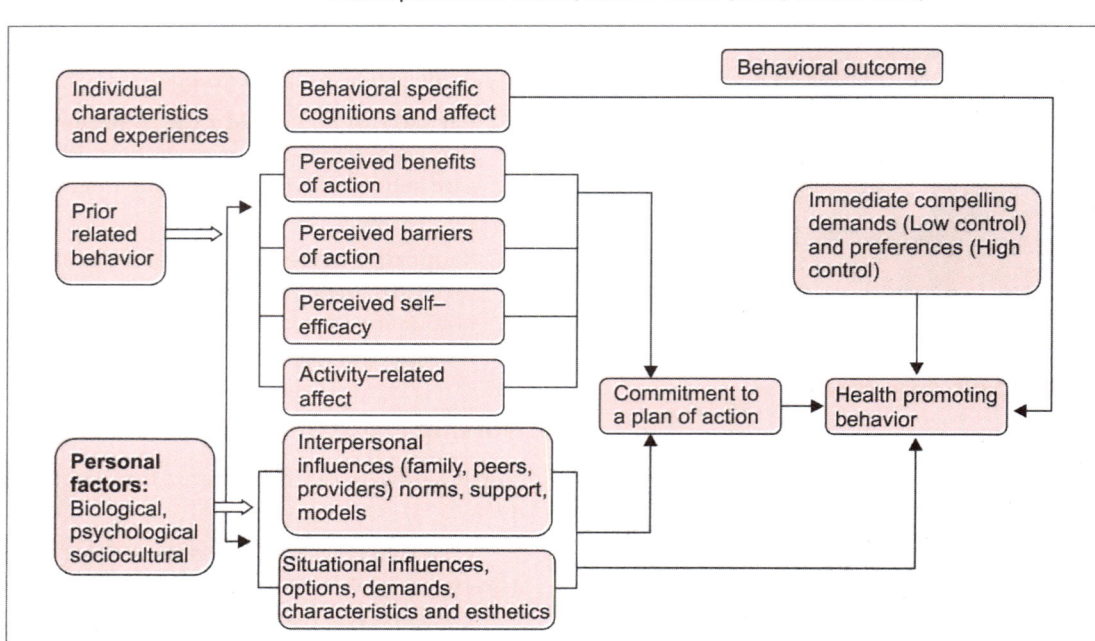

Behavior Specific Cognitive Affect

Perceived benefits of action: Anticipated positive outcomes that will occur from health behavior.

Perceived barriers to action: Anticipated, imagined or real blocks and personal costs of understanding a given behavior.

Perceived self-efficacy: Judgment of personal capability to organize and execute a health-promoting behavior.

Activity-related affect: Subjective positive or negative feeling that occur before during and following behavior based on the stimulus properties of the behavior itself.

Activity-related affect influences perceived self-efficacy, which means the more positive the subjective feeling, the greater the feeling of efficacy.

Interpersonal Influences

Cognition concerning behaviors, beliefs, or attitudes of the others.

Interpersonal influences include—norms (expectations of significant others), social support (instrumental and emotional encouragement) and modeling (vicarious learning through observing others engaged in a particular behavior).

Primary sources of interpersonal influences are families, peers and health care providers.

Situational Influences

This refers to personal perceptions and cognitions of any given situation or context that can facilitate or impede behavior. This may include perceptions of options available, demand characteristics and aesthetic features of the environment in which given health promoting behavior is proposed to take place. Situational influences may have direct or indirect influences on health behavior.

Behavioral Outcome

Commitment to Plan of Action

The concept of intention and identification of a planned strategy leads to implementation of health behavior.

Immediate Competing Demands and Preferences

Competing demands are those alternative behaviors over which individuals have low control because there are environmental contingencies such as work or family care responsibilities. Competing preferences are alternative behaviors over which individuals exert relatively high control, such as choice of ice cream or apple for a snack.

Health-promoting Behavior

Endpoint or action outcome directed toward attaining positive health outcome such as optimal well-being, personal fulfillment and productive living

Assumptions: Each person has unique personal characteristics and experiences that affect subsequent actions. The set of variables for behavioral specific knowledge and affect have important motivational significance. These variables can be modified through nursing actions. Health-promoting behavior is the desired behavioral outcome and is the end point in the HPM. Health-promoting behaviors should result in improved health, enhanced functional ability and better quality of life at all stages of development.

The final behavioral demand is also influenced by the immediate competing demand and preferences, which can derail an intended health-promoting actions.

EPIDEMIOLOGICAL APPROACH

Epidemiology in nursing took strong roots from Florence Nightingale's (1820–1910) time. Nightingale, being a statisticians she had keen interest in knowing more from William Farr (who established medical statistics) about disease classification. Her brilliant statistical representation on preventable deaths among soldiers of Crimean war is an exemplary example of use of epidemiological approach by the nurse many years ago.

Epidemiology gives vision to make scientific questions and that provides the foundation for further construction of this discipline. Epidemiology also absorbs methods from other scientific fields that include but not limited to biostatistics and informatics, biology, economics, social and behavioral sciences. It is a foundational science for public health uses its quantitative abilities to cautiously observe and assess the health-related states and events. However, one should not perceive it as a mere research activity because it is the central component of public health.

Definition

There are many definitions on epidemiology but the most applied practice is:

Epidemiology is defined as "the study of the distribution and determinants of health-related states or events in specified populations, and the application of this study to the prevention and control of health problems." (Last, 1988)

Distribution

Epidemiology studies the frequency and pattern of health events in a population:

Frequency: It is not a mere count of number of health events like the number of cases of hypertension or diabetes in a population, but also the relationship of that number to the size of the population. The results of this allow epidemiologists to compare disease occurrence through different populations.

Pattern: Refers to the occurrence of health-related events by time, place and person.

Time patterns may be annual, seasonal, weekly, daily, hourly, weekday versus weekend, or any other breakdown of time that may influence disease or injury occurrence.

Place: This includes the variations found in geographic region, urban and rural differences and location of work sites.

Personal characteristics include demographic factors which may influence the risk of illness, injury or disability such as age, sex, marital status and socioeconomic status, behaviors and environmental exposures.

Determinants

Determinant is any factor that decides the change in an event, characteristic or other definable entity that contribute to the development of some illnesses. No disease or event occurs in vacuum. There will be some root causes or predisposing factors to trigger disease or condition. Epidemiologists frequently use analytical epidemiology for finding out the causes.

Health-Related States or Events

The original focus of epidemiology was exclusively on epidemics of communicable diseases but later expanded to address endemic communicable diseases and non-communicable infectious diseases. Actually, the term health-related states or events may be seen as anything that affects the well-being of a population.

Specified Populations

The physician in the hospital shows interest on the health of an individual whereas the epidemiologist is concerned about the health of the people in a community or population. The physician's focus is the individual patient; the epidemiologist's "patient" is the community.

The clinician usually focuses on curing and caring for the individual, the epidemiologist focuses on identifying the exposure or source that caused the illness.

Application

Epidemiology does not stop with studying the health of the population. The significant feature of epidemiology is application of the gained knowledge for community-based practice. Diagnosing the health of a community is the major component of epidemiology. This helps to form relevant, feasible and acceptable public health interventions to control and prevent disease in the community.

Using Epidemiological Approach

Disease and Health Status Surveillance

As a practitioner in the field, community health nurse has to have adequate information about the community she serves and she should have the knowledge on new, emerging and re-emerging diseases in the community. Epidemiological measurement and analysis will give an insight about the health status of the community. Health status indicators can help to have a snapshot of the diseases, disabilities and injuries in the community. This would help in planning, prioritizing and for budgeting.

Through surveillance data the community health nurse can estimate the magnitude of health problems in the community, understand the natural history of the disease as well any strange presentation in the disease journey, know endemic disease, and discover any epidemics and help in control of the disease through timely notification and other active measures.

The community health nurse will be able to get surveillance data from existing records, registers or from government sources. Management information system and registries are the best sources of data.

Search for Etiology

Monthly review meetings and audits on perinatal mortality, maternal mortality and under five mortality audits will provide her great information and motivate her to investigate on actual causes of these. Common sources for routinely collected data in India are: data sources of government and private agencies. (Refer unit 3 under vital statistics to have more information)

Evaluating care: Care provided in the health care facilities like sub-center, PHC, etc. can be evaluated using explorative and evaluative studies.

Using Descriptive Epidemiological Approach in Nursing

○ **Defining the population:** Defined population means either the whole population or a representative sample.

○ **Defining the disease under the study:** It is described in terms of time place and person. This would help us to identify whether these characteristics are associated with the presence or absence of the disease.

Disease is examined by asking three questions:

1. When is the disease occurring? Time distribution.

2. Where is it occurring? Place distribution.

3. Who is getting the disease? Person distribution.

○ **Describing the disease by time, place and person:** These characteristics are carefully considered when a disease outbreak occurs, because they provide important clues regarding the source of the outbreak (Fig. 5).

The community health nurse will be able to describe the disease using time, place and person.

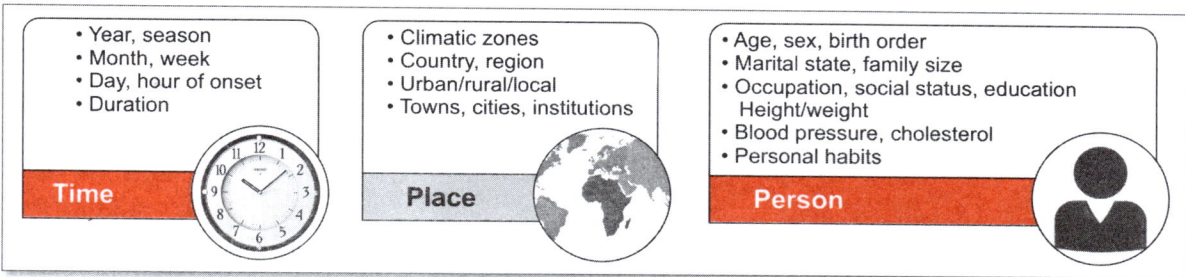

Figure 5: Three pillars of descriptive epidemiology

○ **Comparing with known indices:** This would help her compare the present happening with the past or between the regions/countries.

○ **Formulation of causal hypothesis:** Using the information from the previous steps the community health nurse can formulate hypothesis.

This formulated hypothesis can be tested using analytical epidemiology.

Investigating Food Poisoning

Once the CHN receives the information on food poisoning in a location she will act quickly to contact the person with the symptoms and asks the following questions to run the epidemiological approach:

○ What did they eat?

○ Was there any special event like marriage/festival?

○ Where did they eat prior to illness?

○ When did they eat?

○ What are all the symptoms?

○ Who were all developed the problem?

○ Whether anybody else they ate with also experienced any symptoms?

○ Whether they have been on holiday to other places?

These questions would help in making epidemiological investigation.

Problem-Solving Approach

Experts suggest using a structured or professional approach that involves applying a theoretical model in problem solving and decision making. Decision making is one step in the problem-solving process, an important task that relies heavily on critical-thinking skills (Marquis and Huston, 1995).

Traditional Problem-Solving Approach

The traditional problem-solving model is most well known than the other methods.

The seven steps are:

1. Identify the problem

2. Gather data to analyze the causes and consequences of the problem

3. Explore alternative solutions

4. Evaluate the alternatives

5. Select the appropriate solution (Decision making)

6. Implement the solution

7. Evaluate the results.

Managerial Decision-Making Process

The managerial decision-making model, a modified traditional model, eliminates the weakness of the traditional model by adding a goal-setting step. Harrison (1981) has delineated the following steps in the managerial decision-making process:

○ Set objectives

○ Search for alternatives

○ Evaluate alternatives

○ Choose

○ Implement

○ Follow-up and control.

Nursing Process

The nursing process provides another theoretical system for solving problems and making decisions. Educators have identified the nursing process as an effective decision making model (Pesutand Herman, 1998). The managerial decision-making process flows more or less like the nursing process (Fig. 6).

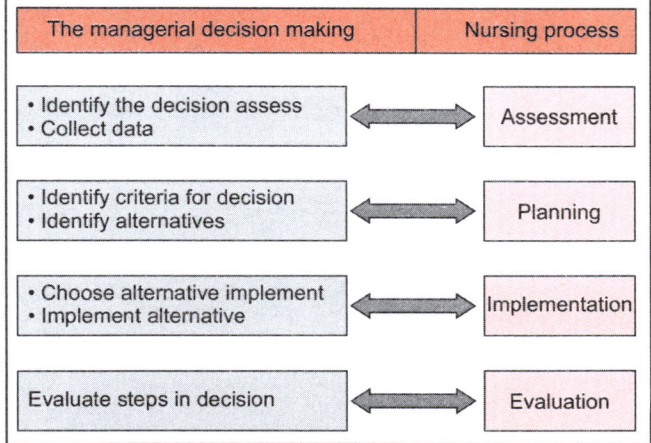

Figure 6: Managerial decision making and nursing process

In day-to-day to practice nurses use nursing process approach for problem solving and decision making.

As a decision-making model, the most significant element of the nursing process is its "feedback mechanism" which other two models lack.

EVIDENCE-BASED PRACTICE APPROACH

Public health decision making is a complicated process because of complex inputs and group decision making. Public health evidence often derives from cross-sectional studies and quasi-experimental studies, rather than the so-called "gold standard" of randomized controlled trials often used in clinical medicine (Fig. 7).

Definition and Meaning

Evidence-based practice (EBP) is "the conscientious, explicit and judicious use of current best evidence in making decisions about the care of the individual patient. It means integrating individual clinical expertise with the best available external clinical evidence from systematic research." (Sackett D, 1996).

Evidence-based practice integrates clinical expertise, patient values and the best research evidence for deciding upon patient care. In community health nursing we equalize clinical expertise to the community health nurse's experience, education and clinical skills. The patient or the client or a person in the community has his personal preferences, concerns, expectations and value system.

Hence, EBP unifies research evidence with clinical expertise and encourages individualization of care through inclusion of patient preferences.

The best research evidence comes from relevant research work that has been conducted using rigorous methodology in the field of community health nursing to adopt into practice.

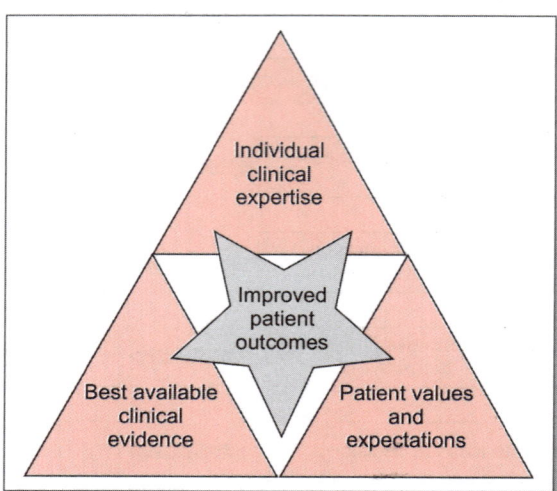

Figure 7: Elements of evidence-based practice

There have been situations in our community health nursing clinical practice where we wondered about the ways of carrying out certain tasks (Why do we do it like this?) and maintained silence by getting known that was the usual way or that was the only way it works." After a long period of silence anyone may end to ask, "Does this make sense?" Here comes the answer: Community health nurses adopting evidence-based practice.

Steps Involved in Evidence-based Practice in Community Health Nursing

○ Evidence-based practice in community health nursing has several steps that includes an initial step of developing a well-constructed clinical question that will drive all the other aspects. Our work environment gives many opportunities for constructing a compelling question, e.g. why do nurses always use a black pen to write their notes? Black ink shows up better than blue when scanning and photocopying.

○ Assess on the amount of evidence available to answer the question.

○ If lot of evidence exists on the question it need not be asked again. If this might be the situation in relation, we need to look for making another question.

○ In contrast, if no evidence is available to support the question, it is really an important question that should be explored.

○ There are many methods used to conduct evidence-based projects in community health nursing. PICO format, presented by Melnyk and Fineout-Overholt (2005).

PICO Method

The PICO stands for:

P—Patient population of interest

I—Intervention of interest

C—Comparison of interest

O—Outcome of interest

Step 1: Defining the patient (population of interest)

Initially we need to define on what population of the community we like to examine: Are we interested in infants, children, adults (women/men) or geriatric individuals? Perhaps we may be interested in antenatal or high-risk pregnancies in the community.

Step 2: Identifying the intervention or process of interest

In this step we need to decide on what intervention or process we need to examine. What do you want to do for this patient population? In other words what are we going to do specifically for this population?

Step 3: Examining the comparison of interest

The comparison of interest is the alternative to intervention that we will decide.

The comparison can be a controlled (Group which receives no treatment) versus a placebo (Group which receives a fake treatment). The comparison can also include measuring the intervention of interest against what is considered as the "gold standard" of treatment for a particular situation or disease process.

Step 4: Outcome of interest

Here the result is examined. In this step we establish the outcome of interest. What will be improved or what do we want to happen in the intervention group? What do we want to accomplish or measure?

Step 5: Time frame

Fine out-Overholt and Johnston (2005) have recommended adding a fifth element to the PICO method, addressing it the PICOT method. The last component "T" stands for time; the time frame in which the question occurs.

Example: Use of PICO method

Does the incidence of protein energy malnutrition among infants (P) of village "A" decrease (O) with the administration of nutritious balls (I) for 6 months compared to infants of village "B" (C)?

Other method:

Schlosser and Costello (2007) proposed the PESICO method, which stands for person, environment, stakeholders, intervention, comparison and outcome.

EMPOWERING PEOPLE TO CARE FOR THEMSELVES

Community empowerment refers to the course of action that would help the communities to develop a greater control upon their lives. It is a known fact that people belong to same community are closely attached in their values through sharing common interests, concerns and identities.

> Enabling implies that people cannot "be empowered" by others; they can only empower themselves by acquiring more of power's different forms (Laverack, 2008).

People's Ownership on their Own Health

○ The concept of people's ownership on their own health carries significant value and importance.

○ The people are their own assets or resources in caring themselves.

○ The external agencies and health care professionals function as catalysts to facilitate the people in acquiring their power to care for themselves. Community health nurses use participatory approaches to enhance knowledge and responsibility of people on their own health.

Community Health Nurses Support Health Literacy

Community health nurses take all efforts in improving people's access to health information. They also engage in helping the patients to improve to use health information effectively, since health literacy is a vital element to empowerment.

The scope of health literacy extends health education, which is a narrow concept. Apart behavioral modification, health literacy also addresses the environmental, political, and social factors that determine health.

Resilient Health System

A well-structured health system with determined goals, excellent staffing, stronger financial base under a good leader is less likely to fail. A system that has universal reach, adequate workforce, mechanisms for community participation, is well-financed, and has leadership and power. Strengthening health systems is therefore a key strategy and priority for health promotion.

India has tried various strategies to improve the health status of the country. The significant health care concepts at various times are presented below.

Comprehensive Health Care

In 1946 Bhore committee introduced the concept of **comprehensive health care** that focused on providing integrated, preventive, curative and promotional health services to all people belong to a defined geographical area.

Features

○ Provision of preventive, curative and promotive health services
○ Services should be close to the beneficiaries
○ Good cooperation between providers and beneficiaries
○ Available to all
○ Concentrate on vulnerable and weaker sections
○ Maintain healthy environment at home and workplaces
○ The concept of Primary health care came into existence in 1978.

Basic Health Services

In 1965 UNICEF and WHO introduced the concept of basic health services. This concept stated that the health services is a coordinated effort between peripheral and intermediate health units with the assurance of availability of competent professional, and auxiliary personnel to carry out the work. In fact, this approach differed only by having different name from the prior approach. Otherwise, both these had the same shortfalls like lack of community participation and inter-sectoral coordination, etc.

CONCEPT OF PRIMARY HEALTH CARE

Primary health care approach had its inception in the year 1978 following an international conference at Alma-Atta in USSR. The primary health care is equally applicable for all the countries from the most to the least developed. The member countries have accepted primary health care as the vital part of the health system.

> The Alma-Ata conference defined primary health care as:
> *"Primary health care is essential health care made universally accessible to individuals and acceptable to them, through their full participation and at the cost the community and country can afford."*

ELEMENTS

○ Education on prevailing health problems and necessary methods to prevent and control them
○ Promotion of food supply and proper nutrition
○ Provision of adequate supply of safe water and basic sanitation
○ Maternal and child health care and family planning
○ Immunization against major communicable diseases
○ Measures to prevent and control local endemic diseases
○ Appropriate treatment to common diseases and injuries
○ Provision of essential drugs.

PRINCIPLES/CONCEPTS

The primary health care includes five main principles/concepts to render appropriate and adequate services to people at basic level (Fig. 8). The principles/concepts are dispersed below:

Equitable Distribution

All people of the country should have access to health services irrespective of their ability to pay (rich/poor) and the kind of resident (rural or urban).

The majority of health services function in the towns and cities doing injustice to the people of rural and urban slum areas. This is addressed as social injustice. The primary health care approach aims at giving a solution for this social injustice. The very simple concept here is health has to be distributed equally. The population of rural India is more vulnerable to the diseases comparing to urban but health services are disproportionately distributed.

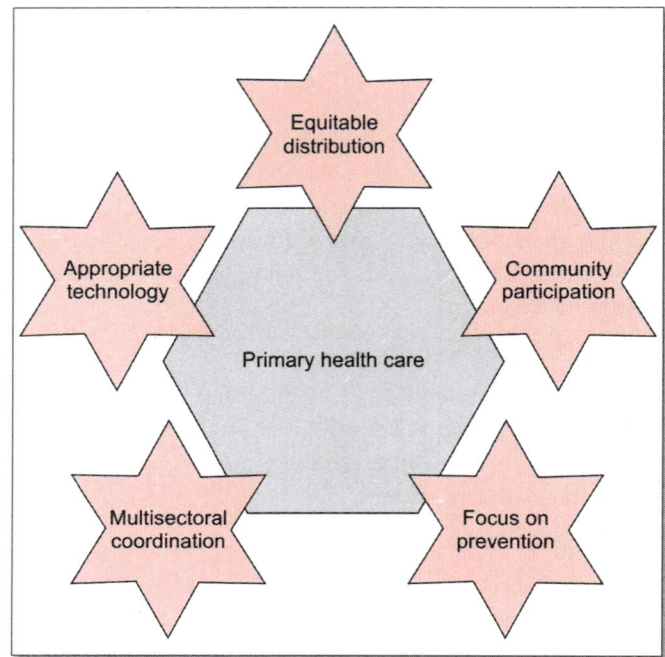

Figure 8: Concepts of primary health care

Community Participation

The health of the people is not just the responsibility of central and state governments alone. It is necessary to involve the individuals, families and communities in the promoting their own health. Taking responsibility for personal health is vital component of primary health care.

It sounds meaningful involving the community in all aspects of planning, implementation and evaluation of health services.

Best example for community participation in India is the introduction of **village health guides scheme** and *Dai training program* using people from local community.

China had set his forefront strategy by introducing community participation in the name of **bare-foot doctors**.

Multisectoral Coordination

The health sector all alone cannot meet the demands of primary health care of the country, it has various elements like community development, in particular agriculture, animal husbandry, food, industry, education, housing, etc. and those to be concentrated by relevant sectors. Planning with the other sectors may help in avoiding the duplication of services and wastage of resources.

Examples for multisectoral approach

Domain: Mother (Women) care

Related activities: Marriage registration, ANC, PNC, case detection and family planning

Departments involved: Public health and family welfare, registrar of vital events and community health nurse

Domain: Child care

Related activities: Institutional delivery, birth registration, early breastfeeding, immunization, treatment of illnesses, and early child care

Departments/people involved: Public Health and Family welfare, trained birth attendant, ANM, Community health nurse, FDA, pharmaceutical and health device industry, pediatric clinics/hospitals, and vaccine industry.

Domain: Communicable diseases

Related activities: Prevention and control activities

Departments/People involved: Water supply and sanitation, urban development, rural development, agriculture, forest, animal husbandry and community health nurse.

Appropriate Technology

Appropriate technology has been defined as "technology that is scientifically sound, adaptable to local needs, and acceptable to those who apply it and those for whom it is used, and that can be maintained by the people by themselves in keeping with the principle of self-reliance with the resources the community and country can afford." It is the tendency of people using the relevant strategies to accomplish the work, no matter whether it is health or other issues. We can see the desired results only when we know the pulse of the people. This approach is addressed as "health by the people" and placing people's health in people's hands.

Focus on Prevention

Prevention is the core strategy of primary health care. Community health nurses focus on health promotion and health maintenance activities for which they engage in primary, secondary and tertiary level of preventive care activities.

The levels of prevention: The levels of prevention occur at various course of disease progression. Leavel and Clark (1965) defined three levels of prevention: Primary, secondary and tertiary.

Primary prevention: Primary prevention focuses on health promotion and protection against specific health problems (e.g. immunization against poliomyelitis). The purpose of primary prevention is to decrease the risk or exposure of the individual or community to the disease.

Primary prevention obviates the occurrence of a health problem; it includes measures taken to prevent illness or injuries from occurring. It is applied to a healthy population and precedes disease or dysfunction.

Examples of primary prevention activities by a community health nurse include:

❍ Encouraging elderly people to install and use safety devices (e.g. hand rails on steps), to prevent injuries from falls

❍ Teaching young adults healthy lifestyle behaviors so that they can adopt changes for a lifetime, for themselves and their children

❍ Working through a local health department to help control and prevent communicable diseases such as rubeola, poliomyelitis, or varicella by providing regular immunization programs.

Secondary prevention: Secondary prevention focuses on early identification of health problems and prompt intervention to alleviate health problems. Its goal is to identify individuals in early stage of disease process and limit future disability.

Secondary prevention involves efforts to detect and treat existing health problems at the earliest possible stage when disease or impairment already exists.

Examples:

❍ Cervical cancer screening through pap smears helps in early detection of cervical cancers.

❍ Hypertension and cholesterol, screening programs in many communities help to identify high-risk individuals and encourage early treatment to prevent heart attacks or stroke.

Tertiary prevention: Tertiary prevention focuses on restoration and rehabilitation with the goal of returning the individual to an optimum level of functioning.

Tertiary prevention attempts to reduce the extent and severity of a health problem to its lowest possible level, so as to minimize disability and restore or preserve function.

Examples:

❍ Treatment and rehabilitation of persons after a stroke to reduce impairment.

❍ Post-mastectomy exercise programs to restore functioning.

❍ Early treatment and management of diabetes to reduce

❍ Problems or slow their progress.

ROLES AND RESPONSIBILITIES OF COMMUNITY HEALTH NURSING PERSONNEL

FAMILY HEALTH SERVICES

Family health is a dynamic state of well-being, which includes the biological, psychological, spiritual, sociological, and cultural factors of individual members and the whole family

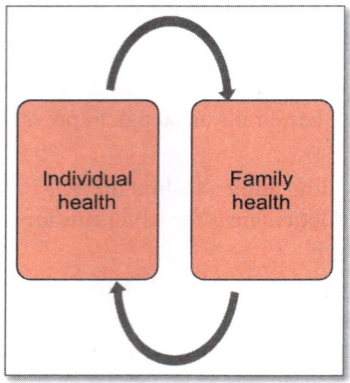

Figure 9: Family health care

system (Hanson, 2005). This definition appropriates that the family is a functioning system and the members of the family as the elements that make system. At any given point of time if the individual member of the family faces an illness or poor health that affects the entire family, the functioning system. When the system malfunctions that again affects the health of the other members too (Fig. 9). Helping a family member may include physical, psychological, social, moral and financial supports.

FAMILY HEALTH CARE NURSING

This is defined as the process of providing for the health care needs of families that are within the scope of nursing practice. This nursing care can be aimed toward the family as context, the family as a whole, the family as a system or the family as a component of society (Hanson, 2005)

Family health services refer to the health services that are available for all the members of the family. The family members may be classified into various categories based on their age like neonate, infant, toddler, school age, adolescent, adult and old age. Again there are special categories that face normal physiological changes those need extra care and attention—antenatal, postnatal women and newborn. The community health nurses function to promote, protect and maintain health; prevent disease and works for rehabilitating people.

Various Roles

Followings are the various roles performed my the community health nurses.

Planner

Recognizes the needs and problems of individuals and families. Prioritizes the problems/needs and plan nursing care.

Care Provider

Community health nurse assumes various roles and responsibilities in providing family health services to provide culturally sensitive and holistic health services to people across their life span.

o   Provision of direct nursing care to sick and diseased and disabled at home.

o   Enhances the family's capacity to care for the sick and disabled of the family.

Coordinator and Collaborator

Community health nurse coordinates with various members of the health team to provide services to individuals, families, and groups.

She would be a key person in helping families to access resources—from inpatient care, outpatient care, home health care and social services to rehabilitation.

Health educator: Community health nurse provides health education based on the needs of the individual and families using appropriate audio-visual aids.

Family advocate: The community health nurse advocates for families. She empowers family members to speak for them. If not the nurse speaks out for the family. An example is the nurse who is advocating for family on safe disposal of waste by supporting legislation that requires the family uses appropriate waste disposal system.

Role model: Community health nurse sets herself as good example of healthful living to the members of the community.

Counselor: Community health nurse functions as counselor for the individual and family. She plays a therapeutic role in helping individuals and families solve problems or change behavior.

"Case-finder" and epidemiologist: The community health nurse is actively involved in case-finding and becomes a tracker of disease. For example, consider the situation in which a family member has been recently diagnosed with tuberculosis. The nurse would engage in investigating the sources of the transmission and in helping other contacts to seek treatment. She is deeply engaged in screening of families and referral of the family members.

Change agent: Motivates in individuals, families, groups and communities to bring about desired changes in lifestyle in order to promote and maintain their health.

Recorder/statistician: Prepares and submits periodic reports and records on family, maintain complete records and reports, prepares statistical data by going through the records and reports.

Researcher: Engages in research work and pursues evidence-based community health nursing practice.

INFORMATION EDUCATION COMMUNICATION

Information education communication (IEC) is defined as a public health approach aiming at changing or reinforcing health-related behaviors in a target audience, concerning a specific problem and within a pre-defined period of time, through communication methods and principles (IEC-Lessons from the past; perspectives for the future").

Being "change agent" community health nurse functions as the orbit of IEC activities in the community. She is involved directly in planning and implementing the activities or she disseminates the IEC materials produced by the IEC department of the government. However, she is expected to be an all rounder in implementing IEC activities.

Community health nurses work with the other members of IEC team (health educator, script writer, creator and designers) in the process of planning, implementing and evaluating the IEC activities.

Community Health Nurse (CHN) in Framing IEC Activities

○ **Problem** should be well defined. It should attempt to focus on a "**specific problem**" (e.g. breastfeeding in teen aged mothers), at a time.

○ Have a clear **objective** that focuses on changing or reinforcing the specific behavior of target **audience** (e.g. antenatal)

○ Set a **time frame** for expected results (change in behavior") to occur

○ Draw a detailed plan for implementation

○ Select the set of indicators for evaluating the course of activity and providing feedback.

Community Health Nursing in Assuring Quality in IEC Materials

Unique: The message should stand out from other materials. Information should be appealing in a novel way.

Appealing: Appealing to both the heart and the mind.

Confidence: Try to win the trust by sending single message in an appropriate manner. In the name of creativity do not spoil the credibility of the material. Trust is founded upon the sender's tone, presentation, realistic images and information.

Benefit: The message provides great benefits to audience.

Community health nurse in evaluating IEC material: Community health nurses should follow some criteria to write IEC material. They are—comprehension, attractiveness, acceptance, involvement, and inducement to action.

Comprehension: The material should have clarity and well presented so that the audience can decode. Complicated or technical vocabulary should be avoided. The print materials should be in easily readable font and size.

Attractiveness: IEC materials should be attractive and eye catching. Visuals are appealing with attractive colors and illustrations. Videos attract us with movement, action, illumination and animation. Sound attracts us with beautiful music.

Involvement: The message should give them a feel, "for you." It should return the characteristics of the target audience.

Stimulus to action: The message should be a stimulus that motivates target audience to do or avoid a particular action.

Piloting the prepared material: It is always advisable to pretest the material by using the above features to check its feasibility.

Community Health Nurse in Developing IEC Activity

Step 1: Define the problem that needs IEC activity. Identify the IEC goals/objectives for the project and prioritize.

Step 2: Select target audience groups, based on the priority.

Step 3: Identify desired changes (in knowledge, behavior and or attitude) to occur in target audience and formulate IEC objectives.

Step 4: Determine the types of IEC activities needed to bring about the expected changes.

Step 5: Outline key messages and delivery plan.

Step 6: Identify the channels, language, and necessary arrangements as per the characteristics of the concerned area/community.

Step 7: Seek help from district/Taluka, government authorities/village authorities/ASHA (NRHM) and anganwadi workers (ICDS).

Step 8: Coordinate with the team.

Step 9: Encourage community participation at all levels of planning implementation and evaluation.

Step 10: Reinforce education on same issue or initiate a new activity based upon the input received from evaluation.

MANAGEMENT INFORMATION SYSTEM (MIS)

Management information systems started to play a vital role since in 1970s for providing efficient and effective patient care in the field of public health.

> A management information is defined "an organized system that manages the flow of information in the proper time frame, and thus, and thus."

Management information system extends help in planning, controlling and operating the health agency.

Purposes of Management Information Systems in Community Health

○ Helps to elicit more information for deciding upon the quantity, quality and cost-effectiveness of health care services

○ Helps in quick reimbursement from third-party payers

○ Helps to satisfy requirements of central and State legislation

○ Helps to plan, control, and organize information

○ Helps in advancing productivity, predicting resource requirements and arriving at meaningful program evaluations.

Steps Involved in MIS in India

In the design of MIS, seven basic sequential stages are to be followed. These are: (1) identification of the information need, (2) collection of information, (3) classification of the information collected, (4) storage of information, (5) retrieval of data, (6) analysis of data and (7) use of data for decision making.

The Role of Community Health Nurse in MIS

Management information system devised four modules to meet its purposes. The modules are: statistical information, billing, patient assessment and community evaluation. The community health nurses takes an important role as assessor of patient's health and progress, care giver, data collector, record keeper, service provider and evaluator of utility of services provided.

Statistical Information Module

This module deals with two types of data: (1) visit information and (2) patient information.

Visit information focuses on the nurse and information on each nursing activity and entered into a daily activity sheet." The patient information focuses on data collected and entered into a "report of service" form on each patient. This module helps in program planning, staffing, and budgeting and in decision-making activities of an agency.

Billing Information Module

This module helps in billing and financial data and improves cash flow. Supports financial process and accounts keeping.

Patient Assessment Module

This module helps to know patient's progress. It starts from initial assessment and proceeds to diagnosis, treatment, subsequent discharge and post-discharge follow-up. This module uses the data generated by the problem-oriented patient record. It relies on definitions for classifying and coding interventions that are appropriate to community nursing practice.

Community Health Service' Evaluation Module

This module provides the important health characteristics and health status indicators of a population for auditing and evaluating the quality nursing practice. It measures the cost effectiveness, the equitable distribution of services, and the long and short-term outcomes of these services.

Uses of MIS

Management information systems serve the growing demands for information.

○ Requires only less number of people to prepare financial information on billings for patient services

○ Enhances cash flow

○ Cut downs the by professorial staff time spent in paperwork

○ Recognizes the significant trends in the utilization of health services

○ Assist in program planning and budgeting

○ Helps in testing the validity of ongoing programs

○ Identifies the new community needs, and

○ Evaluates the effect of nursing practice.

MAINTENANCE OF RECORDS AND REPORTS

Record-keeping is an integral part of nursing and midwifery practice. It is a tool of professional practice and one that should help the care process. It is not separate from this process and it is not an optional extra to be fitted in if circumstances allow. (Nursing and Midwifery Council April 2002). Anything that makes reference to the care of the patient or client is called record.

Functions of Good Record-Keeping

Community health nurses help in various matters by good record-keeping. Good record-keeping helps in:

○ Improving accountability

○ Helps in patient care decisions

○ Supporting effective delivery of health services

○ Making effective clinical judgments

○ Supports patient care and communications

○ Promotes the involvement of client in his/her health care

○ Promotes continuity of care

○ Serves as documentary evidence

○ Helps to communicate and share information among members of health care team

○ Promotes early identification of risks and early detection of complications necessary treatment

- To evaluate the services and allocate resources
- To know about the individual, family and community health and nutritional status
- To elicit the causes of specific mortalities and morbidities
- Helps in planning and budgeting.

Types of Clinical Records

There are various types of clinical records used in the field of community health nursing. They are:

- Handwritten clinical notes (home visit report, individual antenatal, infant, preschooler health record)
- Hand written or electronic health records (including scanned records)
- E-mails
- Official letters from top level health management team
- Laboratory reports and X-rays; printouts from monitoring equipment
- Anecdotes and occurrence (hand written/electronic) reports and statements
- Photographs
- Audio-visual media, e.g. audio and video tapes, digital recordings, CDs and DVDs
- Tape-recordings of telephone conversations
- Text messages.

Some of the Manual Records and Registers Maintained by the CHN

Records

- Newborn health record
- Preschool health record
- Immunization record
- Antenatal health record
- Postnatal health record
- Morbidity record (TB, Hypertension, heart disease, diabetes, etc.)
- Community health nurse maintains the "Register of all activities" that are carried out by different categories health professionals. Some of them are:

Staff Nurse/ANM

- Nurse report book
- ARV/ASV injection register
- TT injection register
- AN clinic register
- PN clinic register
- IP referral register

- RTI/STI clinic register
- IUD register
- Under 5 clinic register
- Laundry register

School Health Program

- Student health appraisal register
- Referral slip and follow-up register
- Home visit register
- Monthly activity report

Registers Maintained by Village Health Nurse

- Family and eligible couples register
- Mother care register
- Child care register
- Vital Events/VPD surveillance register
- Minor ailments treatment register
- Referral register
- Drug stock register
- HSC activities reporting register
- HSC consolidation register
- NRHM related activities register.

Registers Maintained by Male Health Worker—HSC

- Family register
- Disease surveillance register
- Epidemic prevention activity registers
- Program register
- School health register
- Inspection register
- Drugs, consumables/equipment register
- Bimonthly report register and diary
- Birth and death issue register
- Tobacco control activity related registers
- IDSP Activities related reports (Residual chlorine and H_2S Monitoring) disease surveillance register
- ADD/Cholera register
- Register of sanitation
- Register of vital statistics in each panchayat
- Enforcement of health related acts.
- Dangerous and offensive trade register
- Weekly review register
- Report on inspection and case sheets.

Roles of Community Health Nurse in Writing Manual Record or Maintaining Electronic Record

- Be written clearly, legibly in non-erased material and must be dated with time and signature.
- The signatory's name designation/role must be written in the record.
- Be prompt in recording as soon as possible after an event has occurred. If not, the reasons for the delay should be mentioned.
- Records must be factual, complete, consistent, accurate and consecutive.
- Avoid complicated jargon
- Use only internationally accepted abbreviations or follow the organizational policy for internal communication
- Record only relevant and useful information
- Do not overwrite or use erasers or fluid to cancel errors. It is better to strike the word to cancel mistake and initial underneath with sign and date of the person
- It should be visible, readable when photocopied or scanned
- Keep records securely and confidentially
- The information obtained and only shared appropriately and lawfully
- Store under lock and key
- Preserve as per the time mentioned in the institutional policy
- Records must not be in access to unauthorized persons
- Care must be taken to secure confidentiality of electronic records; specifically when it is shared or transferred.

Retention and Disposal of Records

Follow the organizational policy for retaining and disposing of the records.

Records-Auditing

Yearly once or as per the policy of the institution, audit process carried out to assure the quality of record keeping for further planning.

TRAINING AND SUPERVISION OF VARIOUS CATEGORIES OF HEALTH WORKERS

Community Health Workers

"Community health worker" (CHW) is an umbrella term that may include various trained workers (male/female) of community health field who work in the communities where they belong to.

Definition

Community health workers should be members of the communities where they work, should be selected by the communities, should be answerable to the communities for their activities, should be supported by the health system but not necessarily a part of its organization and have shorter training than professional workers. (WHO Study Group (WHO 1989.)

Community health workers carry out one or more functions related to delivery of health care, trained in some way for the interventions and expected to perform the task taught.

Principles of Training

- Provision of comfortable and supportive environment to maintain the interest of the individuals
- Respect and acknowledge past experience of the learners and start building new information
- Appreciate learners with a prompt response in order to improve both skill and confidence
- Sequence and reinforcement
- Initiate with easiest ideas or skills
- Provide information or skills in a structured manner
- Consider reinforcement as a principle measure to strengthen learning
- Introduce learners into real place of work after adequate preparation in a safe environment
- Encourage peer learning and teamwork
- Avoid using high-level jargon, which may hinder learning
- Learning is a cycle
- Give freedom to participants to register their feedback for improvement.

Health Workers at Village Level

Accredited Social Health Activist (ASHA)

Followings are the selection criteria for ASHA

- ASHA must be the resident of the village
- Married/widow/divorced
- Age between 25 and 45 year
- Has effective communication skills and leadership qualities
- Ability to reach out to the community
- Formal education up to eighth standard
- Enough numbers from disadvantaged population
- One ASHA per 1,000 population.

Training

- The **District Health Society** envisaged under NRHM appoints a senior medical officer to function as district nodal officer. Apart, block medical officers appointed as block level nodal officers to facilitate the selection process and organize training for trainers and ASHA as per the guidelines of the scheme.

- Block nodal officer identifies more than 10 facilitators, each covers 10 villages.
- Women from community-based groups, mahila samakhyas, anganwadis or civil society institutions are selected to reach community and create awareness on "ASHA". Gram Sabah will choose ASHA from the shortlist of three.
- ASHA gets training for the period of 23 days in 5 episodes spread over the year.
- During training, ASHA is given learning material. There are 19 themes included in this.
- ASHA is trained to serve and help community at grass root level. She is taught on various aspects of health like, nutrition, pregnancy, breastfeeding, immunization, family planning, etc. She also runs depots in collaboration with national program.

Supervision

Supervision is a facilitating process in which the overseer (supervisor) inspects work in progress in order to remedy rather than punish poor performance.

- ASHA works in liaison with women's committees (self-help groups or women's health committees), village Health, Nutrition and Sanitation Committee (VHNSC) of the gram panchayat, auxiliary nurse midwives (ANMs) and anganwadi workers (AWW).
- ANM or Multipurpose health worker (village health nurse) who works at the village level provides close supervision to ASHA whenever the visits combined. Otherwise, ASHA reports to VHN for providing all the health-related information.
- ASHA also attends monthly review meeting at PHC along with VHN. ASHA is also accountable and answerable to Lady health visitor (Female supervisor/Sector health nurse, female health assistant who works at block/PHC level.

Local Dais

Dais are women traditionally involved in conduction of deliveries at village level. Government took serious efforts in training these untrained birth attendants to reduce maternal and neonatal mortality.

Dais training program (**Refer unit 3 for more information**) was launched under rural health scheme to train all categories of traditional birth attendants (*dais*) in basic concepts of maternal and child health and sterilization.

Supervision

Village health nurses supervise and acknowledge the work of Dais who works in assigned population coverage. Trained Dais gives verbal report to VHNs. The VHN ensures that the *Dai* adopt clean and sterile practices while conducting deliveries. The "*Dai*" reports use of "Sterile -delivery kit" as a witness for following sterile practices during delivery as well to collect her honorarium.

The medical officer, PHC organize training programs continuing education and for the staff of PHC and ASHA as per the guidance of the district health authorities and Health and Family Welfare Training centers.

Areas for Supervision

Supervision of each category (Flowchart 2) is ideally carried out in their work places. It may be antenatal clinic, Well-baby clinic, immunization clinic and during the home visits.

At Antenatal Clinic

The components observed are (not limited to this):

- Health workers approach and interpersonal communication
- Support and guidance
- Assessment and procedure compliance
- Record maintenance
- Information on next visit
- Health education
- Incidental teaching
- Equipment maintenance
- Cleanliness of the unit.

Well-baby and Immunization Clinic

- Assessment on anthropometric measurements (Weight, length/height, chest circumference, head circumference, MAC, etc.)
- Provision of health messages

Flowchart 2: Supervision

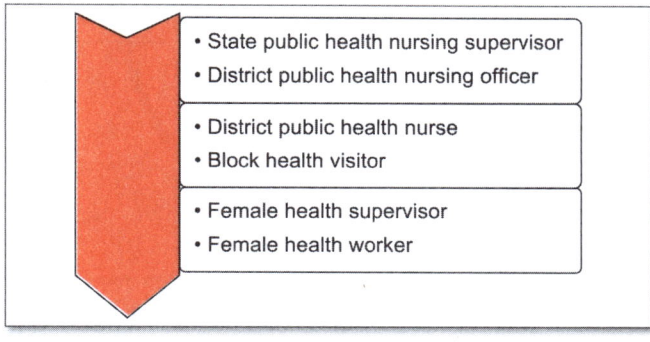

- Plotting measurements in health records
- Incidental teaching
- Health education
- Quick observation on hygiene and other ailments
- Cold chain maintenance in immunization
- Vaccine administration technique
- Recording vaccine in health card.

Home Visits

- Home visit-approaches and appropriate interviewing technique
- Procedures at home
- Reinforcement of messages
- Inviting people to clinic if they are ill and providing treatment to minor ailments
- Respecting the culture and needs of the people.

Anganwadi Workers

Roles and Responsibilities

Anganwadi literally means "courtyard shelter." in Indian languages. **Anganwadi** centers in India were started in the year 1975 for the sake of combating the hunger and malnutrition of mother and children in rural areas.

The curriculum of "Anganwadi worker (AWW)" trains them in various aspects like planning, delivery of services, information, education and communication (IEC) activities, etc.

Learning Goals of the AWW-training

Anganwadi workers are given training for 32 hours in 26 days on various aspects. The main learning goals are (Fig. 10):

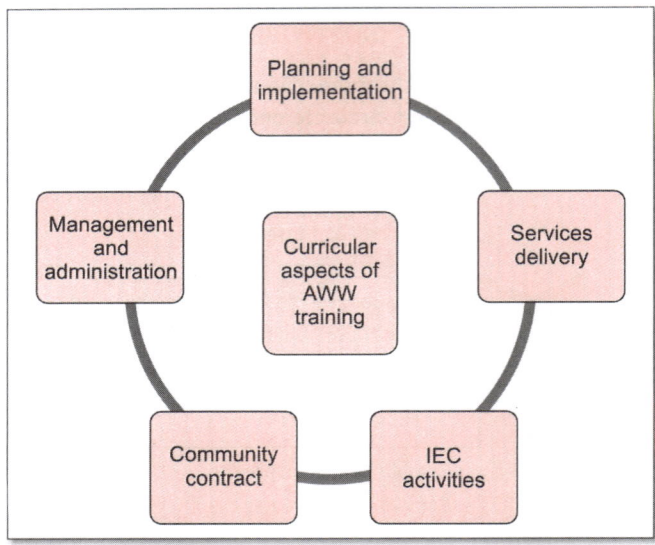

Figure 10: Curricular aspects of AWW training

- Importance of early childhood care and development
- Improved family and community practices in nutrition and health care
- Nutritional assessment and counseling for young children
- Improving parenting skills and behaviors
- Organizing early childhood care and education activities
- Early detection of disabilities
- Management of childhood illnesses
- Communication techniques for behavior change
- Advocacy for child survival and development in the community.

Supervision of AWW

- A Child Development Project Officer (CDPO) is the overall in charge for planning and implementation of Integrated Child Development Scheme (ICDS). In large ICDS Projects, that has more than 150 Anganwadi centers (AWC) in a project, an Assistant Child Development Project Officer works next to CDPO.
- The AWW is selected by a committee at the project level.
- There are 4–5 supervisors who fall under CDPO and responsible for guiding and supervising AWWs.
- Supervisor is responsible for guiding AWW in planning and organizing delivery of ICDS services at AWC. He/she provides spot guidance and training as and when required.
- AWWs also attend skill enhancement and refresher courses.

Supervisor to anganwadi workers

- One supervisor for 20 anganwadi workers in rural projects
- One supervisor for 25 anganwadi workers in urban projects
- One supervisor for 20 anganwadi workers in tribal projects

ENVIRONMENTAL SANITATION

The chains of human activities that occur in the environment turn it as an unsafe atmosphere to live. Some of the major activities those cause unsafe living atmosphere are improper treatment or management of solid waste, waste water, and industrial waste. In addition, it also includes the practice of poor implementation of pollution and noise control measures. Controlling all these factors through proper management of waste water from all sources, pollution control measures refer to **environmental sanitation**.

Community Health Nurses' Role in Protecting the Environment

- Educating public on proper waste disposal methods like dumping, controlled tipping, incineration, manure pits burial, etc.

○ Recommending better drainage system in the villages through village sanitation and health committee under gram panchayat system

○ Participating in town planning activities

○ Participating in planning for necessary arrangements toward forthcoming village melas (celebrations)

○ Encouraging villagers especially youth in monitoring the environment cleanliness

○ Encouraging self-help groups, *mahila mandals*, village committees to conduct environmental awareness sessions

○ Promoting healthful housing by awareness talks

○ Teaching about personal protective measures to prevent the hazards of noise

○ Create awareness on policies on use of loudspeakers and amplifiers especially near silence zones

○ Encourage community to plant coconut, tamarind, and neem trees near to places like hospitals, libraries, schools and colleges. This would help providing quieter atmosphere with reduced levels of noise pollution.

○ Encourage people to use more and more public modes of transportation to reduce air pollution. Also, try to make use of car-pooling

○ Advise community to switch off fans and lights when not in use. Large amount of fossil fuels burnt to produce electricity. We can save the environment from degradation by reducing the amount of fossil fuels burnt.

MATERNAL AND CHILD HEALTH AND FAMILY WELFARE

Mother and child considered belonging to one unit. Hence, the services to mother and child happen in one place. Community health nurse takes up vital role and responsibilities in caring the mother during her antenatal and postnatal period. In addition, she plays a major role in caring and guiding the mother in taking care of her baby from a neonate through all stages like infant, toddler preschooler and school age, etc.

Maternal Health

Antenatal Care

○ Register all pregnancies, before 12th weeks of gestational age. Late comers should be registered and provide care according to gestational age.

○ Minimum 4 antenatal care (ANC) including Registration–12 weeks (1st), 14 and 26 weeks (2nd), 28 and 34 weeks (3rd), (4th) Between 36 weeks and term.

○ CHN makes General assessment on height and weight and other parameters like underweight, overweight, anemia, etc.

○ Providesfolic acid and later iron supplementation and injection Tetanus toxoid.

○ Performs minimum laboratory examination like blood Hb gm%, urine sugar, albumin, etc.

○ Identifies high-risk pregnancies

○ Parenthood preparation

○ Preparation of the mother for breastfeeding

○ Makes appropriate and timely referral when higher level care or opinion needed on further management.

Roles During Intranatal Care

○ Promotes institutional deliveries

○ Encourages home deliveries by skilled birth attendants, if the necessity arise

○ Ensures all births are registered within 14 days

○ Encourages initiation of breastfeeding soon after the birth or within 30 minutes of birth

○ Advises on exclusive breastfeeding for 6 months; weaning from 6 months onwards

○ Timely referral of high-risk cases.

Postnatal Visits

○ Advises on nutrition, adequate sleep and hygiene

○ Performs home visit on 3rd and 7th day and 42nd day following delivery

○ Assess for involution of uterus, measures fundus, checks lochia/bleeding

○ Assesses the breasts for any engorgement or other problems that interfere with breastfeeding

○ Observes for any abnormalities in mother and baby during postnatal visits

○ Advises on suitable contraceptive measures

○ Extra attention paid to low birth weight babies.

Child-Care

○ Ensures that the mother initiates breastfeeding

○ Observes for infection especially on umbilical cord

○ Teaches Kangaroo care to promote bonding feel of security and adequate warmth in neonate to prevent hypothermia

○ Advises on protective clothing

○ Ensures the baby is immunized as per national immunization schedule

○ Alerts the mother to keep the baby health card safely

○ Monitors the growth and development of the baby.

Family Welfare

Community health nurses have a big role in family welfare activities. The main objective of the family welfare program in India is that people should adopt the "small family norm" to stabilize the country's population at the level of 1533 million by the year 2050 AD. Family planning helps individuals and couples to predict and achieve their desired number of children as well to give intervals between their births. A woman's ability to space and limit her pregnancies could directly promote her health and well-being as well as the outcome of each pregnancy.

Community Health Nurses' Roles in Family Welfare

- Assists in spacing and limitation of births
- Provides advice on sterilization for married men and women
- Provides preparenthood education
- Assesses for any illnesses related to reproductive systems and refers
- Refers those mothers who need genetic counseling and premarital consultation and examination.

TREATMENT OF MINOR AILMENTS

Minor ailments may be the symptoms of a disease or the consequences of consumption of some food items, insect bites and stings, accidental injuries, etc.

Most frequently found minor ailments that we may come across in are: Fever, cough, sore throat, eye discharge, ear discharge, vomiting, diarrhea/constipation, foreign bodies in ear/nose in children, stings and burns, etc.

Fever

- Assess the general condition of the child or adult
- Assess temperature, pulse and respiration
- Collect history of the symptoms like sore throat, headache, chills, abdominal pain, diarrhea, vomiting, etc.
- Blood smears need to be collected in case of suspected malaria
- Provide cold applications to reduce fever
- Administer antipyretics as per the policy
- Advice to take plenty of oral fluids
- Patients with continuous fever and not responding to treatment are candidates for referral.

Sore Throat

- In most occasions under-five children happen to report with fever, sore throat and cough.

- Assess vital signs
- Collect history
- Examine the throat thoroughly using a wooden disposable spatula and torch light
- Note for redness, ulcer or and white patches
- Teach how to gargle with saline. Teach how to prepare saline water (Add 1 tsf of salt in a glass of warm water)
- Advise on importance of adequate rest and drinking more water and fluids
- If sore throat persists refer to hospital.

Cough

- Collect the history of cough-since when, related problems, throat irritation, breathing difficulty, etc.
- If sputum is produced, assess the color, odor, and any bloodstain
- Advise steam inhalation in case of cough and cold
- In suspected tuberculosis collect sputum smears on three consecutive days
- Advise to take adequate rest and fluids.

Ear Ache

- Collect thorough history about the pain
- Examine the ear to know the reason for pain before making an attempt to clean
- Assess for the presence of discharge and swollen lymph nodes
- Find out about the associated illnesses
- Clean the ear as the institutional policy. No vigorous syringing advised
- Instill ear drops as per policy
- Administer painkiller.

Foreign Bodies in the Nose and Ears

- Never try to pull. Only trained person is allowed to remove it.
- Do not use any instrument
- Never try to put water or oil into ear or nose
- Refer to hospital with proper advise.

Diarrhea

Collect thorough history about the diarrhea—onset, frequency, duration, had any treatment at home or hospital, major associated complaints and any chronic disease.

Observe for the specific signs and symptoms like dehydration

If dehydrated, start oral rehydration solution and encourage plenty of oral fluids

Use available home remedies based on the availability:

- Parboiled rice kanjee
- Tender coconut water
- Lime juice, filtered tea water leaves water, etc.
- Severe dehydration to be corrected in hospitals
- Refer to hospital with detailed history.

Constipation

- Collect the thorough history and if any associated illnesses
- Assess the pattern of work and mobility and type of diet
- Advise on need for movement in inactive people
- Advise on plenty of fluids, fruits and more vegetables
- Advise fiber-rich foods
- Administer mild laxatives as per the institutional policy.

Bites

Animal Bite

- Wash thoroughly with soap and water
- Apply a loose sterile dressing
- Keep the extremity elevated
- Collect information on last tetanus booster and record
- Refer to physician for evaluation of rabies post-exposure prophylaxis especially in case of dog bite
- Topical antibiotics may be applied.
- The animal should be observed for 10 days.

Human Bite

Human bite is greatly at risk for passing infection:

- Cleanse with soap and lot of water
- Record the date of last tetanus booster. Tetanus booster is not necessary if last shot was within three years
- Collect a detailed history about the person who bit and the context in which this took place
- Refer to physician with a detailed note.

Insect Bite

- Remove the stinger, if seen
- Do not squeeze poison sack found at the end of the stinger
- Clean the area with soap and water
- Apply cold compress. This will help to relieve pain and reduce swelling

- Observe for generalized allergic reaction like urticaria, swelling, difficulty in breathing and anaphylaxis
- Keep skin clean to prevent infection
- There need to be well-developed referral system to refer the case if needed.

Conjunctivitis

In community there are many culturally believed practices for treating conjunctivitis, they are: instillation of breast milk, giving hot fomentation, covering the affected eye with a cloth dipped in turmeric powder, etc. We advise:

- Irrigating eyes with saline water
- Application of ointment or drops as per the institutional policy
- Protecting eyes from small flies to prevent transmission of infection
- Advice to wear eyeglasses
- Painkillers to relieve pain.

Cuts and Abrasions

- Assess the cut or wound
- Wash it with soap and water
- If it is a small abrasion just touch with Gentian violet and leave open to dry
- If it is big in size clean with providon iodine and apply sterile dressing or apply sterile dressing with tincture benzoin.

Severe Bleeding

- Apply pressure firmly with a clean bandage to stop bleeding
- Keep the injured area elevated (above the level of the heart)
- In case of suspected fracture, provide support to the part and elevate as appropriate
- Be cautious that the bandage does not disturb the circulation
- If blood oozes more, try to apply more dressing. However, never try to remove original pressure dressing
- Refer for higher level care
- If bleeding is more and patient is under shock and some part is severed due to accidental injuries do the following:
  - Never leave the patient alone till you reach for appropriate medical care
  - Do not attempt to wash/scrub, or apply any medicine to the part that has been severed partially or fully
  - Put the severed part in a plastic bag and tie. Place this bag in a container which has ice water. Reach the bag to the hospital with the patient

❏ Never try to put the severed part directly on ice.

❏ In case of partially severed, splint it in a functional position and cover it with a dry sterile dressing. Cool-ant bags applied over the outer part of the dressing.

Convulsions

○ Make the patient lie with head turned to one side

○ Keep a spoon wrapped in cloth or a bandage roll between upper and lower teeth line to prevent from tongue biting

○ Inform relatives/care taker to be with the patient

○ Advice the relatives not sprinkle water on the face and not to pour water into mouth

○ Do not allow people getting crowded around.

Collect the Detailed History

○ Is he a known case of convulsions?

○ Is he a defaulter?

○ Write detailed report and refer to higher level of care for further management.

SCHOOL HEALTH SERVICES

Role of Community Health Nurse in School Health Services

The school nurse identifies health-related barriers to learning, serves as a health advocate for children and families, and promotes health while preventing illness and disability (NASN, 1999).

Responsibilities of the School Nurse

○ Further, the role of the school nurse includes that of care provider, change agent, teacher, manager and educator.

○ The main responsibilities are illness prevention, promotion and maintenance of the health in the school community.

○ School nurse is responsible for taking care of the health of individuals, families and groups in school. Apart from this, she also serves all staff members of the school

Three main responsibilities of school health nurses include:

1. Health services

2. Health education, and

3. Promotion of a healthy school environment

Health Services

○ Anthropometric measurements (weight, height, etc.)

○ Monitoring of vital signs

○ Promoting oral hygiene

○ Screening for diseases (TB, Leprosy)

○ Immunization services/clinics

○ Administration of medication

○ Meeting the health care needs of children with special needs

○ Conducting first aid clinics

○ Thorough assessment on any acute health problems

○ Periodic health examinations

○ Advising on selection of students for athletic participation or school entry)

○ Health education

○ Referrals whenever needed

○ Health record maintenance

○ Meeting with teachers and parents.

Role in Health Education

○ Health education is a vital component of school health

○ School health nurses provides health education with a written plan; However incidental teaching becomes essential when school nurse happens to see a student with problem other than the planned teaching

○ School health is responsible for developing curriculum that includes classes in health science and healthful living with appropriate use of educational media, library resources and community facilities.

○ The health messages helps students develop positive attitudes toward health and adopt sound health practices.

Promotion of Healthy School Environment

○ Emphasizes on healthy school environment that may include proper selection of location, organization and maintenance of the physical infrastructure

○ Student safety measures are the most priority

○ Visual, thermal and acoustic factors, aesthetic values, sanitation and safety of the school bus system and food services are advised.

○ There need to be provision to observe classroom experience and activities: Emotional climate, program and methods of teaching.

○ It also includes reporting of suspected child abuse and violations of environmental health standards, etc.

○ Promote the physical, mental and emotional health of school personnel by being a resource to teachers and staff regarding their own health and safety.

○ School health nurse coordinates with other members (Psychologist, counselor, principal, teachers and physical education masters and teachers) to plan and execute school health.

NOTE: Students are advised to read the content on school health services in unit-3 to get better understanding on services.

OCCUPATIONAL HEALTH NURSING

Earlier it was addressed as "Industrial Nursing."

In occupational health nursing the community health nurse applies nursing principles for the purposes of protecting, promoting and maintaining the health of workers at the workplace.

Major objectives are:

- Health assessment and monitoring
- Health promotion and maintenance
- Prevention of disease
- Promoting safe work environment

Role of Community Health Nurse in Occupational Health (Fig. 11)

WHO defined occupational health as "the promotion and maintenance of the highest degree of physical, mental and social well-being of workers in all occupations" (Harrington and Gill,1992).

The Occupational Health Team

The occupational health nurse works in a team (Box 1).

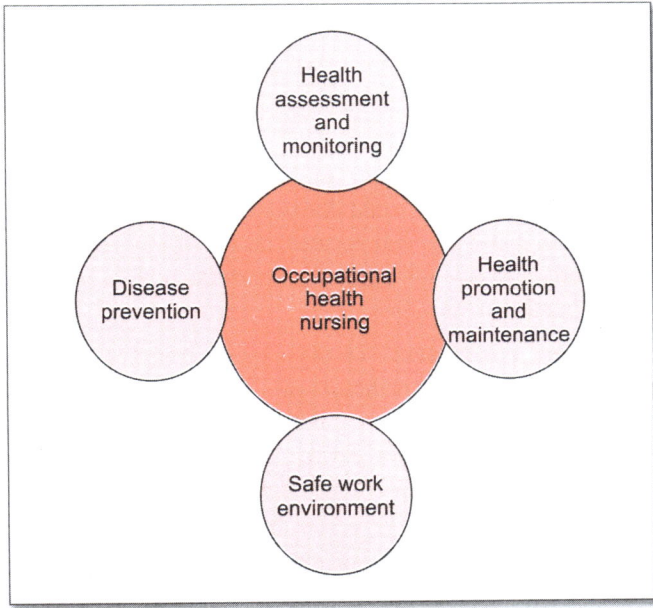

Figure 11: Roles of occupational health nurses

> **Box 1: The occupational health team**
>
> The professionals involved in the occupational health team includes, some or all of the following:
> - Occupational health nurses
> - Occupational health physicians
> - Industrial hygienists
> - Safety engineers
> - Work organization specialists
> - Psychologists
> - Counselors
> - Physiotherapists.
> - Ergonomists
> - Health economists
> - Academic researchers and others.

The occupational health nurse need to play many inter-related and complimentary, roles:

As a Clinician

- Capable of assessing human behavior and habits that are closely related to actual working practices
- Identification and correction of work factors
- Advise on protective equipment
- Prevention of industrial injuries and diseases
- Advice on protection of the environment.

As a Specialist

- Provides emergency care to injured workers prior to transfer to hospital or the arrival of the emergency services
- Provides the level of support that goes beyond the one that is provided by the first aider
- In some countries occupational health nurses provide curative (treatment) services too
- Use of nursing diagnosis helps in providing holistic care
- Makes general health assessment and provides advice accordingly
- Uses research information of many fields to support the general health of the working population
- Plays a vital role in health assessment:
  - Fitness to work
  - Preemployment or preplacement examinations
  - Periodic health examinations
  - Health assessments for lifestyle risk factors
  - Undertaking routine health surveillance procedures
  - Has knowledge of working environment of the workers
  - Planned rehabilitation strategies to ensure safe return to work.

Manager

- At times performs managerial role to guide the multidisciplinary occupational health team
- As an administrator maintains medical and nursing records, staffing levels and monitors expenditure
- Plays a vital role in budget planning
- The occupational health nurse takes actively observes quality assurance and improvement initiatives
- Keeps her knowledge and skills current to render quality services.

Coordinator/Team Player

The occupational health nurse acts as a coordinator by bringing together all the professionals of the team.

- Educate and train workers on protection from occupational hazards, and preventable diseases.
- Reports on environmental health.

Adviser

Advises to staff and management to develop workplace health policies and procedures.

Health Educator

Health education is the most essential element of occupational health nursing. Inculcates most acceptable behaviors and lifestyle practices that can help in keeping away the diseases.

Counselor

Ensures that the individuals are referred to appropriate care.

Researcher

- Conducts thorough health needs assessment carries out research in order to perform evidence-based practice.
- She needs to update herself on principles and different research methods used in epidemiology.
- Organization of clinics, camps: Types, preparation, planning conduct and evaluation.

CLINIC

Clinic is a place, as in connection with a medical school or a hospital, for the treatment of nonresident patients, sometimes at low cost or without charge.

Dictionary definition

Clinics conducted with many purposes but the primary goal is treating outpatients.

We usually witness many specialty clinics conducted in hospitals like ortho clinic, neuroclinic, dental clinic, etc. In community too we have different clinics conducted.

Clinic in the Community

The major purpose of setting a clinic is mainly to help the needy in community. It is not always possible for all sick individuals of the community to attend hospital because of affordability, time and accessibility matters.

Usefulness

- Women who cannot find time to seek treatment from hospitals located in far off places
- Sick children who cannot walk and have no caretakers to carry
- Old people with severe illnesses
- Physically challenged
- Poor people who are unaffordable to seek treatment from bigger hospitals due to high cost.

Determinants of the Service Size

Following are the factors that determine the service size, i.e. number of people of the clinic.

Population: People from local community and nearby residents utilize clinic services and it is natural seeing attendees from the defined local areas. It is advisable to assess the needy by making a small survey to decide upon clinic size while planning to establish clinic services.

Training of health workers: Efficient health workers are capable of serving the community at doorsteps. She not only focuses on treating minor ailments but also concentrates more on health promotive and disease preventive behaviors of people. This could bring down the clinic attendance.

Affordability and number of doctorruns clinics in the location: Rich people would like to attend doctor clinics that run on regular basis and located near to their residences. Therefore, it is not ideal to run nonprofit, service oriented clinics in such areas.

Winning the confidence of the community: For running any kind of clinic, one should gain the trust of people. A clinic that routinely greets patients, attend immediate minor medical needs, provides advice and makes appropriate referrals may win public interest and survive longer even if there are competitors.

Cost to service: People always look for the cost. If more charges collected, they may not like to attend. On the contrary if anything given free of cost, it loses its value.

Prerequisites for Setting a Clinic

Location: Clinic should be located in the center part of the village if it serves one single village. One need to choose a neutral place in case if it serves more than one village making convenient for all people. The distance between the residents' houses and clinic should be within "an hour" travel.

Meeting with community leaders: It is always good to have a preliminary meeting to get suggestions from the leaders of the community.

Layout: Health subcenters were established in all the villages (1/5000 population) by government of India. These subcenters also provide clinic services.

> *Private/nongovernmental agencies run health clinics to provide services under two categories—(1) for profit and (2) not for profit.*

Permission from statutory bodies: Obtaining necessary permission to run a clinic in the community.

Organizing clinical activities:

Reception and registration area/room: Registration takes place in reception area where people wait for their turn after receiving a small token following registration. Initial registration fee is paid here.

Weight measurement place/room: The weighing area is next to registration. A range of measurement-activities performed here, head circumference, like weight, height, mid-arm and chest circumference, length of the baby. After weighing, temperature and BP are checked. All these measurements recorded in the health chart/health card or under-fives/adult accordingly.

Consultation room: Consultation, advising diagnostic tests and prescribing treatment are part of clinic doctor's job. After consultation the patient moves to laboratory room.

Laboratory: It has the provision to test blood, sputum, urine, skin test for leprosy, etc.

Procedure room: First aid, dressing, injection, examination by doctor and one-to-one health education provided here.

Dispensing: Preferably, this should be located near to registration. Dispensers are responsible for dispensing and stocktaking. The dispenser explains the dosage, frequency, duration and route. The dispenser labels all the envelopes and bottles. If the patient is illiterate symbols are used on the cover and bottles.

Patient records and registers: These are maintained as per the policy of the institution. Examples include:

- Antenatal record
- Postnatal record
- Baby health card/Immunization card
- Antenatal register
- Postnatal register
- Immunization register
- Oral contraceptives register
- Morbidity register
- Surveillance register
- Birth register
- Death register
- Marriage register

Types of Clinics

General clinic: In this clinics all cases are seen.

Antenatal clinic: Meant for pregnant women.

Postpartum clinic: Meant for postnatal mothers and the babies and under-five who come with the mother.

Well-baby clinic: Services like health assessment, immunization, feeding, growth monitoring and health education are the various components.

First aid clinic: First aid is provided to anyone who comes with a need.

Under-five clinics: Services like health assessment, immunization, feeding, growth monitoring and health education are the various components.

Morbidity clinic: Chronic noncommunicable diseases like diabetes, asthma, cardiac disease, hypertension and epilepsy are treated. Dosage and change of drugs are advised by the doctor.

Tuberculosis (TB) and Leprosy clinics conducted separately: In almost all the places *directly observed treatment shortcourse (DOTS)* centers are established to provide treatment and investigations free of cost for treating TB.

Evaluation of the Clinic Services

Evaluation of the clinic services are conducted by evaluating the following aspects like—

- Staffing of the clinic
- Accessibility of the services
- Utilization of clinic services
- Client satisfaction
- The beneficiaries
- Changes in the behavior
- Morbidity and mortality

Desirable outcome indicators are set before initiating the clinic services. Following which the achievements are compared with the outcome criteria by conducting formative and summative evaluations.

ORGANIZATION OF HEALTH CAMP

Health camps are organized for various purposes.

Types of Camps

General Health Camps

General health camps aim to help, treat and refer people for the prevailing diseases. The government or the concerned agency decides upon the frequency and duration of the camps. Usually, the camps are organized once in 6 months or annually. Most general health camps attend the areas where people do not have adequate health care facilities.

Disease Screening Camps

The screening camp focuses to screen for specific diseases. The general population is screened for specific diseases using a specific test or method. This also could be from government or from nongovernmental agencies or from research centres. E.g. Screening for cervical cancer using pap- test.

Health Camps for Old Aged People

The camp attends old aged people on many occasions the focus is on noncommunicable diseases.

Reproductive Health Camps for Women

Only female reproductive health related problems are treated.

Immunization Camps

Where people (children/adult/old aged) are immunized against specific diseases.

Organizing Health Camp

Community Meeting

Conduct a meeting with the community leaders and the health workers (ANM/Village health nurse, ASHA and Anganwadi worker, link workers, sanitation health guide, etc.)

- Identify the problem or need to plan health camp
- If the camp is a planned or ready to go project explain the guidelines of the government to the members and seek their support.

Community Participation

Encourage community participation to know their responsibility.

Venue Selection

- The venue selected should be in easy access to the beneficiaries
- Choose a building which has adequate facilities to run the camp
- Most often community halls or school building or panchayat building is chosen for running the camp
- Obtain permission from concerned authorities
- Temporary sanitary toilet facilities should be established if there are no such facilities available in the premise
- Mobilize the equipment, medicine and other items required for the camp.

Public Announcements

- Public announcements (PA) should be made at railway stations and bus stops (where ever PA facility is available) for a period of 1 month
- Public announcements can also be made through mike, and "Tom, Tom" (person verbally announces with drum by walking through the areas)
- Conduct pre-camp folk shows (Puppet show, skit, drama etc) in all four directions at different places to attract the attention of the community
- Issue brochures or notice door to door
- Utilize ASHA, anganwadi workers and *dais* for providing information and guide people to camp area.

Medicine and Staff

- Adequate number of doctors, nurses, laboratory technicians and other field staff should be available
- Prepare duty roster for staff who are involved in the camp
- Determine the expected number of patients who may attend the health camp and plan accordingly
- Check for the availability of medicines, kits, consumables and others
- Inform patients on follow up procedures, if needed.

Referral

- Perform general health check up for everyone who attend the clinic
- Develop a proper referral system to refer patients for further diagnosis and management.

BIOMEDICAL WASTE

Biomedical waste means any waste, which is generated during the diagnosis, treatment or immunization of human beings or animal or in research activities pertaining thereto or in the production or testing of biological, including categories mentioned in the Schedule of the Biomedical Waste (Management and Handling) Rules, 1998.

Categories of Biomedical Waste

Category 1: Human anatomical waste—this includes human tissues, organs and body parts.

Category 2: Animal waste—this includes animal tissues, organs, body parts, carcasses, bleeding parts, fluid, blood and experimental animal used in research; waste generated by veterinary hospitals and colleges: Discharge from hospital and animal houses.

Category 3: Microbiology and biotechnology waste—this includes waste from laboratory cultures, specimens of microorganism, live or attenuated vaccines, etc.

Category 4: Waste sharps—this includes needles, syringes, scalpels, blades, glass, etc. that may cause puncture and cuts.

Category 5: Discarded medicines and cytotoxic drugs—wastes of outdated, contaminated and discarded medicines.

Category 6: Soiled waste—it comprises of item contaminated with blood, and body fluids including cotton, dressings, soiled plaster casts, linens, beddings, other material contaminated with blood.

Category 7: Solid waste—this includes wastes generated from disposable items, other than the waste sharps, such as tunings, catheters, intravenous sets, etc.

Category 8: Liquid waste—this includes waste generated form laboratory and washing, cleaning, housekeeping and disinfecting activities.

Category 9: Incineration ash—this consists of ash form incineration of any biomedical waste.

Category 10: Chemical waste—this contains chemical used in production of biological and chemical used in disinfection, insecticides, etc.

Diseases Spread through Infectious Waste

There may be variety of pathogenic microorganisms present in the infectious waste. Pathogens select different routes to enter the human body. The routes are:

○ Through a puncture, abrasion or cut in the skin. Examples are: HIV, HBV and HCV.

○ Through the mucous membranes for example: Anthrax and skin infections

○ By inhalation, for example: Respiratory infections

○ By ingestion, for example: Gastrointestinal infections.

Table 1: Categorization and color coding of wastes

Categories	Types of container	Color coding
Human anatomical waste	Plastic bag	Yellow
Animal waste	Plastic bag	Yellow
Microbiology and biotechnology waste	Plastic bag	Yellow/Red
Waste sharp	Plastic bag, Puncture-proof container	Blue/White/ Translucent
Discarded medicines and cytotoxic wastes	Plastic bag	Black
Solid waste (plastic)	Plastic bag	Yellow/Red
Incinerator ash	Plastic bag	Black
Chemical waste solid	Plastic bag	Black

Biomedical Waste Management

Segregation of Waste

○ It is segregated as per categories (Table 1). The generator of biomedical waste like doctors, nurses and technicians should take up the responsibility.

○ Nurses play a vital role throughout all the stages of waste disposal from center, clinic or hospital.

Collection of Biomedical Waste

○ There need to be separate containers placed at the waste generation points for disposing general wastes by municipal authority.

○ Items sent to incinerator/deep burial (Categories. 1, 2, 3 and 6)—yellow colored bags.

○ Biomedical waste to be sent for microwave/autoclave treatment-red colored bags. (Categories 3, 6)

○ Waste sent to shredder after autoclaving/microwaving/ chemical treatment-packed in blue/white translucent bag.

Labeling: All the bags/containers must be labeled with "Biohazard or cytotoxic" symbols according to the rules (Schedule III of biomedical Waste Rules, 1998)

Bags

○ Ensure that waste bags are filled up to three-fourth capacity, tied securely and removed from the site of the generation to the storage area.

○ The categories of waste—4, 7, 8, and 10 should be removed from the site of generation only after pretreatment (decontamination/disinfection).

○ Document the quantity of waste collected. Clean garbage bin with disinfectant regularly.

Storage of Waste

- Storage refers to the holding of biomedical waste for a certain period of time at the site of generation till its transit for treatment and final disposal.
- No untreated biomedical waste shall be kept stored beyond a period of 48 hours.
- The person authorized need to obtain permission from concerned authority to store the waste beyond 48 hours providing reason.

Transportation of Waste within Community Centers/Hospital

- Avoid the passage of waste through patient care areas by pre-deciding its route of transportation
- Assign different timings for transporting general waste and biomedical waste
- Use labeled containers or carts for transportation
- The trolleys should be cleansed and disinfected after use
- Transport the wastes in authorized and labeled vehicles to the site of disposal.

Treatment of Hospital Waste

General Waste

These are nonhazardous, nontoxic, noninfectious. Safe disposal of general waste is by the resident through local municipal authority.

Biomedical Waste

This needs strict monitoring of incinerator/autoclave/microwave that have been used.

Incineration

The facility should be authorized by the prescribed authority for the management and handling of biomedical waste including installation and operation. Chlorinated plastics bags should not be incinerated.

Autoclave and Microwave Treatment

The waste under categories 3, 4, 6 and 7 can be treated by these methods.

Shredding: The plastics (IV bottles IV sets syringes, catheters, etc.) sharps (needles, blades, glass, etc.) should be shredded after chemical treatment/microwaving/autoclaving, ensuring disinfection.

Needles destroyers can be used for disposal of needles directly without chemical treatment.

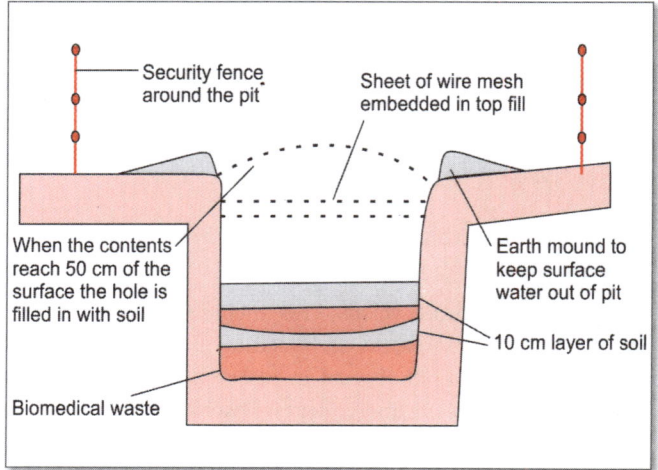

Figure 12: Deep burial pit for biomedical waste management

Secured landfill: Wastes like incinerator ash, discarded medicines, cytotoxic substances and solid chemical should be treated by this (categories 5, 9 and 10).

Liquid (Categories 8) and Chemical Waste (Categories 10)

These are generated mainly from Laboratories. Treat with 1% hypo chlorite solution before disposal

Deep Burial

The cities having less than 5 lakhs population can go for deep burial for wastes under categories 1 and 2.

Standards for deep burial pit as per biomedical waste (management and handling) rules, 1998 (Fig. 12):

- Dig a pit of 2 m deep
- Start filling the waste to its half
- Cover it with lime for 50 cm surface
- Fill the rest of the pit with soil
- Cover it with galvanized iron/wire meshes to keep away animals
- Add a layer of 10 cm of soil after each disposal of waste into it
- The deep burial site should be relatively impermeable
- There should be no shallow wells close to the site
- The pits should be away from habitation; it should not be at a place where there is high-risk of flood.
- The location of the deep burial site should be authorized.

Personal Protection

Followings are the protective equipment to be used by the personnel while handling the biomedical waste.

- Heavy duty rubber gloves (should cover till elbows) for cleaners
- Masks: Simple and cheap mask to prevent health care workers against: Aerosols splashes and dust.
- Protective glasses
- Plastic aprons
- Special foot wear, e.g. gum boots for hospital waste Handler.
- Immunization Hepatitis B and Tetanus shall be given to all hospital staff.

HOME VISIT: CONCEPT, PRINCIPLES, PROCESS

Home visit refers to identification and prioritization of health needs of the individual and family at their door steps and provision of care using available resources. In natural setting (home) of people, the nurse not only provides care but prevents disease, promotes health and plans for health maintenance using her knowledge, technical and analytical skills and decision-making abilities. Home is not like hospital where you find ready sets of items/equipment to perform procedures or provide care. As a community health nurse you are carrying your own articles, your smart brain and skilful hands. Community health nurse uses a bag which contains the necessary items to provide care at home.

SMART PRINCIPLES OF WORK FOR HOME VISIT

- Learn your community by collecting relevant information and that would help in diagnosing the community
- Identify the resources of the community and use them efficiently
- Be one among the community by establishing a good rapport with community
- Learn policies and procedures of your agencies that would allow you to perform your duties freely as well to protect you legally
- Conducts need analysis that provides the platform for planning home visits. Need analysis avoids wastage of manpower, time, money and material
- Prioritizes the identified needs and plan further
- Prior to home visit know about the family by collecting information from the family folder or from "information system" available in the agencies
- Empathize and be patient in listening
- Respect the individual, culture and family
- Your procedures and health messages must have scientific rationale

- Never try to present in a way that you are the only one who knows everything. Nowadays people have many opportunities to come across health messages from various sources like newspaper, radio and television, etc.
- Involve family in planning and executing the care; work collectively toward the goal
- Though you may go with a need-based plan for home visit, problems identified and require immediate attention takes up the priority
- While assessing and caring an individual, your observation must also be on other members of the family
- Need-based plan concentrate on vulnerable group (women, children and elderly)
- Problem-based plan concentrates on morbidities
- Write a note in your diary or individual record; as per the institutional policy the data may be kept in the family folders or fed to the system
- Evaluate the work to assure quality for further improvement.

ADVANTAGES OF HOME VISIT

- It helps in prevention of disease, promotion of health and maintenance of health, early detection of disease, surveillance and follow-up
- It is possible to meet all the members of the family at a time in their natural setting
- Family tends to develop confidence in the subsequent visits of the community health nurse
- Helpful in assessing the individual and family in action
- Helps in assessing the existing relationship between the family members
- Family members will be relaxed and at ease in their home environment
- Older people of the family can be contacted and their influence on the family members can be observed
- Family members' attitude and practices can be observed in natural setting
- Helps in referring the people who are in need for higher level care
- Governmental agencies and nonprofit voluntary agencies do not charge the patients
- Patient can get health messages in their houses itself
- Home visits help community health nurses to learn the culture of the family and to provide culturally sensitive care
- Community health nurse can assess the progress or growth of the family
- Home visit helps in identifying the new problems and plan needed care accordingly.

PURPOSES OF HOME VISIT

Community health nurse visits the home with various purposes. Some of the usual purposes are:

- To fulfill the planned or scheduled visits
- Family seeks help from the nurse to visit one of the members who is sick or injured or has some other problem
- To visit the antenatal or high-risk mother who needs continuous support
- To assess the postnatal mother and newborn to assess their health status
- To alert the mother on immunization that is due for her or for her baby or child
- To assess the nutritional status and conduct physical examination
- As a follow-up measure
- To check the treatment compliance of patients with communicable diseases like tuberculosis and noncommunicable diseases like hypertension, diabetes, etc.
- To screen the contacts for communicable diseases
- To provide health education and reinforce previous teaching
- To lead and supervise the other health workers.

STEPS INVOLVED IN HOME VISIT

Planning for a Home Visit

- Before proceeding to plan get to know the day's issues (like political issues, very hot day, heavy rain or road blocks or any fairs and festivals) in the area to be visited
- Stick on to agency or institution's policy in scheduling the home visits
- Elicit the due visits from institution's information system or manually from the family folders and individual records
- Plan to visit group of houses located in the same area to save energy and time unless there is an emergency or problem or need from other streets or areas
- Plan the approximate duration of time to be spent for each family based on the required care
- Planning of the care includes activities related to health promotion and health maintenance, disease prevention, early detection of disease and rehabilitation
- Individual care is planned may fall in one of the above levels of care
- Fill the community health bag with adequate supplies to perform the procedures at home
- Plan and arrange for the transport to reach the area

- The community health nurses who have the teaching responsibilities for nursing students should schedule her time for that too
- Community health nurses should give preference to cotton saris or salwar suits (as per agency policy) and suitable footwear to walk in the area
- Carrying an umbrella and a water bottle is a must to protect health.

Locating the House

- Once you reach the area it is your duty to locate the house or family to be visited
- Identify the address from family folder or from the information system list from the institution and note down the landmarks (like near to school, opposite to temple, next to rice mill, etc.) to locate the house
- If you are new to the area you can very well ask people by respectfully presenting the name of the head of the family of the house to be visited.

Establishing Rapport with the Family

- When you reached the house to be visited and if the door is opened and the family members are standing out you do not have the job of knocking the door but make sure that the people are from that house only
- If the door is closed look for the availability of calling bell, if so you can press the bell and wait-do not ring the bell continuously, this may annoy the family
- If there is no calling bell, give a decent knock on the door
- When people are out greet them and tell the purpose of your visit by introducing yourself and your agency. For the subsequent visits, greeting alone can help to enter into the house
- Leave your footwear and enter into the house
- Show your respect and cheerful face to all the members of the family
- When family offers a seat accept it cheerfully
- Be friendly and show your respect humbleness in all your doings.

Observation

- Make a note of family's response; you need to be a good observer of the verbal and nonverbal cues of the family to initiate further action
- Observing the house and the surroundings will help you to get to know the strong and weak factors that promote or demote the health of the individuals
- Initiate conversation with the members of the family to know about each individual of the family. Get to know

their concern about the prevailing health problems or any other issues about the family and its members

- During the conversation community health nurse also observes for any person with acute or chronic illnesses, woman who is pregnant, children with watering nose or with skin rashes or eruptions or injuries and anyone crying in pain at home
- Encourage a discussion with the members and get to know their previous and further plans to tackle the prevailing situation (like water stagnation and mosquito breeding in front of the house)
- She also observes the attitude and practices of family members.

Interviewing Technique

An interview is a conversation where questions are delivered with a purpose to a person who willingly answers to the same. Family interview will reveal more information about the individual and family health. Although an understanding of the health care values of various cultures are helpful, community health nurses should remember that persons within a culture are different from each other.

Principles of Interviewing

- Develop trust with the client/family
- Choose appropriate environment. Provide environment free of distractions
- Provide privacy
- Be confidential
- Make the patient as comfortable as possible
- Maintain personal distance level of 3 feet
- Maintain good eye contact and interact at eye level
- Community health nurse should be a good listener
- No preconceived ideas about the client or family
- Time and duration should be planned
- Recording the interview
- Evaluation of the interview
- Set essential follow-up goals.

Phases of Interview

There are three phases of interview. They are:

1. Introduction or initial phase
2. Focus or working phase
3. Termination or recapitulation and transition phase.

Introduction or Initial Phase

- Introduce yourself
- Respect the client and family

- Make the client comfortable
- Watch for signs of client discomfort; do not overtire the client or family
- Use polite, humble and professional tone through the interview
- Thoroughly explain the interview procedure
- Always initiate the interview with general concerns, then move on to specific ones.

Focus or Working Phase

- Take notes only needed. Do not write throughout
- Use effective communication techniques
- Control the process of interview, but do not monopolize
- Be flexible
- Treat the individual and the family with respect
- Do not contradict the views or beliefs of the individual or family
- Never try to impose your own moral standards upon the individual
- Be compassionate and empathetic
- Create conducive atmosphere.

Termination or Recapitulation and Transition Phase

- Recap the interview results
- Set further goals and discuss about the follow-up plans or care
- At the end find out from the individual if anything else he/she wishes to discuss.

Community Health Nurse in Action at Home

- Assessment of individual and family for existing health problems. Assessing the knowledge, attitude, beliefs and practices of people
- Involving family members in goal setting to prevent disease and promote health
- Reinforcing the previous health educational topic
- Providing the planned care at home. For example, checking temperature of the baby
- Conducting planned health teaching sessions
- Improvization and use of equipment at home for various procedures. For example, using indolium paladai in place of feeding bottle. Stainless steel paladai spout will be very sharp, so indolium is better
- Demonstrating home remedies: Preparation of oral rehydration solution at home.

Closing the Visit

Here the community health nurse concludes her visit by giving out the summary of the visit. She also conveys her plan for next visit (within how many days, weeks, or months) and confirms their availability. Community health nurse completes the day's visit by thanking the family.

Community Health Nurses Bag

Community health nurses use a bag that contains necessary items to provide care at home in the community. Usually these bags have an iron or aluminium frame to provide structure to the bag. Using the frame bags are made out of khaki cloth or any washable, durable cloth material most often preferred color is found to be blue. These bags also come in leather or rexine mixed material. Furthermore, some institutions use improvised vanity boxes as community bags. Again, the shape of the bag differs from institution to institution. But traditionally the community health nursing bags are made out of cloth material. Whatsoever could be the material, shape and size of the bag, the basic idea is it should be smartly designed to follow the principles in performing procedures at home.

Traditional Cloth Bag: Checking Oral Temperature

Purpose

- As part of physical examination
- As a requirement prior to carrying out some procedures like baby bath
- After immunization
- As one of the diagnostic criteria.

Needed Articles from the Bag

- Newspaper to spread on the floor
- Rectangular shape newspaper to make paper bag
- Soap dish with soap
- Towel pack
- Oral thermometer
- Two cotton balls
- Long layer of cotton strip to disinfect thermometer
- Spirit container.

Steps Involved in the Procedure

- After greeting the family members, find a clean area to place the bag
- Explain the procedure

- Take out the newspaper from the outer cover, spread it on the flat surface, and place the bag on it. Even a plastic square can be used to place the bag
- Get a newspaper from the family or from the outer cover and make a paper bag for discarding the soiled cotton and dressing material
- Explain the importance of paper bag to the family and keep the paper bag stand at one corner of the newspaper
- Remove your watch and pin it in your sari
- Unbutton the outer lining of the bag or open the bag in case of nonbuttoned bags by touching only the outer part of the bag
- Remove the soap and towel pack from the bag
- Identify suitable washing area with the help of the family member and keep your towel and soap dish there
- Wash your hands with soap and water and scrub for 3–5 minutes following hand washing technique. If tap water is available it is easy to wash. Otherwise you can use a mug from family and help yourself. Be economic in using the water especially in places that have water scarcity
- Air dry or use towel to dry your hands
- Open the outer layer by touching the inner part
- Open inner lining by rolling the left and right flaps toward concerned sides and keep the folds stay aside
- This step can be improvised according to the design of inner lining of the bag
- Now take out the items from the bag for performing the specific procedure (oral temperature)
- Items needed for checking oral temperature: Oral thermometer, two cotton balls and a long layer of cotton to disinfect thermometer
- Go with the oral thermometer to the place where your wash items are placed
- Wash the oral thermometer in running cold water or wash by pouring water
- Take a cotton ball that is placed on the newspaper and wipe the thermometer from bulb to stem and have it in your hand
- Slowly rotate thermometer at eye level to read mercury level
- Mercury is to be below 96°F (35.5°C). Thermometer reading must be below patient's actual temperature before use
- If mercury is higher than desired level, shake thermometer downward
- By explaining the procedure with client's permission keep the thermometer under the tongue and ask the patient to close the mouth carefully and use lip grip over the thermometer.

○ Give a 3 minutes period of time

○ After 3 minutes remove the thermometer read the temperature at eye level and wipe from stem to bulb with the same cotton used for drying the thermometer. Discard the used cotton into paper bag

○ Apply soap into long strip of cotton, wrap thermometer in it, and leave safely

○ Wash hands and come back to the place where bag is kept

○ Now you can use the time effectively to collect history or health educate individual or do physical or nutritional assessment

○ After around 10–15 minutes of time pickup the thermometer wrapped in the soapy cotton, provide spiral motion toward the bulb and pullout the thermometer with the other hand

○ Now rinse the thermometer with water, dry it with a cotton ball, clean it with alcohol, and replace it in its case

○ Now discard all the used cotton into paper bag including the soapy swab used for disinfecting the thermometer, close the flap of the paper bag, and give to family for disposal by burning

○ Now wash your hands with soap and water wipe your hands and return to bag. Open the bag, replace all the articles (thermometer and spirit bottle) and button the bag. Half close the inner lining. Improvise this step according to the type of bag used

○ Now bring soap dish and the towel pack replace them in the outer pocket

○ Now close bag by touching the outer part of the outer lining and close the bag

○ Now pickup the paper and fold it in such a way, so that the side, which contacted the floor surface, goes inside

○ Do not forget to dry your towel.

> For rest of the community health nursing procedures please refer to "**Procedure Manual, Community Health Nursing by Shyamala D Manivannan**"

Principles of Community Health Nursing

Before we getting to know about the **qualities of a community health nurse** we must have a good understanding about the principles of community health nursing.

Community health nurses build their expertise in a specialty area and demonstrate skills using following principles:

○ Promote, protect and preserve health, prevent disease and injury

○ Promote, protect and preserve the environment that contributes to health

○ Advocate for healthy public policy

○ Lead the integration of comprehensive and multiple health promotion approaches that build the capacity of clients

○ Respect the diversity of clients and caregivers, focus on the linkages between health and illness experiences and enable clients to achieve health

○ Provide evidence-informed care in a variety of settings such as the client's home, school, office, clinics, on the street, communal living settings or workplace

○ Cooperate, coordinate and collaborate with a variety of partners, disciplines and sectors

○ Recognize that healthy communities and systems that support health contribute to health for all. Engage a range of resources to support health by coordinating care, and planning services, and programs

○ Work with a high degree of autonomy to initiate strategies that will address the determinants of health and positively impact people and their community.

Qualities of Community Health Nurse

She needs to be adaptable with resourcefulness: Community health nurse goes to people and works with people. She needs to know how to adapt to hard situations. Since she works in various settings she should be alert about the hierarchy and functions and whom to approach.

Well organized with excellent leadership and management skills: She must be well organized to manage and lead the community in to an appropriate directions.

Culturally sensitive: She should have a thorough assessment about her culture and community culture. She needs to be culturally sensitive while providing care.

Coping abilities: She needs to possess good coping skills to manage stressful situations. Community health nurses may have to walk from house-to-house and street-to-street. One must have patience to increase coping abilities.

Caring is core: The main core of community health nursing is the caring quality of the community health nurses.

There need to be a call from within to care for the community.

Compassionate: Stealing the hearts of people through mere relationships equals the word compassion.

Compassion takes its platform tacitly designed on empathy, respect and dignity. Some address compassion as intelligent kindness.

Competent: Competence is the technical skills, which the community health nurse must possess. Thus the ability to understand client's health and social needs and provide effective care using his/her expertise, clinical and technical knowledge based on research and evidence.

Communication skill: Communication is one of the tools of community health nursing. It is vital for successful caring relationships and effective team working. Communication, collaboration and contracting are primary tools for community health nurses. They form the basis for effective relationships and for the protection and promotion of aggregate health.

Courageous: Courage provides great foundation for our personal strength and vision. Courageous community health nurse will be able to help her community with assertive notion, correct decisions and prompt action.

Commitment: Community nurses are committed to individual family and community. All the achievements seen community is the results of someone's committed services.

Current knowledge: "Not outdated" but, "updated"—always with current knowledge and essential and desirable skills to practice the profession.

JOB DESCRIPTION OF COMMUNITY HEALTH NURSING PERSONNEL

Job Description of Health Worker—Female (ANM)

According to National Health Mission (NHM) health worker female (ANM) is responsible for health promotion, disease prevention, delivery of prescribed treatment and assigned rehabilitative tasks. She holds specific responsibilities to work for achieving the goals of various national health programs.

She is responsible to work in different programs like maternal and child health family planning, medical termination of pregnancy, nutrition, universal program on immunization (UIP), communicable diseases (leprosy, malaria, endemic areas of filarial, kala-azar is endemic, dengue/chikungunya and JE). In addition, her job also includes working in control programs of noncommunicable diseases, collection and reporting of vital events. Record keeping, treatment of minor ailments, team activities, house-to-house surveys and as a facilitator of accredited social health activist (ASHA).

Maternal and Child Health Related Job Responsibilities

- Early identification and registration of pregnant mothers and provision of 4 antenatal visits during antenatal period
- Provision of care during antenatal period
- Testing antenatal mothers for urine albumin and sugar and blood hemoglobin levels
- Refer antenatal mothers to **PHC/CHC for testing** blood for grouping and **RPR** test for syphilis

- Referring the abnormal cases of antenatal and mothers with medical problems to primary health centre
- Conduction of deliveries in Sub-centre and at home
- Supervise deliveries conducted by dais and assist them whenever called for
- Referring the complicated cases to hospital
- Referring newborns with abnormalities to get institutional care
- Carrying out the formalities to help the beneficiaries for the disbursement of money under Janani Suraksha Yojana (JSY) scheme
- Conducting weekly/fortnightly meetings with all ASHAs of her area to guide and monitor them
- Visit postnatal mothers at home on 0, 3, 7 and 42nd day for those who delivered at home
- Visit postnatal mothers on 3, 7, and 42nd day at home for those who had institutional deliveries
- Provide advice on care of the mother and care and feeding of the newborn
- Accountable to make six postnatal visits to low birthweight babies (on 0, 3, 7, 14, 21 and 28th day) to screen for congenital abnormalities and appropriate referral
- Responsible to motivate mothers to initiate early breast-feeding (within one hour of birth, exclusive breastfeeding for 6 months) and timely weaning at 6 months
- Monitors growth and development under 5 children and makes necessary referral
- Provides treatment to diarrhea, respiratory infections and other minor ailments and refer cases as per national guidelines
- Health educates mothers on maternal and child health, family planning, nutrition, immunization, control of communicable diseases, personal and environmental hygiene
- Assists in conducting antenatal and postnatal clinics at the Sub-centre.

Family Planning-Related Job Responsibilities

- Maintains eligible couple and child register for the family planning program
- Motivates couples for family planning
- Distributes oral contraceptives to the couples and extends necessary help to prospective acceptors of family planning services
- Helps through arranging the dai/ASHA to accompany them to hospital
- Provides follow-up services to female family planning acceptors

- Inserts intrauterine device (Cu T) at subcentre
- Helps in training of the depot holders for distribution of conventional
- Build rapport with acceptors, village leaders, ASHA, dais and others and utilize them for promoting family welfare program
- Identify women leaders and train them with help of the health assistant female (HAF)
- Participate in mahila mandal meetings and use the opportunity for educating women in family welfare program.

Medical Termination of Pregnancy-Related Job Responsibilities

- Create awareness on the consequences of unsafe abortion and inform about the availability of services for medical termination of pregnancy.
- Identify the women requiring help for medical termination of pregnancy and refer them to the nearest approved institution.

Nutrition Related Job Responsibilities

- Identify low birthweight, malnourished infants and young children (zero to five years) and refer to the primary health centre
- Administration of iron and folic acid tablets to pregnant, nursing mothers and **adolescent girls** and syrups to young children (up to five years), as per the guidelines
- Administer Vitamin A solution to children as per the guidelines
- Health educate the community about nutritious diet
- Coordinate with anganwadi workers.

Universal Program on Immunization-Related Job Responsibilities

- Immunization of pregnant women with tetanus toxoid
- Immunization of infants and children against diphtheria, pertussis, tetatnus, measles, TB, poliomyelitis, hepatitis and meningitis as per the national immunization schedule and ensure injection safety and safe disposal
- Recording, reporting and management adverse event following immunization (AEFI)
- Submission of monthly reports UIP, weekly surveillance reports and any epidemic should be reported immediately
- Cold chain maintenance for vaccines during fixed and outreach immunization and safe disposal of waste generated during immunization as per guidelines
- Preparation of expected beneficiaries list with the help of anganwadi worker and ASHA ensuring their vaccination through adequate mobilization of vaccines.

- Tracking of immunization dropouts
- Surveillance and reporting of vaccine associated paralytic poliomyelitis (VAPP)
- Indent vaccines and logistics weekly in as per due beneficiary list.
- Display the time schedule in subcentre that consists of name of the village, venue, date and time of immunization session. It also indicates the names of ASHA and AWW.
- Posters/Paintings that hold key messages, positioning during vaccine administration, safe injection practices and vaccine vial monitor (VVM) should be displayed in subcentres.

Communicable Diseases

- Notifying about any unusual occurrence of cases of diarrhea, fever with rigors, etc to the medical officer and information to the health assistant
- Involve in HIV/STI counseling
- Engage in HIV/STI screening

Leprosy-Related Job Responsibilities

- Health educate community on leprosy and availability of treatment
- Refer suspected leprosy cases and those with complications to PHC
- Administration of doses of MDT to patients
- Ensure regularity and completion of treatment
- Assist in self-care practices and refer to PHC when required
- Assist the health worker (male) in maintaining records on patients who are on treatment for malaria, tuberculosis and leprosy
- Administer oral rehydration solution to diarrheal cases
- Refer suspected cases of blindness and refer to medical officer of PHC.

Malaria-Related Job Responsibilities

- Identify fever cases in ANC, immunization clinic and during home visits and make blood smears. Refer seriously ill to PHC for immediate treatment
- Provide treatment to positive cases as per the drug policy
- Maintain records of blood smears collected and patients provided with anti-malarial treatment
- To ensure compliance of radical treatment (Pf – 45 mg and PV – 15 mg) for 15 day
- To adopt universal precautions to collect blood smears.
- Ensure that the pregnant women of endemic areas receive insecticidal-treated mosquito nets.

In Filarial Endemic Area-Related Job Responsibilities

o Identification of cases like lymphedema and hydrocele and refer to PHC/CHC

o Training of patients with lymphedema elephantiasis on "care of feet"

o Train ASHAs and community health guides for mass drug distribution of DEC + Albendazole on National Filarial Day.

In Kala-Azar Endemic Area-Related Job Responsibilities

o Identify and refer fever cases with history of fever for more than 15 days. Collect the history about the migratory status of the family/guest during last three months

o Ensure that the patients complete the treatment

o Follow-up of the cases for treatment compliance

o Assist the male health worker in supervision of the spray activities

o Health education activities to create community awareness and encourage their involvement.

In Dengue/Chikungunya Endemic Areas—Job Responsibilities

o Assess for people who have fever with rashes and joint pain and refer such cases to PHC

o Supervise the source reduction activities during anti-dengue month

o Coordinate the activities of village health sanitation and nutrition committee

o Conduct health education activities to create awareness on elimination of Aedes breeding sources and proper water storage practices.

In JE Endemic Areas—Job Responsibilities

o Enquire for presence of any fever with meningeal signs and refer such cases to the nearest PHC

o Conduct health education activities to create community awareness.

Noncommunicable Diseases-Related Job Responsibilities

o Information, education and communication Activities are conducted for prevention and early detection of harmful consequences of tobacco, mental illnesses, iodine deficiency disorders (IDD), diabetes, CVD and strokes.

o Conduct surveys for early identification and refer cases of hearing and visual impairment

o Conduction of screening camps

o Sensitization of ASHA/AWW about the non-communicable diseases

o Identification and referral of care of common mental illnesses and epilepsy for treatment and follow them up in community

o Greater participation/role of community for primary prevention of NCD and promotion of healthy lifestyle.

o Promotion of healthy lifestyle to prevent non-communicable diseases

Vital Events Related Job Responsibilities

Record and report of the vital events including births and deaths to the health authorities.

Record Keeping Related Job Responsibilities

o Maintenance of all records concerning mothers, children and eligible couples

o Submit weekly/monthly reports to the health assistant (Female).

o Maintain passive surveillance register for malaria cases.

Treatment of Minor Ailments Related Job Responsibilities

Provision of treatment for minor ailments and referral to PHC or nearest hospital when required.

Team Activities Related Job Responsibilities

o Attend staff meetings at PHC/Community Development block or both

o Coordinate her activities with the other health workers and health volunteers like ASHA and *dais*

o Coordinate with "village health sanitation and nutrition committee."

o Draw **village health plan** with the help of health worker (Male) and VHSC

o Dispose medical waste as per the guidelines

o Organize "VHN Days" at anganwadi centers.

House-to-House Surveys Related Job Responsibilities

Conduct annual surveys with the help from HW (male), ASHAs, anganwadi workers, community volunteers, panchayat members and village health sanitation and nutrition committee.

As a Facilitator of ASHA-Related Job Responsibilities

Guide ASHA in the following activities:

- Conduct weekly/fortnightly meeting with ASHA and discuss the activities
- Functions as a resource person to train ASHA
- Takes the help of ASHA to bring the beneficiaries during the outreach session
- Provides guidance in organizing the Health Days at Anganwadi Centres.
- Coordinates with ASHA to update eligible couple register
- Involves ASHA in motivating antenatal to come for initial checkups and motivates ASHA to bring married couples to subcentre for adopting family planning methods.
- Guides ASHA in motivating antenatal for taking full course of IFA Tablets and TT injections
- Educate ASHA on important signs of pregnancy and labor and dose schedule and side effects of oral pills to provide timely help to mothers
- Provides initial and periodic training to ASHA with a compensation for performance and TA/DA.
- Trains ASHA in salt testing using salt testing kits.

Job Functions of Health Worker Male

Male health worker's job responsibilities are more are less the same like female health worker. However, the male health workers are not utilized in maternal health related activities. They concentrate more on environmental health and many national control programs like malaria, filaria, leprosy, dengue, chikungunya, temporary and permanent contraceptive methods for male.

Job Responsibilities of Staff Nurse

- Involves herself in all reproductive and child health (RCH) related activities and conduction of deliveries, episiotomy, etc.
- Supervises and facilitates immunization activities
- Supervises and facilitates the work of health workers (female and male)
- Provides training to the subordinates
- Takes responsibility of conducting sub-centre OPD
- Ensures and promotes quality in all services delivered

Job Responsibilities of Health Educator

It is desirable that every PHC have one health educator. Nonetheless, at least, one health educator must be available in each block. He/she functions under the immediate administrative control of the PHC medical officer.

Job Description

- Uses the information on development activities of the block for program planning, specifically for health and family welfare
- Develops work plan in consultation with the Medical Officer of his/her PHC and the Block Extension Educator
- Collect, analyze and interpret the data in respect of extension education work
- Maintenance of records of educational activities and tour programs
- Assists the medical officer in conducting training of health workers and ASHAs
- Organizes the health days and weeks and publicity programs
- Conducts orientation training for health and family welfare workers, opinion leaders, local medical practitioners, school teachers, *dais* and other involved in health and family welfare work
- Assist in the organization of mass communication programs
- Supervises the field workers performance in the area of education and motivation
- Verifies the eligible couple register
- Checks the available stock of conventional contraceptive with the depot holders and the kits with HWs and ASHAs
- Help field workers to overcome the resistant cases and drop-outs in the health and family welfare programs
- Maintain a complete set of educational aids on health and family welfare for training purpose
- Public education and health educational sessions in schools
- Maintains a list of acceptors of family planning methods
- Sends a monthly report about the progress of educational activities in the block to the higher authority
- Participates actively in health promotion and related IEC Activities.

Job Responsibilities of Health Assistant Female (LHV – Lady Health Visitor/Female Supervisor)

Health assistant female covers a population of 30,000 in plain areas and 20,000 in tribal and hilly areas. She is responsible for six sub-centres.

The health assistant female will carry out the following duties:

Supervision and Guidance

- Supervises and guides the health worker female, dais and ASHA in the delivery of health care services to the community
- Strengthens the knowledge and skills of the health worker female
- Help and guide the health worker female in planning and organizing her programs of activities
- Visits sub-centre once a week on a fixed day to supervise and guide the health worker female in her day-to-day activities
- Assesses the work of the health worker female through reports
- Supervises the health worker female during home visits
- Supervises the referral of all pregnant women for RPR testing at PHC.

Team Work

- Helps the health workers to work as part of the health team.
- Coordinate her activities with those of the Health Assistant male and other health personnel including the dais.
- Coordinate the health activities of agencies and attend meeting at PHC level.
- Conducts regular staff meetings with the health workers in coordination with the health assistant (Male).
- Attends staff meetings at the PHC.
- Assist the medical officer of the PHC.
- Participates in mass camps and campaigns in health programs
- Facilitate and Participate in activities of village health and nutrition day.

Supplies, Equipment and Maintenance of Subcentres

- Works in collaboration with the health assistant male
- Checks the stores in subcentre at regular intervals toward procurement of supplies and equipment
- Drugs and supplies at the subcentre are checked properly
- Ensures that the health worker female maintains her general kit, midwifery kit and Dai kit in the proper way
- Ensures cleanliness of the subcentre
- Records and reports
- Scrutinizes and guides the record maintenance of the health worker female.
- Reviews and consolidates the reports of the health workers female.

Where Kala-azar is endemic, additional duties are:

- Randomly checks the minimum of 10% of the houses to verify whether those houses were visited by health worker female
- Checks the suspected Kala-azar cases and ensures complete treatment.
- Accountable for ensuring complete treatment of Kala-azar.
- Ensuring complete coverage of the spray activities and search operation.
- Health education activities.

Training

- Organize and conduct training for Dais/ASHA with the assistance of the health worker female.
- Assist the medical officer of PHC in conducting training program for various categories of health personnel.

Maternal and Child Health

- Conduct MCH clinics at each subcentre
- Provide necessary help to health worker female and male, the health guides and the trained dais.
- Conduct deliveries when required at PHC level and provide domiciliary and midwifery services.

Family Welfare and Medical Termination of Pregnancy

- She will ensure through spot checking that health worker female maintains up-to date eligible couple registers all the times
- Conduct weekly family planning clinics along with the MCH clinics at each subcentre with the assistance of the health worker female
- Personally motivate resistant case for family planning
- Provide information on the availability of services for medical termination of pregnancy and for sterilization
- Refer suitable cases for MTP to the approved institutions
- Guide the health worker female in establishing female depot holders for the distribution of conventional contraceptives and train the depoth olders with the assistance of the health workers female
- Provide IUCD services and their follow-up
- Assist medical officer PHC in organization of family planning camps and drives.

Nutrition

- Ensure that all cases of malnutrition among infants and young children (0-5 years) are given the necessary treatment and advice and refer serious cases to the PHC
- Ensure that iron and folic acid vitamin A are distributed to the beneficiaries as prescribed
- Educate the expectant mother regarding breastfeeding UIP
- Supervise the immunization of all pregnant women and children (0–5 years)
- She will also guide the MPW (M) and MPW (F) to procure supplies organize immunization camps provide guidance for maintaining cold chain, storage of vaccine, health education and also in immunizations
- Supervise the immunization of all pregnant women and infants
- Follow the directions given in manual of health worker (female) under national immunization program.

Acute Respiratory Infection

- Ensure early diagnosis of pneumonia cases
- Provide suitable treatment to mild/moderate cases of ARI
- Ensure early referral in doubtful/severe cases.

School Health

- Assist medical officer of PHC in school health services.
- Ensure treatment for minor ailments, provide ORS and first aid for accidents and emergencies and refer cases beyond her competence to the PHC or nearest hospital.

Health Education

- Carry out educational activities related to MCH, family welfare, nutrition and immunization, control of blindness, dental care and other national health programs like leprosy, tuberculosis and NCD programs with the assistance of the health worker female.
- Arrange group meetings with the leaders and involve them in spreading the message for various health programs.
- Organize and conduct training programs for women leaders with the assistance from the health worker female.
- Utilize members of mahila mandal, teachers, ICDS workers and other women of the community in the activities related to family welfare programs.

Job Responsibilities of Health Assistant Male

Health assistant male covers a population of 30,000 in plain areas and 20,000 in tribal and hilly areas. There is one male health assistant for every six subcentres.

The job responsibilities of Health Assistant Male include:

Supervision and Guidance

- Responsible to supervise and guide the Male Health Workers of the Subcentres under his population coverage.
- Helps in enhancing the knowledge and skills of the Health Worker Male.
- Guides the Health Worker Male to plan and organize various health activities.
- Visits each Health Worker Male once a week on a fixed day for the supervision and guidance.
- Submits the report on progress of work of the Health Worker Male to the Medical Officer-Primary Health Centre.

Team Work

- Coordinate his activities with the health assistant female, dais and health guides
- Coordinate the health activities with other departments and agencies
- Conduct staff meetings once in 15 days at one of the subcentres (by rotation) with the health workers in coordination with the health assistant female
- Attend staff meetings at the PHC
- Assist the medical officer in various health services
- Takes part in mass camps and campaigns in health programs
- Assist the medical officer in conducting training programs for various categories of health personnel.
- Facilitates and participates in village health and nutrition day.

Supplies, Equipment and Maintenance of Subcentres

- Collaborates with the health assistant female, and places indent for procuring the supplies and equipment on time.
- Ensures the maintenance of drugs and equipment at the subcentre
- Checks for the maintenance of general kit male health worker
- Monitors and guides the maintenance of records by the health worker male
- Submits reports to the Medical officer by reviewing the records of the health worker male.

Malaria

- Supervises the work of the "Male Health Worker" by concurrent visits to a minimum of 100 houses
- During the visit, he may collect thick and thin smears of suspected fever cases
- He is responsible for providing radical treatment to positive cases of malaria. Supervises the spraying of insecticides in the area.

In Kala-Azar Endemic Areas

- Checks a minimum of 10% of the houses to verify the visit of male health worker to those houses
- Checks on identification and complete treatment of kala azar by male health worker
- He carries all relevant records, diary and guidelines for identifying suspected kala-azar cases
- Responsible for ensuring complete coverage treatment to kala-azar patients in his area
- Responsible for complete coverage of the spray activities and search operation
- Responsible for health education.

In Endemic Areas of Japanese Encephalitis

- Supervises the work of male health worker.
- Checks a minimum of 10% of the houses to verify the work of the male health worker.
- Performs health education activities.

In Endemic Areas of Lymphatic Filariasis

- Supervises the work of health worker (male)
- Checks a minimum of 10% of the houses to verify the work of health worker (male)
- During mass drug administration ensures the coverage and drug-compliance > 80%
- Conducts health educational activities.

Communicable Disease

- Needs to be alert on epidemics of diseases, such as diarrhea/dysentery, acute eye infections, etc and take immediate measures

- Control of stray dogs with the help of the health worker male and local authorities.

Leprosy

- Ensure regular and complete treatment by all cases and recovery of defaulter
- Assess and monitor grade 1 and 2 disability for leprosy disabled patients.

Tuberculosis

Check if any defaulters and inform the medical officer, PHC.

Noncommunicable Diseases

Health assistant male is responsible for health promotion and IEC activities.

He is responsible to motivate people on (1) Environmental sanitation (2) community sanitation (3) safe water sources (4) soakage pits (5) kitchen gardens (6) manure pits (7) compost pits (8) sanitary latrines (9) smokeless chullas and supervise their construction and supervise the chlorination of water sources including wells.

Universal Immunization Program-Responsibilities

- Conducts immunization sessions for children with the help of the health workers
- Family welfare personally motivates resistant case for family planning
- Guide the health worker male in establishing family planning depot holders and supervise the functioning
- Assist MO PHC in organization of family planning camps
- Provide information on services for medical termination of pregnancy and refer suitable cases to the approved institutions
- Follow-up of all cases of vasectomy, tubectomy, IUCD and other family planning acceptors.

Summary

Community health nurses use various approaches to provide care in the community. Some of them are: Nursing theories and nursing process, epidemiological approach, evidence based approach and empowering people to care for themselves.

Theory is a set of systematically interrelated concepts or hypotheses that seek to explain or predict phenomena. Model is a description or analogy used as a pattern to enhance our understanding of something that is known.

Theories:

○ Identify standards for nursing practice

○ Identify settings in which nursing practice should occur

○ Identify distinctive nursing processes and technologies to be used

○ Direct the delivery of nursing services

○ Serve as the basis for clinical information systems including the admission database, care plan, discharge summary, etc.

○ Guide the development of client-classification systems

○ Directs quality assurance program.

Nightingale's theory of environment: She strongly believed nursing should focus on healthy as well as the ill. She also had recognized health promotion as an activity in which nurses should engage. Florence Nightingale believed that "pure air, pure water, efficient drainage, cleanliness and light" are five essentials to have healthful house. She maintained that "nature alone cures" and healthy environment is essential for sick to heal.

Betty neuman's systems theory: This theory shows interest on how a patient/client system responds to actual or potential environmental stressors. The focus is also on the use of primary, secondary, and tertiary level of nursing interventions toward the prevention for retention, attainment and maintenance of patient system wellness.

Each patient system is tuned with a normal set of responses to its environment refers to normal line of defence and this serves as the reference scale to identify if any deviation.

When a person experiences stress, the flexible line of defence gets an "alarm" to protect the normal (solid) line of defence thereby to keep the system free from stressor reactions. On the other hand, the exposures to stressors on continuous basis will make the flexible line of defence to fail, unable to cope up with the stressors. As a result, the normal line of defence alters. Threat occurs to the wall that protects the basic structure of the individual causing instability to the person's system leading to development of illness.

The Roy's adaptation model: Sister Callista Roy developed this model, closely related to systems theory. The major goal of this model is to allow the client to reach his or her highest level of functioning through adaptation. Man is a dynamic entity with both input and output.

Inputs are stimuli arise from internal (from within) and external (physical surroundings, family, and society) environments. Output equals the behavior that the client may demonstrate consequent to the stimuli that are affecting him or her. Generally, the output (behavior) is modified by the client's internal attempts to adapt to the inputor stimuli.

The Orem's self-care model: Dorothea E Orem's model of nursing on self-care believes that health care is each individual's own responsibility. She described people who need nursing care as those who lack ability in self-care (Orem, 2001).When self-care demand exceeds the client's ability, the condition of self-care deficit arises. This situation calls for nursing intervention. The major goal of nursing intervention is to help people know their self-care demands and limitations and increase their self-care ability.

Health promotion model (HPM): Each person has unique personal characteristics and experiences that affect subsequent actions. The set of variables for behavioral specific knowledge and affect have important motivational significance. These variables can be modified through nursing actions. Health promoting behavior is the desired behavioral outcome and is the end point in the HPM. Health promoting behaviors should result in improved health, enhanced functional ability and better quality of life at all stages of development. The final behavioral demand is also influenced by the immediate competing demand and preferences, which can derail an intended health promoting actions.

Epidemiological approach: Epidemiology is defined as "the study of the distribution and determinants of health-related states or events in specified populations and the application of this study to the prevention and control of health problems." As a practitioner in the field, community health nurse has to have adequate information about the community she serves and she should have the knowledge on new, emerging and reemerging diseases in the community. Epidemiological measurement and analysis will give an insight about the health status of the community. Health status indicators can help to have a snapshot of the diseases, disabilities and injuries in the community. This would help in planning, prioritizing and for budgeting.

Problem-solving approach: Experts suggest using a structured or professional approach that involves applying a theoretical model in problem solving and decision making. Decision making is one step in the problem-solving process, an important task that relies heavily on critical-thinking skills (Marquis and Huston, 1995).

Nursing process: The nursing process provides another theoretical system for solving problems and making decisions. Educators have identified the nursing process as an effective decision making model (Pesut and Herman, 1998). The managerial decision-making process flows more or less like the nursing process. EBP integrates clinical expertise, patient values, and the best research evidence for deciding upon patient care. In community health nursing we equalize clinical expertise to the community health nurse's experience, education and clinical skills. PICO format, presented by Melnyk and Fineout-Overholt (2005).

PICO Method

The PICO stands for:

P - Patient population of interest

I -Intervention of interest

C- Comparison of interest

O- Outcome of interest

Primary health care: Primary health care approach had its inception in the year 1978 following an international conference at Alma-Atta in USSR.

The Alma-Ata conference defined primary health care as below:

"Primary health care is essential health care made universally accessible to individuals and acceptable to them, through their full participation and at the cost the community and country can afford."

Elements of Primary Health Care

○ Education on prevailing health problems and necessary methods to prevent and control them

○ Promotion of food supply and proper nutrition

○ Provision of adequate supply of safe water and basic sanitation

○ Maternal and child health care and family planning

○ Immunization against major communicable diseases

○ Measures to prevent and control local-endemic diseases

○ Appropriate treatment to common diseases and injuries

○ Provision of essential drugs

The principles/concepts include: Equitable distribution, community participation, multisectoral coordination, appropriate technology and focus on prevention.

Family health: Family health is a dynamic changing state of well-being, which includes the biological, psychological, spiritual, sociological, and culture factors of individual members and the whole family system (Hanson, 2005). The community health nurses function to promote, protect, and maintain health; prevent disease and works for rehabilitating people. Community health nurse plays various roles like: Planner care provider, coordinator and collaborator, health educator, family advocate; role model counselor, "case-finder" and epidemiologist, change agent, researcher and recorder/statistician.

Information education communication: "IEC" is defined as a public health approach aiming at changing or reinforcing health-related behaviors in a target audience, concerning a specific problem and within a predefined period of time, through communication methods and principles (IEC-Lessons from the past; perspectives for the future").Being "change agent" community health nurse functions as the orbit of IEC activities in the community.

Management information system (MIS): Management information systems started to play a vital role since in 1970s for providing efficient and effective patient care in the field of public health. A management information is defined as "an organized system that manages the flow of information in the proper time frame, and thus, assists the decision making process."

Maintenance of Records and Reports

Record keeping is an integral part of nursing and midwifery practice. It is a tool of professional practice help the care process. Good record keeping helps in various ways: Improving accountability, helps in patient care-decisions, supporting effective delivery of health services, making effective clinical judgments, etc. Community health nurse maintains the "register of all activities" that is carried out by different categories health professionals. Yearly once or as per the policy of the institution, audit process carried out to assure the quality of record keeping for further planning.

Community health workers (CHW) should be members of the communities where they work, should be selected by the communities, should be answerable to the communities for their activities, should be supported by the health system but not necessarily a part of its organization, and have shorter training than professional workers (WHO Study Group (WHO 1989). CHWs carry out one or more functions related to delivery of health care, trained in some way for the interventions and expected to perform the task taught.

Environmental sanitation: The chains of human activities that occur in the environment turn it as an unsafe atmosphere to live. Some of the major activities those cause unsafe living atmosphere are improper treatment or management of solid waste, wastewater and industrial waste. In addition, it also includes the practice of poor implementation of pollution and noise control measures. Controlling all these factors through proper management of wastewater from all sources, pollution control measures refer to *environmental sanitation*.

Maternal and Child Health and Family Welfare

Mother and child considered belonging to one unit. Hence, the services to mother and child happen in one place. Community health nurse takes up vital role and responsibilities in caring the mother during her antenatal, postnatal period. In addition, she plays a major role in caring and guiding the mother in taking care of her baby from a neonate through all stages like infant, toddler preschooler and school age etc.

Treatment of minor ailments: Minor ailments may be the symptoms of a disease or the consequences of consumption of some food items, insect bites and stings, accidental injuries etc.

Most frequently found minor ailments that we may come across in are: Fever, cough, sore throat, eye discharge, ear discharge, vomiting, diarrhea/constipation, Foreign bodies in ear/nose in children, stings and burns etc.

Role of community health nurse in school health services: The school nurse identifies health-related barriers to learning, serves as a health advocate for children and families, and promotes health while preventing illness and disability (NASN, 1999). The role of the school nurse includes that of care provider, change agent, teacher, manager and educator. The main responsibilities are illness prevention, promotion, and maintenance of the health in the school community. School nurse is responsible for taking care of the health of individuals, families, and groups in school. Apart from this, she also serves all staff members of the school.

Role of community health nurse in occupational health: WHO defined occupational health as "the promotion and maintenance of the highest degree of physical, mental and social well-being of workers in all occupations" (Harrington and Gill, 1992).

Major objectives include health assessment and monitoring, health promotion and maintenance, prevention of disease and promoting safe work environment.

Clinics in the community: The major purpose of setting a clinic is mainly to help the needy community. It is not always possible for all sick individuals of the community attend hospital because afford ability, time and accessibility matters. The clinics are useful to women who cannot find time to seek treatment from hospitals located in far off places. Sick children who cannot walk and has no caretakers to carry, old people with severe illnesses, physically challenged and poor people who are unaffordable to seek treatment from bigger hospitals that charges more.

The achievements are compared with the outcome indicators through formative and summative evaluations.

Waste management in the center and clinics: Biomedical waste means any waste, which is generated during the diagnosis, treatment or immunization of human beings or animal or in research activities pertaining thereto or in the production or testing of biological, including categories mentioned in the schedule of the Biomedical Waste (Management and Handling) Rules, 1998. There may be variety of pathogenic micro-organisms present in the infectious waste. Pathogens select different routes to enter the human body. Waste management process uses series of steps: collection, transportation, storage and treatment.

Home visit: Concept, principles, and process: Home visit refers to identification and prioritization of health needs of the individual and family at their doorsteps and provision of care using available resources. In natural setting (home) of people she not only provides care but prevents disease, promotes health and plans for health maintenance using her knowledge, technical and analytical skills, and decision making abilities. Home is not like hospital where you find ready sets of items/equipment to perform procedures or provide care. As a community health nurse you are carrying your own articles, your smart brain and skilful hands. Community health nurse uses a bag, which contains the necessary items to provide care at home.

Community health services rendered by community health nursing personnel working at various levels. They are trained to serve the community. Every job has a job description with expectation that the staff performs accordingly.

Assess Yourself

I. Multiple Choice Questions (Choose the Correct Answers)

1. Which of these following theories focuses on pure air, water and ventilation?
   a. Betty Neuman's theory   b. Florence Nightingale's theory
   c. Callista Roy's theory   d. Orem's theory

2. Which of these following theories categorizes nursing care based on dependency?
   a. Environmental theory   b. Roy's adaptation theory
   c. Neuman's theory   d. Orem's self care deficit theory

3. Which of these following theories states that man responds to internal and external stimuli?
   a. Environmental theory   b. Roy's adaptation theory
   c. Neuman's theory   d. Orem's self-care deficit theory

4. Which of these following states that "every person has unique personal characteristics and experiences that affect subsequent actions"?
   a. Health promotion model   b. Health belief model
   c. Orem's model   d. Adaptation model

5. Which of these following is *not* an element of primary health care?
   a. Provision of maternal and child health care
   b. Provision of immunization
   c. Provision of essential drugs
   d. Provision of employment

6. Primary prevention activities of a community health nurse includes all *except:*
   a. Encouraging elderly people to install and use safety devices
   b. Teaching young adults healthy lifestyle behaviors
   c. Larva control measures for prevention of malaria
   d. Teaching a postsurgery patient to walk with crutches at home

7. Minimizing disability and restoring or preserving function equals:
   a. Primary prevention   b. Secondary prevention
   c. Tertiary prevention   d. Early detection

8. ASHA covers the population of
   a. 1000   b. 2000
   c. 3000   d. 4000

9. In rural areas what is the supervisor to Anganwadi worker (AWW) ratio?
   a. 1:20   b. 1:25
   c. 1:30   d. 1:35

10. Which of the following weeks before which antenatal mothers should be registered?
    a. 10   b. 12
    c. 14   d. 16

II. Write Short Answers:

1. Mention four qualities of community health nurse.
2. Write purpose of standing order.
3. Define occupational health.
4. Define epidemiology.
5. Write four importance of maintaining records and reports.
6. List down four functions of female health worker.
7. List down four functions of male health worker.
8. List down four functions of "Male health assistant/Male supervisor".
9. List down four functions of "Female health assistant/Female supervisor".
10. Write four uses of management information system.
11. Principles of home visit.
12. List down four principles of primary health care.
13. Write any two qualities of community health nurse.

III. Write Short Notes on:

1. Epidemiological approach
2. Home visit
3. Components of school health program
4. Role of community health nurse at maternal and child health center.
5. Roles and responsibilities of community health nurse in school health services.
6. Treatment of minor ailments
7. Maintenance of records and reports
8. Problem solving approach
9. Concepts of primary health care
10. Evidence based approach
11. Empowering people to care for themselves.

IV. Write Essays on:

1. List various health committees of India. Describe Bhore and Mudaliar committee.
2. Explain in detail about home visit. Write the job description of community health nurse.
3. Define occupational health. Discuss in detail the role of occupational health nurse.
4. Define occupational health services. Explain in detail about occupational hazards and role of community health nurse in its prevention.
5. Explain in detail about the various approaches used by community health nurses in caring practice.

ANSWERS

I. **1.** b   **2.** d   **3.** b   **4.** a   **5.** d   **6.** d   **7.** c   **8.** a
  9. a   **10.** b

Assisting Individuals and Groups to Promote and Maintain their Health

5
Unit

Learning Objectives

At the end of this unit the learners will be able to:

❏ Develop skills in assessing self and family
❏ Develop skills in promoting community to seek for health services
❏ Maintains health records for self and family
❏ Develop skills in assisting individuals and families to continue medical care and follow-up for various diseases and disabilities
❏ Demonstrate skills in carrying out therapeutic procedures
❏ Guides people in waste disposal from family and community
❏ Sensitize to handle social issues affecting health and development of self and family
❏ Assist self and family to utilize community resources effectively

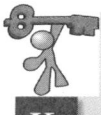

KEY TERMS

- Empowerment for self-care
- Monitoring growth and development
- Measurements to assess normal growth status
- Weight
- Height
- Head circumference
- Pubertal growth
- Newborn
- Motor development
- Speech development
- Anthropometric measurements
- Uses of growth chart
- Mean or median
- Percentile or centiles
- Mid-arm circumference (MAC)
- Gomez classification
- Waterlow's classification
- Parental guidance
- Menstrual cycle
- Breast self-examination (BSE)
- Testicular self-examination (TSE)
- Warning signs of various diseases
- Warning signs of breast cancer
- Testing for urine sugar
- Albumin (cold method)
- Blood glucose/sugar testing
- Routine health checkup
- Immunization

Contd…

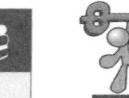

KEY TERMS

- Counseling
- Diagnosis and treatment and follow-up
- Medical care and follow-up
- Intramuscular injection
- Nasal drops instillation
- Blood-hemoglobin test
- Skin suture removal
- Waste management
- "Three–Rs"
- Incinerator, pyrolysis
- Dumps and landfills
- Bangalore method
- Mechanical composting
- Integrated solid waste management (ISWM)
- Disposal into sea
- Women empowerment
- Women and child abuse
- Convention on the rights of the child (CRC)
- Abuse of elders
- Maintenance and Welfare of Parents and Senior Citizens Act, 2007
- National program for health care for elderly (NPHCE)
- Pensions portal
- Commercial sex workers
- Food adulteration
- Bureau of Indian Standards (BIS)
- Food safety and standards authority of India (FSSAI)
- Substance abuse
- Resources for self and family
- Trauma services
- Old age homes
- Help age India
- Homes for physically and mentally challenged
- Destitute

EMPOWERMENT FOR SELF-CARE OF INDIVIDUALS, FAMILIES AND GROUPS

Self-care is a vital strategy to promote health and prevent disease. Though it is vital, the advancing world of medical technology did not emphasize or implement much on self-care. At the regional conference (2008) on "revitalizing primary health care", Jakarta came out with a new definition of health for all: "A stage of health development, whereby everyone has access to quality health care or practices self-care protected by financial security so that no individual or family experiences catastrophic expenditure that may bring about impoverishment".

Self-care should be the core of promotive, preventive, curative and rehabilitative care. The role of community health nursing is fundamental for empowering people to implement self-care. Health information may need to be demystified to make self-care easily understood by all people.

On day-to-day practice, many health-related goods and services line up in the market. The public receive information through various sources gets into dilemma, and becomes indecisive on many occasions. Health or health-related services always must reach individuals in an appropriate, acceptable, and affordable form. As we have learnt, we use four principles in implementing primary health care like universal coverage, community participation, multisectoral collaboration, and use of appropriate technology. Fortunately, self-care embraces all of these principles. Appropriate strategies are essential in empowering the community: Self-care is found basic to bring down the load on our health systems, reduce cost, and ease our efforts in achieving universal coverage.

Self-care should be a continuum of care with a developmental approach from birth through childhood, adolescent, adulthood and elderly. Experts look at self-care as a translation of community participation in health development. To strengthen community participation, the first activity is the empowerment of women. Women empowerment is the biggest strategy for revitalizing and shaping the interest on self-care in the community. Information is wealth. However, having access to information from various sources alone will not help. The kind and quality of information is very important to enrich and promote self-care activities among people.

There need to be well-developed policies for promoting self-care activities that include self, families, groups, and communities. Some of the examples of community empowerment plans are: health capacity building in the community, national health campaigns, health clubs, and peer support activities. Some examples of healthy public policy include: (1) establishment of health promotion fund, (2) National Health Act, (3) Tobacco Consumption Control Act, and (4) Alcohol Consumption Control Act.

Definition: Self-care

WHO/SEARO Working Definition 1991(6)

"Self-care in health is behavior where individuals, families, neighborhoods, and communities undertake promotive, preventive, curative and rehabilitative action to enhance their health".

Self-care Promotion at Various Levels

Self-care is everyone's responsibility. However, it is government's responsibility to provide necessary framework to promote self-care at various levels.

National and Sub-national Levels

- Policy and legislative support
- Adequate budget provision for self-care plans
- Self-care intervention to be included in all relevant programs and projects.

Community Level

- Provision for adequate fund to support self-help groups
- Adequate representation by women.

Family and Individuals

- Continuing education
- Support and follow-up including self-care advice on discharge from hospital.

Institutions for Self-care Promotion

Enhance communication skills of health workers through pre-service education and in-service reorientation:

- Services from local government and other relevant public sector offices/organizations
- Faith-based groups
- Self-help groups
- CBOs/NGOs/professional associations
- Private sector schools
- Multisectoral sectors like education; information; industry and the media.

ASSESSMENT OF SELF AND FAMILY

Assessment and monitoring of growth and development is the most important and primary activity of community health nurses. We generally able to witness many changes occur in shape and size of our body, as we grow.

Growth

Growth is an increase in physical size of the whole body or any of its parts.

This change (in size and length) is measured in quantitative terms. The units of measurement used for measuring the increase in size: Grams, kilograms and pounds. The units of measurement used for measuring the increase in length: meters, centimeters, foot and inches.

Development

Development refers to a progressive increase in skill and capacity of function.

This refers the functioning ability of the child as it grows and this can be assessed qualitatively through continuous observation.

Factors Affecting Growth and Development

Genetic inheritance: The features and characteristics of the parents passed to the child before birth itself. Examples are the color of the skin and eyes, the height, intellect, etc.

Prenatal environment: This refers to the mother's womb where the fetus grows. Mother's poor nutritional status, stress, smoking, certain diseases, all these can adversely affect the growing fetus.

Under nutrition of mother during pregnancy: Mothers who are undernourished may have energy imbalance, anemia and leading to placental insufficiency and intrauterine growth retardation (IUGR) babies.

Nutrition of the child: Poor nutrition causes growth retardation in child, which is the fact to be considered before and after the birth.

Age: Growth rate is high during fetal, infancy and pubertal periods comparing to other periods.

Sex: Growth spurt occurs in girls at the age of 10–11 years. Whereas in boys growth spurt occurs a little later, that is between 12 and 13 years.

External environment: Sunshine, good ventilation and healthful housing all influence growth.

Psychological factors: Parenting style and child parent relationship highly influences the psycho social and intellectual development of the child.

Infections and parasitosis: Certain mother to child infection (e.g. rubella, syphilis) retards the fetal growth. After birth, the infections like diarrhea, measles, and the intestinal parasites (e.g. round worm) hamper child's health.

Economic factors: The socioeconomic standards of the child greatly influence his/her health. For example, children from rich background have good weight and height comparing to the children born of the poor family.

Other factors: Some of the other factors like birth order, birth spacing, birthweight, education and income of parents all have considerable influence on child's growth and development.

Monitoring Growth and Development

Principles of Growth and Development

○ Growth is an orderly sequence, happening in systematic way.

○ Rates and patterns of growth are specific to certain parts of the body.

○ Big individual differences exist in growth rates.

○ Growth and development influenced by a multiple factors.

○ Development proceeds from the simple to the complex and from the general to the specific.

○ Development occurs in a **cephalocaudal** (head-to-toe direction) and a **proximodistal** (inward to outward pattern) progression.

○ There are critical periods for growth and development.

○ Rate of development vary.

○ Development continues throughout the individual's life span.

Human being passes through series of growth and developmental stages (Table 1).

Importance of Growth and Development

○ Community health nurse (CHN) is clear about what kind of growth and developmental changes to expect of the child at any given age.

○ CHN gains adequate knowledge on reasons behind illnesses.

○ She can formulate appropriate plan of care for the given age.

Table 1: Stages of growth and development

Age	Phase	Stage
Conception to 8 weeks	Embryonic	Perinatal
8–40 weeks	Fetal phase	Perinatal
Birth to 28 days	Neonate	Newborn
28 days 1 year	Late neonatal phase	Infancy
1–3 years	Toddler	Early childhood
3–6 years	Preschool	Early childhood
6–11 years	School age	Middle childhood
11/12–18/19 years	Adolescent	Late childhood
18/19–40 years	Adult	Early adulthood
40–60 years		Middle age
60 and above		Old age

○ Her knowledge helps her educate parents on growth and development in order to achieve optimal growth and development at each stage.

Community health nurse plays an important role in assisting the parents to know what changes to expect during each stage of development. Parents easily capture these points and apply in everyday life. Parents assess their child for any developmental delays or deviation and seek help appropriately.

Measurements to Assess Normal Growth Status

Weight: Assessing and calculating the rate of weight gain is the most considered method to assess the physical growth. Periodic measurement to assess the children of 1–5 years of age is very important because this group is at high-risk for growth faltering.

Height: Height is a stable measurement of growth. Height points out the events took place in the past. When the child's height is low for the said age, it is "nutritional stunting." This reflects the past malnutrition. The cutoff point is 90% of height for age values. The average expected height increase is given in Table 2.

Head circumference: The head circumference is about 34 cm at birth. The posterior fontanele closes after 2 months.

The anterior fontanele widens after birth and closes at the age of 18 months. The head circumference increases to 44 cm at 6 months and 47 cm by 1 year.

Table 2: Weight and height increase

Age	Weight increments/week
0–3 months	200 g
4–6 months	150 g
7–9 months	100 g
10–12 m	50–75 g
	Weight increments/year
1–2 years	2.5 kg
3–5 years	2.0 kg
	Length increments per year
1st year	25 cm
2nd year	12 cm
3rd year	9 cm
4th year	7 cm
5th year	6 cm

The circumference of the head is bigger than that of the chest at birth, but at the age of 1 year, they become equal. Chest circumference crosses the head circumference at 18 months.

Teeth: Twenty deciduous teeth appear between the age of 6 months and 2½ years. The first tooth appears at about 6 months. Prior to tooth eruption the child has excessive drooling and tries to bite. The deciduous teeth fall between 6 and 12 years of age, permanent teeth erupting. At the age of 12 years, the child should have 28 permanent teeth. The wisdom teeth come up after the age of 18 and they are four in number. One must remember that the teething does not follow same pattern in all children. Even some babies have tooth when they are born and is considered normal.

Pubertal growth: This happens at around 10 years, but it is expected to occur any time from 8 to 13 years of age. In boys, puberty begins occurs between 11 and 13 years.

STAGES OF DEVELOPMENT AND NEWBORN

As a transition, the fetus of intrauterine environment enters to extra uterine environment as a newborn baby. Newborn stage refers to the first 4 weeks or first month of life.

○ *A baby should gain at least 500 grams of weight per month in the first 3 months of life.*

○ *On an average, a healthy baby doubles his birthweight by 5 months, triple it by the end of 1st year and quadruple by the age of 2.*

Motor Development

○ Keeps hands fisted while sleeping on back
○ Grasps our finger firmly (the grasp reflex)
○ Takes a few steps when made to stand on firm flat surface (the walking reflex)
○ The grasp reflex and the walking reflex disappear in about 2 months.

Perception and Social Response

○ Wrinkles forehead to sound
○ Blinks to strong light
○ Stops crying when someone cuddles
○ Sucks at the breast with satisfaction
○ Feels of secured, while sucking.

Speech Development

The lusty cry for hunger or any discomfort is the sign of development of speech.

At the Age of 1 Month

Motor Development

o When put on back he kicks his legs in joy.

o When put on stomach, he lifts head, and turns to protect his nose.

o Able to bring his hand within the range of his eyes.

Perception and Social Response

o Gazes at colored rattle when moved at 20 cm distance

o Follows it when moved from midpoint to one side

o Attentive black and white pictures

o Able to differentiate between sounds

o Manages to have eye contact with mother while sucking.

Speech Development

The child may make some throaty sounds like 'ah' and 'coo'.

Role of Community Health Nurse in Guiding the Parents of 1 Month Infant

Parental Guidance

o Begin to expose infant to different household sounds

o Change crib location in room

o Use bright-colored clothing and linen

o Put infant to sleep on back until old enough to roll

o Keep infant nearby

o Play with infant when awake

o Hold during feeding.

At the Age of 2 Months

Motor Development

When lying prone, lifts head at 45° and can holds for about 10 seconds.

o Able to keep the head up for a little longer.

o The fist is kept open more often.

Perception and Social Response

o Listens to sounds more attentively

o Does not blink or cry on hearing sounds

o Social smile at 6 weeks.

Speech Development

Makes a few throaty sounds like 'goo', 'ab' and 'coo'.

Role of Community Health Nurse in Guiding the Parents of 2 Months Infant

Parental Guidance

o Talk to infant and smile; get excited when infant coos.

o Place infant seat on a secure surface (e.g. floor, center of a table—never near edge of table) near mother's activities.

o Put infant in prone position in bed or on floor.

o Expose infant to different textures.

o Exercise infant's arms and legs.

o Sing to infant.

o Provide tactile experience during bathing, diapering, and feeding.

At the Age of 3 Months

Motor Development

o Holds head erects and steady

o Opens or closes hand loosely

o Holds object put in hand.

Role of Community Health Nurse in Guiding the Parents of 3 Months Infant

o Take outdoors with proper clothing (similar warmth as that of adults), hat, and PABA-free sunscreen

o Bounce on bed

o Play with infant during feeding

o Rattles can be used effectively for visual following and for hand play

o Encourage older siblings to "make faces," sing and talk to infant.

At the Age of 4 Months

Motor Development

o Roll over from front to back

o Hold head erect and steady while in sitting position

o Bring hands together in midline and plays with fingers

o Grasp objects with both hands.

Perception and Social Development

Turn head toward the direction of the sound.

Language Development

Listening and communicates by laughing loudly.

Role of Community Health Nurse in Guiding the Parents of 4 Months Infant

- Be certain button eyes on toys and other small objects cannot be pulled off
- Hold rattle, let infant reach, and grasp it
- When infant is in high chair, strap in
- Move mobile out of reach—infant may grab it and cause injury
- Repeat child's sounds
- Talk in varying degrees of loudness
- Begin looking at and naming pictures in book
- Begin rough housing play by both parents
- Give space in playpen or on sheet on floor to practice rolling over
- Place on abdomen for part of playtime.

At the Age of 5 Months

Motor Development

- Balances head well while sitting
- Sits with support
- Pulls feet up to mouth when supine
- Grasps objects with whole hand
- Holds one object while looking at another.

Perception and Social Response

- Differentiates strangers from close ones
- Able to make out if you are angry by the tone of the voice.

Language Development

He may now try to join a few syllables and say "da-da" or may use them separately as "ma", "goo" or "da".

At the Age of 6 Months

Motor Development

- Sits alone briefly
- Turns completely over (abdomen to abdomen)
- Lift chest and upper abdomen when prone
- Holds own bottle
- Palmar grasp—uses entire hand to pick up an object.

Perception and Social Response

- Hearing is now more sensitive
- Smiles when sees his own reflection in a mirror
- Very conscious of strangers.

Language Development

Joins a few syllables and say 'da-da' 'ma', 'goo' or 'da'.

At the Age of 7 Months

Motor Development

- Sits alone
- Holds cup
- Imitate simple acts of others.

Perception and Social Response

- When an object falls on ground follows until he locates
- Plays games like 'peek-a-boo.'

Role of Community Health Nurse in Guiding the Parents of 5–7 Months Infant

- Play as long as you can
- Tie toys to chair with short string
- Play with extra spoon at feeding
- Give soft finger foods, because infant puts everything in mouth, use safety precautions
- Keep small items away from infant as they could choke in his throat
- Show excitement at achievements
- Supply safe kitchen items for toys.

At the Age of 8 Months

Motor Development

- Sit alone steadily
- Drink from cup with assistance
- Eat finger food that can be held in one hand.

Perception and Social Response

When you hide a toy under a cloth the child will try to find it.

At the Age of 9 Months

Motor Development

- Rise to sitting position alone
- Crawl (i.e. pull body while in prone position)
- Hold one bottle with good hand-mouth coordination
- Pincer grasp—can grasp small objects using thumb and forefinger.

Perception and Social Response

- Shows interest in soft sounds like a watch
- Enjoys dropping objects and someone picks it
- Likes to play "hide-and-seek".

Language Development

Joins two syllables and say "dada", "mama", or "baba".

At the Age of 10 Months

Motor Development

- Creep well (use hands and legs)
- Walk but with help
- Bring the hands together.

Perception and Social Response

- Claps, copies "ta-ta" or "bye-bye,"
- Likes to see pictures in books
- Understands the meaning of 'No'.

Language Development

Repeats "da-da" or "ma-ma" when you say.

Role of Community Health Nurse in Guiding the Parents of 7–10 Months Infant

Protect from dangerous objects—cover electrical outlets, block stairs, remove breakable objects from tables.

- Have child with family at mealtime
- Offer cup
- Talk and sing to infant.

At the Age of 11 Months

Motor Development

- Walks holding on furniture
- Stands erect with minimal support.

Perception and Social Response

Repeats the action when we appreciate.

Language Development

Uses some jargon less likely to use words with meaning.

At the Age of 12 Months

Motor Development

- Stands-alone for variable length of time
- Sits down from standing position
- Walk in few steps with help or alone (hands held at shoulder height for balance)
- Pick up small bits of food and transfers them to his mouth.

Perception and Social Response

- Shakes her head for 'No'
- Enjoys playing simple games.

Speech

- Imitates words like "dada" or "mama" spoken by you.
- Says 1 or 2 words with meaning.
- Red flag indicators indicates the deviation

Role of Community Health Nurse in Guiding the Parents of 10–12 Months Infant

- Allow self-directed play rather than adult-directed play.
- Continue to expose to foods of different textures, taste, smell and substance. Offer cup.
- Show affection and encourage child to return affection.
- **Safety teaching:** Child gets into everything within reach. Place medications in safe and locked place.
- Create a safe environment for child.

At the Age of 1–1½ Year-old

Motor Development

- Walks without support and with balance
- Falls less frequently
- Throws ball
- Stoops to pick up toys
- Turns pages of book.

Red flag indicators during infant development
- Unable to sit alone by age of 9 months
- Unable to transfer objects from hand to hand by age of 1 year
- Abnormal pincer grasp by age of 15 months
- Unable to walk alone by 18 months
- Failure to speak recognizable words by 2 years

Cognitive and Emotional Development

- ○ Has vocabulary of 10 words that have meanings
- ○ Uses phrases and imitates words
- ○ Points to objects named by adult.

Role of Community Health Nurse in Guiding the Parents of 1–1½ Year-old Child

- ○ Begin to teach tooth brushing to establish good dental habits; however, continue to brush child's teeth
- ○ Establish limits to give toddler sense of security, but encourage exploration
- ○ Reinforce safety teaching.

At the Age of 1½ –2 Years

Motor Development

- ○ Walks up and down stairs
- ○ Opens doors, turns knobs
- ○ Has steady gait. Holds drinking cup well with one hand
- ○ Uses spoon without spilling food (may prefer fingers)
- ○ Kicks a ball in front of him without support
- ○ Builds a tower of 4–6 blocks
- ○ Scribbles
- ○ Rides tricycle or kiddie car (without pedals).

Cognitive Development

- ○ Has 200–300 words in vocabulary
- ○ Begins to use short sentences
- ○ Refers to self by pronoun.

> **Red flags indicators in preschooler**
> - Inability to perform self-care tasks, handwashing simple dressing, daytime toileting
> - Lack of socialization
> - Unable to play with other children

Role of Community Health Nurse in Guiding the Parents of 1½ –2 Year-old Child

- ○ Has need for peer companionship, although displays immaturity by inability to share and take turns
- ○ A decrease in appetite normally occurs at this stage
- ○ Toilet training should be started (each child follows own pattern)
- ○ Begin to have child eat meals with family, if not already doing so
- ○ Child begin to read. Child likes storybooks with large pictures.

At the Age of 2–3 Year-Old

Developmental Milestones for 2–3 Year-old

Motor Development

- ○ Shows affection for others
- ○ Able to play by himself or herself
- ○ Continues to explore world around him
- ○ Begins to being more helpful
- ○ May also begin to show challenging behavior
- ○ Runs forward
- ○ Uses two or three word sentences
- ○ Speech is understood by familiar listeners
- ○ Follows two step directions
- ○ Helps dress and undress themselves
- ○ Jumps in place with one foot
- ○ Kicks a ball
- ○ Climbs on to things with ease
- ○ Bends over

Cognitive Development

- ○ Responds to simple directions
- ○ Groups objects by their category
- ○ Observes and imitates more complex actions and gestures
- ○ Typically egocentric, or self-centred, in their thinking
- ○ Understands differences in meanings (i.e. stop and go or up and down)
- ○ Holds a pencil in a writing position

Role of Community Health Nurse in Guiding the Parents of 2–3 Year-old Child

- ○ From 2–3 years, the child develops a seeming maturity; do not expect more than child is able to do
- ○ Arrange first visit to the dentist to have teeth checked
- ○ Be aware that negativistic and ritualistic behavior is normal
- ○ Be consistent in discipline
- ○ Control temper tantrums
- ○ Begin to teach traffic safety
- ○ Supervise outdoor play.

At the Age of 3–4 Years

Motor Development

- ○ Drawings have form and meaning but not detail
- ○ Copies a circle and a cross

- Buttons front and side of clothes
- Laces shoes
- Bathes self, but needs direction
- Brushes teeth
- Shows continuous movement going up and down stairs
- Climbs and jumps well
- Attempts to print letters.

Cognitive Development

- Awareness of body is more stable; child becomes more aware of own vulnerability. Child is less negativistic
- Learns some number concepts
- Begins naming colors.

Issues Observed in Toddlers

- Stranger anxiety—should dissolve by age 2½–3 years
- Temper tantrums: Disappears by age of 3
- Sibling rivalry: Shows aggressive behavior toward new infant: peak between 1 and 2 years and this may prolong indefinitely
- Thumb sucking
- Toilet training.

Role of Community Health Nurse in Guiding the Parents of 3–4 Year-old Child

- Base your expectations within child's limitations
- Provide limited frustrations from environment to assist in coping
- Give small tasks to do around the house (putting silverware on table, drying a dish)
- Expand child's world with trips to the zoo, to the supermarket, to restaurant, etc. Prevent accidents
- Provide for brief nonthreatening separation from parents and home
- Reinforce correct use of language
- Use opportunities for simple sexual education as child's needs arise
- Accept masturbation as a normal phenomenon to be discouraged in public
- Provide consistent discipline, motivated by love rather than anger
- Consider nursery school.

At the Age of 4–5 Years

Motor Development

- Hops two or more times
- Dresses without supervision

- Has good motor control—climbs and jumps well
- Walks up stairs without grasping handrail
- Walks backward
- Washes self without wetting clothes
- Prints first name and other words
- Adds three or more details in drawings
- Draws a square.

Cognitive Development

- Has 2,100-word vocabulary
- Talks constantly
- Uses adult speech forms
- Participates in conversations
- Asks for definitions
- Knows age and residence.

Role of Community Health Nurse in Guiding the Parents of 4–5 Year-old Child

- Parental guidance
- Child no longer takes an afternoon nap
- Prepare child for kindergarten
- Tell him stories
- Provide opportunities and reassurance for group play; have his friends visit for lunch and an afternoon of playing
- Prevent accidents
- Encourage child's participation in household activities.

METHODS OF GROWTH MONITORING

Methods used for growth monitoring are:

- Growth charting
- Anthropometric measurements—height for age, weight for height and mid-arm circumference.

Growth Charting

Growth charts were first designed and introduced by David Morley. World Health Organization took efforts to modify these charts and put it into practice. Growth chart is otherwise known as "road-to-health" chart. It displays the growth and development of the child.

Under integrated child development services scheme (ICDS) a joint mother and child protection card developed separately for boys and girls.

This card accommodates the following:

Family identification and registration, birth record, pregnancy record, preparation for delivery, registration under *Janani Suraksha Yojana*, details about immunization procedures, breastfeeding and introduction of supplementary food, miles stones of the baby, birth spacing and reasons for special care.

Basic Features of Growth Chart

- In weight for age chart the height of the child is not considered
- Weight is more sensitive measure of growth
- Deviations can be detected easily by comparison with reference curves
- A child can lose weight but not height
- Effective, if plotted correctly
- Flattening or falling of the child's weight curve signals growth failure that alerts on PEM (Protein energy malnutrition).

Uses of Growth Chart

- **Growth monitoring:** It is of great value in child care. It is very simple and inexpensive to monitor weight gain and child health.
- **Serves as diagnostic tool:** Helps in identifying high-risk children, e.g. malnutrition.
- **Planning and policy making tool:** It provides an objective basis for planning and policy making in child health related issues.
- **Educational tool:** Being a visual tool it easily attracts even the uneducated parents to learn about the various aspects of growth and development monitored by it. Hence, it serves as a tool to educate mothers and encourage her participation in child health related sessions and discussions.
- **Tool for action:** Helps the health worker efficiently on type of interventions needed. It also makes referrals easier.
- **Tool for teaching:** It is used as a teaching tool, e.g. importance of feeding, effects of diarrhea, etc.
- **Evaluation:** It helps in measuring the effectiveness of interventions provided in improving the growth and development of children.

Anthropometric Measurements for Children

Weight, height, head and chest circumference (CC), mid-arm circumference and (MAC) skin-fold thickness are used to assess the growth and nutritional status of the children. These measures are compared with the reference standards using three methods:

- Mean or median
- Percentile or centiles
- Weight for age and weight for height.

Mean or Median

A variation of 2 standard deviations from either side of the mean or median is considered as within normal limits.

Percentile or Centiles

- Percentile refers to the percentage of individuals falling below a particular level. By definition, 3% of children are below the 3rd percentile and a 3% are above the 97th percentile. The remaining 94% of individuals (between 3rd and 97%) is regarded as being within normal level.
- The individuals falling below 3rd percentile (3) and above 97 percentile (3), a total of six cannot be considered as abnormal if their growth is parallel to centile lines.

Weight for Height/Length

- An expected weight for height is used as reference value for comparison. World Health Organization's reference value guides us in assessing the weight to corresponding height.
- A child who is less than 70% of expected weight for height is considered as severely malnourished. Measurements to assess nutritional status.

Weight

- Assessing and calculating the rate of weight gain is the most considered method to assess the physical growth.
- Periodic measurement at intervals is vital to assess the children of 1–5 years of age because this group is at high risk for growth faltering.

Height

- Height is a stable measurement of growth
- Height points out the events those took place in the past. If a child is low in height for age it is known as nutritional stunting
- This reflects the past malnutrition. The cutoff point is 90% of height for age values. The average expected height increase is given in (Table 3).

Table 3: Waterlow's classification

Nutritional status	Stunting (% of height/age)	Wasting (% of weight/height)
Normal	>95	>90
Mildly impaired	87.5–95	80–90
Moderately impaired	80–87.5	70–80
Severely impaired	<80	<70

Head and Chest Circumference

- At birth, the baby's head circumference (HC) measures 34 cm.
- Normally the head circumference (HC) of the baby measures about 2 cm more than that of the chest circumference (CC) at birth. By 6–9 months, the two measurements become equal.
- Later, as the baby grows the CC overtakes the HC.
- There will be a delay in overtaking by 3–4 years in severely malnourished children due to inadequate development of the thoracic cage.
- Measure HC by placing the inch tape on the forehead over the frontal eminences and bring it around over the occipital protuberance. Measure CC by placing the inch tape over the nipple line and bring it around the chest.

Percentile Interpretation of HC

- Less than 3: Microcephaly
- 3 and <97: Normal head circumference
- ≥97: Macrocephaly

Mid-arm Circumference

- Mid-arm circumference is considered as the reliable estimation of body's muscle mass. Any reduction in this tells that the body is adjusting the inadequate energy intakes.

Grading Malnutrition based on Mid-arm Circumference

- MAC >13.5 cm: Satisfactory nutritional status
- MAC 12.5–13.5 cm: Moderate malnutrition
- MAC <12.5 cm: Severe malnutrition
- Gomez classification of malnutrition is given in (Table 4).

How to Measure MAC

- Let the arm hang onside
- Measure the distance between the tip of acromion process (a part of scapula found over the shoulder) and olecranon process (a part of "ulna bone" found in elbow) and locate the midpoint by placing the finger then bring around the inch tape and note the reading.

Table 4: Gomez classification

Percent of reference weight for age	Interpretation
90–110%	Normal
75–89%	Grade I: Mild malnutrition
60–74%	Grade II: Moderate malnutrition
<60%	Grade III: Severe malnutrition

- Field workers assesses MAC using "Shakir's tape and "Bangle test." Shakir's tape is based on Arnold, classification.
- Shakir's tape is designed with three color zones on a plastic tape. The zone above 13.5 cm is green and represents normal MAC.
- The zone with 12.5–13.5 is "orangish-yellow" indicates borderline malnutrition. The zone colored in "red" and measuring less than 12.5 cm indicates malnutrition. Bangle test—Bangle is of 4 cm internal diameter.
- If the bangle passes easily above the elbow and to the child's upper arm the child has severe malnutrition.

Growth Monitoring and Grading Malnutrition

There are many classifications available to grade malnutrition. Some of them are:

Gomez classification: In this, child's weight is compared to that of a normal child (50th percentile) of the same age. It is useful for population survey and community health interventions (Table 4).

Percent of reference weight for age

$$= \frac{\text{Weight of the child}}{\text{Weight of the normal child of the same age}} \times 100$$

Waterlow's classification: Chronic malnutrition can result in stunting. Malnutrition also affects the child's body proportions eventually resulting in body wastage (Table 3)

Percent (%) weight for height

$$= \frac{\text{Weight of the child}}{\text{Weight of normal child of the same age}} \times 100$$

Indian Academy of Pediatrics (IAP): The classification was given by Indian academy of pediatrics (IAP) and this is also based on weight for age but the cut off level to separate the malnourished children is 80% of the standard. Severely malnourished children are placed under grade III and grade IV malnutrition.

- Grade-I—70–80%
- Grade-II—60–70%
- Grade-III—50–60%
- Grade-IV—<50%

Moderate acute malnutrition (MAM) is defined by WHO/UNICEF as:
Weight-for-Height Z-score <–2 but <–3
Severe acute malnutrition (SAM) is defined by WHO/UNICEF as:
Mid upper arm circumference (MUAC) <11.5
Weight-for-Height Z-score <–3
Has bilateral pitting edema
Marasmic-kwashiorkor (both wasting and edema)

Measuring Weight Using Salter Weighing Scale

Salter, a spring hanging scale (Salter) is widely used for checking weight of preschoolers. This scale can weigh up to 25 kg. This is calibrated by 0.1 kg (100 g) increments.

Steps for Measuring the Weight of a Child Using Salter Scale

○ Hook the scale to a strong horizontal, metal or wooden bar at eye level or tie it with the bar using a strong rope.

○ Hang the weighing pants to the lower hook of the scale and readjust the scale to zero. Explain the procedure.

○ Undress the infant and place him/her in the weighing pan.

○ If you want to weigh a toddler or a preschooler advise the mother to dress him with light clothes.

○ If possible these clothes can be weighed separately and subtracted from the weight-taken with dress of the child to know the accurate weight of the child.

○ You also must enquire the mother about the previous weight measuring procedure used. This is mainly done to compare the present weight with the old weight.

○ Ensure that parent or any other person should not touch the pan or the scale while weighing.

○ Ensure that the child hangs freely without holding onto anything.

○ You should record weight only when the child settles properly and the weight record looks stable.

○ The weight is recorded to the nearest 100 g.

○ Inform the weight to the parent from the scale.

Purpose

○ To assess the growth of the child

○ To assess the health status. To calculate drug dosages

○ To calculate body mass index to rule out obesity or underweight.

Articles Required

○ Weighing machine

○ Health card and pen to mark.

Steps Involved

○ Establish a rapport with parent and child

○ Explain the procedure

○ Ask for health card to know the previous weight and glance at weight gain

○ Place the scale on firm surface or floor like tile or wood. Do not place the scale in uneven place

○ Have the child remove shoes and any heavy clothing, such as sweaters

○ Have the child or teen stand with both feet in the center of the scale

○ Record the weight to the nearest decimal fraction

○ Inform the mother about child's weight and gain over the previous weight using road to health card (if mother has one such and handed to you)

○ Compare the actual weight with the expected weight and provide health education accordingly

○ Record weight as per agency policy (In the health card or individual record).

Measuring Weight at Home

Where Salter weighing scale is not available weight of the toddlers and preschoolers can be checked by using electronic-weighing machine.

MEASURING VITAL SIGNS

Oral Temperature Using Community Health Nursing Bag

Steps Involved

○ Take out the newspaper from the outer opened flap, spread it on the flat surface, and place the bag on it.

○ Even a plastic square can be used to place the bag.

○ Get a newspaper from the family or from the outer cover and make a paper bag for discarding the soiled cotton and place it at one corner of the newspaper since you need to have the clean space on your paper to place other articles.

○ Explain the importance of paper bag to the family and keep the paper bag stand at one corner of the newspaper.

○ Remove your watch and pin it in your sari. Students who use salwar-kameez as uniform can pin accordingly.

○ Identify suitable washing area with the help of the family member and keep your towel and soap dish there.

○ Wash your hands with soap and water and scrub for 3–5 minutes following hand washing technique. If tap water is available it is easy to wash. Otherwise, you can use a mug from family and help yourself.

○ Be economic in using the water especially in places with water scarcity.

○ Air dry or use towel to dry your hands.

○ Go to working area where your bag is placed. Lift the unzipped outer covering of the upper compartment of your bag using your elbow.

- Now open the inner cardboard lining by holding the small piece of cloth attached at the center of the cardboard lining.
- Now take out the items from the bag for performing the specific procedure (oral temperature).
- Items needed for checking oral temperature: Oral thermometer, two cotton balls, a long layer of cotton to disinfect thermometer and spirit. Place these on the newspaper.
- Now close inner cardboard lining of the bag to avoid contamination.
- Go with the oral thermometer to the place where your wash items are placed.
- Wash the oral thermometer in running cold water or wash by pouring water.
- Take a cotton ball while is placed on the newspaper and wipe the thermometer from bulb to stem and have it in your hand.
- By explaining the procedure with client's permission keep the thermometer under the tongue and ask the patient to close the mouth carefully and use lip grip over the thermometer.
- Give a 3 minutes period of time.
- After 3 minutes remove the thermometer, read the temperature at eye level and wipe it from stem to bulb with the same cotton used for drying the thermometer.
- Discard the used cotton into paper bag.
- Now take long strip of cotton and thermometer to washing area. Apply soap to long strip of cotton, wrap the thermometer in it and leave safely for 10–15 minutes.
- Wash hands and come back to the place where bag is kept.
- Now you can use the time effectively to collect history or health educate individual or do physical or nutritional assessment.
- After around 10–15 minutes of time pickup the thermometer wrapped in the soapy cotton and provide spiral motion toward the bulb and pull out the thermometer with the other hand.
- Now rinse the thermometer with water, dry it with cotton ball, clean it with spirit, and replace it in its case, leave it on newspaper. Wash your hands thoroughly.
- Replace thermometer and spirit.
- Close the inner cardboard lining and do not zip upper lining. Take the paper bag to wash area and discard soapy swab into paper bag.
- Close the paper bag with its flap and give it to family member for discarding (burning).
- Bring soap dish and the towel pack replace them in the outer side pocket and zip.
- Now close bag's upper lining and pull the zips from both the sides so that the zips remain in the middle.

- Now hang the bag on your shoulder and pickup the paper and fold it in such a way so that the side which contacted the floor surface goes inside.
- Do not forget to dry your towel once you return back to center.

Measuring Blood Pressure

Purpose: To assess systolic and diastolic arterial blood pressure.

Equipment: Sphygmomanometer with cuff, stethoscope, antiseptic solution to clean the diaphragm or bell of the stethoscope and paper bag.

Procedure

- Explain the procedure to the patient or relative.
- Locate a place to assemble the equipment at a convenient work area.
- Expose the patient's arm above the elbow.
- Tell the patient to be at ease and keep his or her arms relaxed.
- Place the compression bag over the inner aspect of the arm, approximately 1 inch above the elbow. (Before the application squeeze and expel excess air out.)
- Firmly secure the strap of VELCRO sleeve band. Adjust the manometer at eye level.
- Palpate for the pulsation of brachial artery at the antecubital area.
- Tighten the screw that is located on the bulb.
- Squeeze the bulb to inflate the pressure cuff until the brachial artery can no longer be palpated.
- Now inflate the cuff to a mercury reading of 20–30 mm Hg above the point where the pulse disappeared.
- Place the diaphragm or bell of the stethoscope over the patient's brachial artery where the pulse was palpated. (The bell transmits low-pitched arterial blood sounds more effectively than the diaphragm.)
- Place the tips of the stethoscope in your ears, with the tips pointing down and forward.
- Slowly release the pressure valve of the inflation bulb, permitting the mercury to fall at a rate of 2–3 mm Hg per second.
- Listen for pulse sounds.
- Note the reading where the first pulsation sound is heard. It is the systolic pressure.
- Continue to release the pressure slowly, until the last pulsation is heard. This is the diastolic pressure.
- Allow the pressure to fall rapidly to zero, and remove the cuff.

○ Wipe the bell or diaphragm of the stethoscope with an antiseptic solution to prevent cross-contamination.

○ Discard the soiled swab into paper bag and dispose it safely.

MENSTRUAL CYCLE

○ Many health concerns in women are closely related to normal changes or abnormalities of the menstrual cycle. Many of these problems occur as a result of lack of awareness on (1) menstrual cycle, (2) developmental changes, and other factors that may have an impact on the pattern of the menstrual cycle.

○ Community health nurses have a responsible role in educating women about the menstrual cycle and the changes that may occur over time. She also focuses on adolescent girls who have inadequate or no knowledge about menstrual cycle.

○ The appropriate time to start teaching should be prior to menarche. Therefore, the adolescents will be adequately prepared about the menstruation and the lifelong changes in the menstrual cycle. This teaching would gain their confidence prepare them to anticipate and accept the changes as normal physiological process and part of any girl's life.

○ Menstruation is a cyclic process of vaginal flow from tissue that lines the uterus. It occurs about every 28 days during the reproductive years.

○ Normal cycles can vary from 21 to 42 days. The flow usually lasts 4–5 days, during which time 50–60 mL of blood is lost.

Definitions

Menstruation: Sloughing and discharge of the lining of the uterus, if conception does not take place.

Menarche: Beginning of menstrual function.

Estrogen: Hormone that develops and maintains the female reproductive system.

Progesterone: Hormone produced by the corpus luteum.

○ **Follicle-stimulating hormone (FSH):** Hormone released by the pituitary gland to stimulate estrogen production and ovulation.

○ The two **gonadotropic hormones** released from the pituitary gland, FSH and LH.

○ Follicle-stimulating hormone (FSH) stimulates the ovaries to secrete estrogen. Luteinizing hormone (LH) stimulates progesterone production.

○ Elevated estrogen levels in the blood reduce FSH secretion but promote LH secretion, whereas elevated progesterone levels reduce LH secretion.

○ In addition, gonadotropin-releasing hormone (GnRH) from the hypothalamus affects the rate of FSH and LH release.

Phases of Menstrual Cycle (Fig. 1)

○ During **proliferative phase**, just after menstruation, FSH increases in levels → stimulating estrogen secretion → Endometrium thickens and become more vascular.

○ In the **secretory phase** (day 14 in a 28–day cycle) LH increases, → stimulating **ovulation**.

○ Combined stimulus from estrogen + progesterone → Endometrium thickens more with increased vascularization.

○ The **luteal phase** → secretion of progesterone from the corpus luteum occurs. → If the ovum is fertilized → estrogen and progesterone levels remain high → hormonal changes of **pregnancy** occurs.

○ If the ovum has not been fertilized → FSH and LH level falls → estrogen and progesterone secretion falls → the ovum disintegrates → endometrium is thick and congested, become hemorrhagic. This is actually the old blood, mucus, and endometrial tissue → Flows through the cervix and into the vagina.

○ After the menstrual flow stops, the cycle begins again.

Psychological Preparation

○ Not to feel bad it is only a physiological period not a sickness

○ Every girl has this.

○ Breast tenderness and fullness before menstruation begins

○ Some may have fatigue, discomfort in the lower back, legs, and pelvis on first day

○ On the first day, mood changes are common.

Community Health Nurse as Care Provider

○ Menstruation has many cultural-related issues so she needs to be culturally sensitive

○ Community health nurse needs to understand about the beliefs, attitude and practices of the community.

Advise by Community Health Nurse

○ Regular exercise

○ Low-fat vegetarian diet

○ Heating pads may be very effective for cramps

○ Nonsteroidal anti-inflammatory drugs (NSAIDs).

○ Any woman with excessive cramping or dysmenorrhea is refer to hospital to get consultation from gynecologist.

○ Hygiene
  ▫ Advise all ladies to keep self and her genitals clean
  ▫ Use clean cotton cloth pieces or cotton pads for better absorption of the blood and to maintain hygiene
  ▫ Take bath at least twice a day
  ▫ Not to use soiled cloth
  ▫ Change cloth/pads, based on the need and amount of bleeding

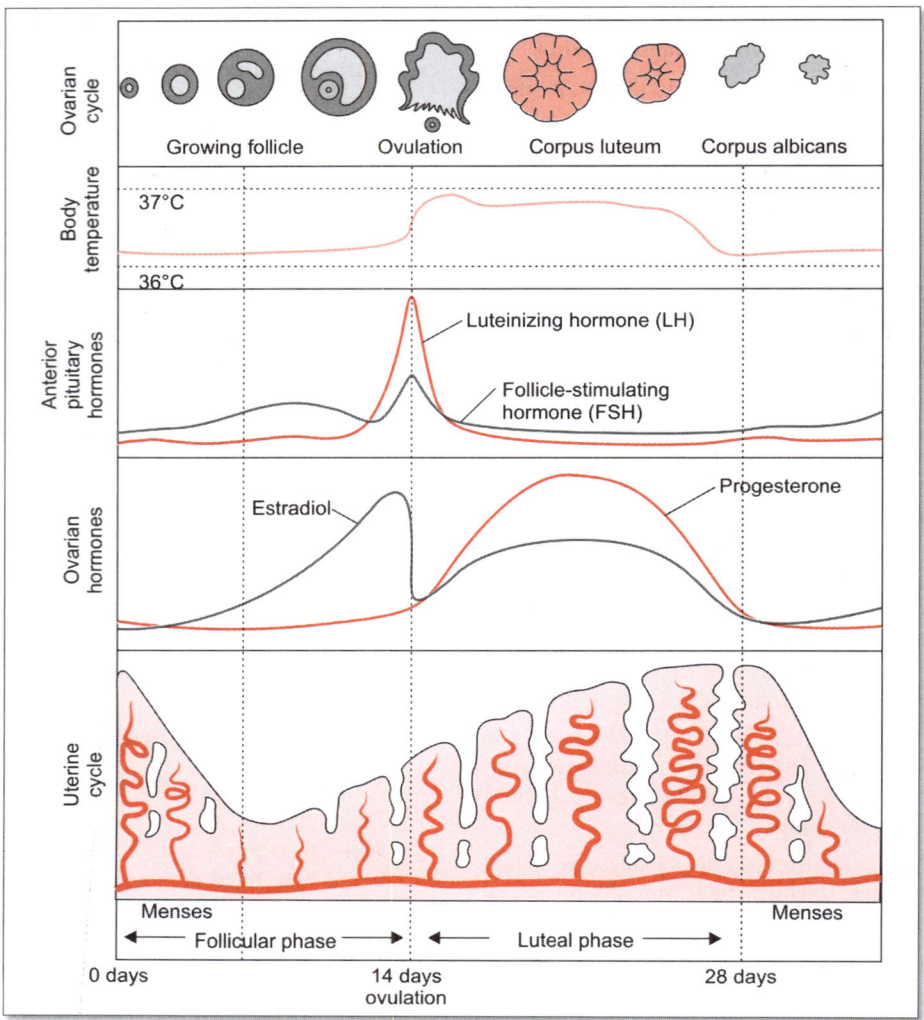

Figure 1: Phases of menstrual cycle

- Wash perineum with clean water before changing the pad
- Wash hands with soap and water after changing
- Use clean underwear and garments
- Dispose used cloth/pad by wrapping it in paper into a dustbin
- Do not dispose the soiled pads into the toilet and drains it may get blocked
- Do not throw the blood soaked cloth pieces here and there. Instead dispose it properly.
- Clean your bathroom, wash your clothing and dry under the sun.

Breast Self-Examination (BSE)

Breast self-examination (BSE) is performed to detect the carcinoma of breast at early stage itself. Therefore, the woman can undergo an appropriate treatment.

Ideally, it is advisable to perform a BSE between 7 and 10 days after the first day of menstrual period. As the breasts are less lumpy and tender at this time to perform self-examination. Pregnant women or others who have no longer menstrual cycles, can perform BSE at any time, but they need to perform this at same time each month. Breastfeeding women should perform BSE monthly at the same time of each month. Any time of the day is okay for BSE and it takes only a few minutes. A woman should somehow find time and privacy to do this.

Following are the steps to follow while performing breast self-examination

- Stand undressed from the waist up in front of a full-length mirror with your arms relaxed at your sides. Even this can be performed in sitting position. Any changes can be noted on the breast by mating a visual screening. Any changes noticed should be notified to health care provider.

○ Compare both breasts by turning from side-to-side. Look for any change in breast size, shape, skin texture or color. Any redness, dimpling and retraction should be noted.

○ Look for nipple changes, like scaliness, pulling to one side, or a change in direction.

○ Place your hands on your waist and press inward then turn from side-to-side to note any changes. One who is unable to place her hands on waist, try clasping hands together in front of the body that helps in tightening the chest muscles.

○ Try different positions, such as putting your hands above your head and turning side-to-side as you look.

○ Place your hands at your waist and stoop toward the mirror, letting your breasts fall forward. Note any changes in breast shape.

○ Look for any nipple discharge by assessing your bra or clothing. Do not squeeze the nipple or do not try to expel any secretions. Notify your health care provider if you notice any discharge.

○ Feel with your fingers for pea- and bean-sized lumps or thickening above or below your collarbone. Use skin cream or lotion to make it easy.

○ Check for lumps or thickening under your arm while relaxing your arm at your side. Reach across with your other hand to feel the area. Check deeply up and down the inside of the armpit, and up and forward toward your chest. Note any changes from previous self-exams.

Lie on the bed to perform the followings:

○ Place a pillow or folded towel under your left shoulder to help your breast tissue spread evenly across your chest wall. Bend your left arm behind your head. Reach across with your right hand to your left breast.

○ Examine your armpit by moving your three middle fingers together using light, medium and deep pressures.

○ Your hand should move in straight rows to cover all the breast tissue from the line where your blouse seam would fall (mid-axillary line) to the bra line, the breastbone (sternum) and collarbone (clavicle). Then, repeat on the other side.

Breast Cancer Screening Guidelines

For women with no unusual risk factors or breast problems:

○ A monthly breast self-examination for woman of age 20–39 years

○ A clinical breast examination every 1–3 years by a trained health professional

For women age 40 and older

○ A monthly breast self-examination

○ A yearly clinical breast examination by a trained health professional

○ A yearly screening mammogram starting at age of 40 years.

TESTICULAR SELF-EXAMINATION

Testicular self-examination (TSE) plays a major role in the early detection of testicular cancer.

Purposes: To find testicular cancer at an early stage itself.

Steps in Performing TSE (Fig. 2)

○ Choose a separate room for privacy where there is a full-sized mirror.

○ Undress and stand in front of the mirror.

○ Use both hands to palpate the testis. The normal testicle is smooth and uniform in consistency.

○ Place your index and middle fingers under the testis and the thumb on top, roll the testis gently in a horizontal plane between the thumb and fingers. Feel for any small lump or abnormality.

○ Now palpate upward along the testis using same said procedure.

○ Familiarize yourself by locating and palpating the epididymis, a cord-like structure on the top and back of the testicle that stores and transports sperm. Also locate and palpate the spermatic cord. This is to avoid suspecting as lump; it is natural structure.

○ Repeat the examination for the other testis, epididymis, and spermatic cord. It is normal to find that one testis being larger than the other.

○ If you find any small, pea-like lump or if the testis is swollen (possibly from an infection or tumor), consult your physician.

Frequency of Performing TSE

Perform TSE once in a month. The test is neither difficult nor time consuming.

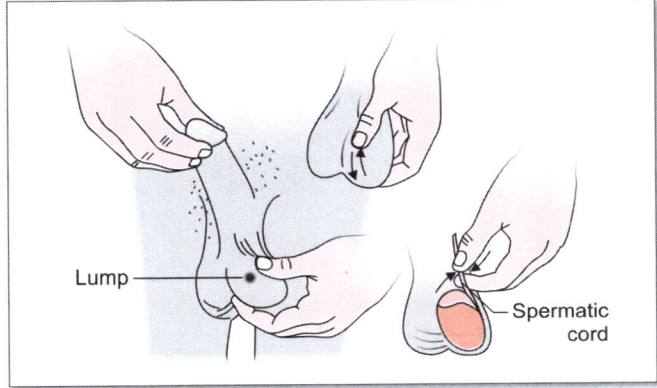

Figure 2: Performing testicular self-examination

WARNING SIGNS OF VARIOUS DISEASES

Breast Cancer

- Lump, hard knot or thickening
- Swelling, warmth, redness or darkening
- Change in the size or shape
- Dimpling or puckering of the skin
- Itchy, scaly sore or rash on the nipple
- Pulling in of your nipple or other parts
- Nipple discharge that starts suddenly
- New pain in one spot that does not go away.

Diabetes

- Increased thirst
- Increased hunger (especially after eating)
- Dry mouth
- Frequent urination or urine infections
- Unexplained weight loss (even though you are eating and feel hungry)
- Fatigue (weak, tired feeling)
- Blurred vision
- Headache

Cancer

To remember the seven early warning signs of cancer, think of the word CAUTION

1. **C**hange in bowel or bladder habits
2. **A** sore that does not heal
3. **U**nusual bleeding or discharge
4. **T**hickening or lump in the breast, testicles or elsewhere
5. **I**ndigestion or difficulty swallowing
6. **O**bvious change in the size, color, shape, or thickness of a wart, mole, or mouth sore
7. **N**agging cough or hoarseness.

Mouth Cancer

- Mouth ulcers which are sore and not getting healed for weeks
- Long-term lumps in the mouth with no obvious cause
- Long-term lumps in the lymph glands in the neck
- Difficulty in swallowing (dysphagia)
- Voice changes
- Speech problems
- Unexplained weight loss
- Unexplained bleeding in the mouth
- Feeling of numbness in the mouth
- Problems in moving the jaw.

Ovarian Cancer

Although ovarian cancer rarely produces symptoms in its earliest stages, eventual the warning signs may include:

- Persistent back and pelvic pain
- Swollen abdomen with persistent pain
- Persistent bloating
- Difficulty eating, feeling full up quickly
- Feeling nauseous
- Urinating more often
- Change in bowel habits
- Extreme fatigue
- Abnormal vaginal bleeding
- Weight loss.

Cervical Cancer

- Excessive irregular bleeding per vagina
- Irregular periods
- Bleeding after sex
- Pain or discomfort during sex
- Postmenopausal bleeding
- Unusual and/or unpleasant vaginal discharge
- Persistent lower backache.

Dengue

- Abdominal pain or tenderness
- Persistent vomiting
- Mucosal bleeding
- Lethargy/restlessness
- Liver enlargement.

Tuberculosis

- Cough lasting for more than 2 weeks
- Unintentional weight loss
- Fever and night sweat
- Loss of appetite.

In advanced cases:

- Chest pain, or pain with breathing or coughing
- Coughing up blood.

Severe Hypertension

- Feeling confused or other neurological symptoms
- Nosebleeds
- Fatigue
- Blurred vision
- Chest pain
- Abnormal heartbeat.

Cardinal Symptoms of Pregnancy-Induced Hypertension

- Pedal edema
- Proteinuria
- Increased blood pressure.

Preeclampsia

In addition to edema, proteinuria, and hypertension, pre-eclampsia will show the following cardinal symptoms:

- Abdominal pain
- Severe headache
- Rapid weight gain due increase in bodily fluid
- Change in reflexes
- No urine or low urine output
- Dizziness
- Excessive vomiting
- Vision changes.

LAB INVESTIGATIONS

Testing for Urine Sugar

Though all the lab-related works are specifically carried out in labs and by lab technicians some of the basic procedures are carried out by community health nurse to help people at home.

Purpose

- As a diagnostic procedure to identify new cases with certain disease symptoms.
- To perform as s routine urine test in acute and chronic conditions like diabetes.
- To identify gestational diabetes.

Articles Required

Benedict's solution, test tube, test tube stand, test tube holder, match box, dispensing plastic cup (ounce cup) filler and a spirit lamp, and a specimen bottle from the house with clean-catch urine.

Steps Involved

- Take out the newspaper from the outer opened flap, spread it on the flat surface, and place the bag on it.
- Even a plastic square can be used to place the bag.
- Explain the importance of paper bag to the family and keep the paper bag stand at one corner of the newspaper.
- Remove your watch and pin it in your sari.
- Explain the procedure of catching clean urine specimen by getting a small bottle or a plastic container from the family.

- Unzip the upper compartment, do not open it.
- Unzip the lower compartment.
- Unzip the side pocket and remove the soap from a soap dish and towel.
- Identify suitable washing area with the help of the family member and keep your towel and soap dish there.
- Wash your hands with soap and water and scrub for 3–5 minutes following hand-washing technique.
- If tap water is available it is easy to wash. Otherwise, you can use a mug from family and help yourself.
- Be economic in using the water in especially in places that have water scarcity.
- Air dry or use towel to dry your hands.
- Go to working area where your bag is placed. Lift the unzipped outer covering of the upper compartment using your elbow.
- Now open the inner cardboard lining by holding the small piece of cloth attached at the center of the cardboard lining.
- Take out the Benedict's solution and place it at one corner of the newspaper and close the cardboard lining of the upper compartment.
- Unzip the lower compartment and take out test tube, test tube stand, dispensing cup to measure the Benedict's solution, spirit lamp, match box and a small mackintosh.
- Measure 5 mL of Benedict's solution using dispensing cup and pour into the test-tube.
- Keep the test tube with solution in the stand.
- Take and arrange these items at the backyard or the place away from the living area or locate the area to place items with the help of family members.
- Fix the test tube in the holder and keep in the stand.
- Light the spirit lamp.
- Holding the test tube with the holder, heat it over a spirit lamp till the Benedict's solution boils without over-flowing. After heating a while, if there is any color change seen, discard the solution and re-do with solution from other bottle.
- Now take urine from the specimen container using a filler.
- Add 8 drops of urine into the Benedict's solution that is boiling.
- Boil the mixture again and allow it to cool under tap water.
- While cooking, the mixture changes color.
- The change of color of the mixture serves as a guide to the amount of sugar present in the urine. The guidelines to interpret urine sugar is shown in the Figure 3.

- Blue—sugar absent
- Green—0.5% sugar
- Yellow—1% sugar
- Orange—1.5% sugar
- Brick red—2% or more sugar.

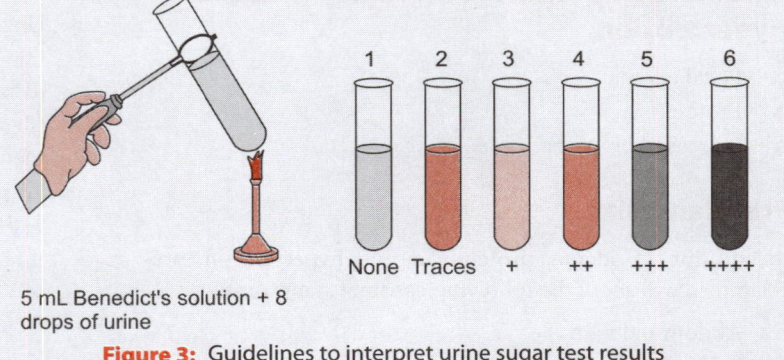

The guidelines to interpret the result
1. No change in color i.e. blue: Absence of sugar.
2. Pale green with slightly cloudy: Trace
3. Definite cloudy green: 1+
4. Yellow: 2 +
5. Orange: 3 +
6. Brick red: 4 +

5 mL Benedict's solution + 8 drops of urine

None Traces + ++ +++ ++++

Figure 3: Guidelines to interpret urine sugar test results

❍ Show the reading to the patient and tell the results.

❍ Wash your articles and dry.

❍ Wash your hands thoroughly and air dry.

❍ Take the Benedict's solution container and replace it into the upper compartment by lifting the inner lining of the cardboard.

❍ Cover the upper lining and zip it.

❍ Collect the articles test tube, test-tube stand, filler, spirit lamp, match box, etc. from the wash area and place it in the lower compartment and close the zip.

❍ Now go and wash your hands and bring back the towel and soap and replace into the side pocket and zip it.

❍ Give if any instructions and tell about your plan for next visit.

❍ Now take the bag and pickup the newspaper by touching the outer portion and fold it in such a way so that the surface that came in contact with the floor goes in.

❍ Refer the patient to hospital, if needed, based on the report.

Testing for Urine Albumin (Cold Method)

Normally, healthy people's urine does not contain protein. But protein may be found to get excreted in the urine when the kidneys do not function properly or due to some other diseases. Community health nurses can opt for testing albumin in urine based on the presented signs and symptoms.

Purposes

❍ As a diagnostic measure to assess the amount of protein present in urine

❍ As a part of routine urinalysis

❍ To assess pregnant mothers.

Articles Required

Sulpha salicylic acid, test-tube, test-tube stand, test-tube holder, match box, dispensing plastic cup (ounce cup) filler and a spirit lamp and a specimen bottle from the house with clean-catch urine.

Steps Involved

❍ Take out the newspaper from the outer opened flap, spread it on the flat surface and place the bag on it.

❍ Even a plastic square can be used to place the bag.

❍ Explain the importance of paper bag to the family and keep the paper bag stand at one corner of the newspaper.

❍ Remove your watch and pin it in your sari.

❍ Explain the procedure of catching clean urine specimen by getting a small bottle or a plastic container from the family.

❍ Unzip the upper compartment, do not open it.

❍ Unzip the lower compartment.

❍ Unzip the side pocket and take out from a the soap soap dish and towel.

❍ Identify suitable washing area with the help of the family member and keep your towel and soap dish there.

❍ Wash your hands with soap and water and scrub for 3–5 minutes following hand-washing technique.

❍ If tap water is available it is easy to wash. Otherwise you can use a mug from family and help yourself.

❍ Be economic in using the water and especially in places of water scarcity.

❍ Air dry or use towel to dry your hands.

❍ Go to working area where your bag is placed. Lift the unzipped outer covering of the upper compartment using your elbow.

❍ Now open the inner cardboard lining by holding the small piece of cloth attached at the center of the cardboard lining.

❍ Take out the sulphur salicylic acid and place it on the newspaper and close the cardboard lining of the upper compartment.

❍ Unzip the lower compartment and take out test tube, test-tube stand, filler, sulphur salicylic acid and a small mackintosh.

❍ Take equal small amount of sulphur salicylic acid and urine in the test-tube (each one finger height in the test tube by measuring with your finger).

- Allow it stand for 5 minutes and observe the turbidity.
- If there is no change in the mixture it indicates the absence of albumin.
- If the mixture turns turbid at the upper portion, it indicates the presence of albumin.

> **Grading of turbidity:**
> Assess against dark background
> 1+ Dense cloudiness.
> 2+ Cloudiness with granules and definite flocculation.
> 3+ Cloudiness with flocculation.
> 4+ Cloudiness with precipitation.

- Show it to the patient and convey the result and follow-up measures.
- Wash the articles and dry it. Wash your hands.
- Go to your working area and place the sulphur salicylic acid in upper compartment using the principles.
- Close inner and outer lining and zip the upper compartment.
- Go to wash area and collect test tube, stand and mackintosh and place it into the lower compartment and close the zip.
- Wash and wipe your hands and place in side pocket.
- Record the findings and perform a related health teaching session.
- Tell about your next visit.

Blood Glucose/Sugar Testing

In more recent years, self-care management of diabetes became comparatively easy because of improved technology, various campaigns on diabetes, interest from governmental and nongovernmental organizations and involvement of community health nurses in causing awareness and promoting self-care abilities of people in the community. Earlier, primarily diabetes was identified by measuring urine sugars, which were very unreliable. Nowadays, most people /patients in the community check their blood glucose levels using self-administered devices.

Purposes of Monitoring Blood Sugar at Home

- To diagnose or as a part of routine check (master checkup)
- To check the glucose levels of patients with diabetes
- To prevent the occurrence of hypoglycemia (low blood sugars) during the night.
- To improve sugar control
- To know effects of some food items and exercises on blood glucose levels
- To have the sense of control on foods

- To check blood glucose in pregnancy as a prophylactic measure.

Guidelines for Testing Blood Sugar/Glucose Level

Fasting blood sugar (FBS), drawn after at least an 8-hour fast, to evaluate circulating amounts of glucose; postprandial test, drawn usually 2 hours after a well-balanced meal, to evaluate glucose metabolism; and random glucose, drawn at any time, nonfasting.

- **Fasting glucose:** Advise patient to maintain 8-hour fast overnight; can have sips of water.

  Advise patient to avoid smoking before the blood-glucose sampling as this affects the test results.
- **For postprandial test:** Advise patient that not to eat during the 2-hour interval.
- **Random blood glucose:** Note the time and content of the last meal.

Procedure

- Check the physician's order.
- Provide privacy and explain the procedure.
- Wash hands; hand washing decreases the spread of microorganisms.
- Do not clean gloves as a protective barrier.
- Select suitable site to puncture.
- In adults mostly the outer aspect of side of finger is selected since it is most vascular and has only fewer nerve endings. Heels and toes are more frequently used sites for infants.
- Choose site for finger stick and massage toward puncture site to increase blood flow to site.
- Cleanse with alcohol swab and leave to dry to reduce bacteria on skin surface from invading puncture site.
- Place automated lancet firmly against side of finger, and gently press the activating button.
- Wipe away the first drop of blood since it has more serum, which can dilute blood and may alter results.
- Stroke from base of finger, toe, or heel to puncture site. Do not squeeze puncture site.
- Stroking in a massaging motion will increase blood flow; squeezing will increase serum and dilute specimen.
- Now fill capillary tube with blood by placing tip of tube at base of drop of blood; or if using reagent strip, place next to blood drop, making sure that enough blood is absorbed by the strip for accurate results.
- Apply pressure to puncture site for 15–30 seconds with gauze to stop bleeding.

- If using a glucose meter, allow blood to stay on strip for specified time and then place in meter for digital readout.
- Compare patient's value with normal lab values.
- Inspect puncture site for further bleeding.
- Record the finding as per agency's policy and inform the results to the patient.

Note: Glucometers come to market with different styles and techniques.

Teaching patient: General steps are:

- Ask patient to wash his hands thoroughly; air dry.
- Insert a test strip into glucometer. While inserting keep the glucometer on.
- In some glucometers we have to an on-off the switch.
- Select the side of your fingertip near the fingernail to avoid soreness at the end of your finger.
- Using a lancet, prick your fingertip.
- Gently squeeze or massage your finger until a drop of blood forms.
- Touch and hold the edge of the test strip to the drop of blood.
- Glucometer will "beep" when there is enough blood.
- Blood sugar result will appear on the glucometer-display.
- If glucometer has storing facilities—set date and time and store results.
- Show your record when you visit hospital.

Interpretation of Blood Values as Diagnostic for Diabetes Mellitus

- FBS greater than or equal to 126 mg/dL on two occasions
- Random blood sugar greater than or equal to 200 mg/dL and presence of classic symptoms of diabetes (polyuria, polydipsia, polyphagia, and weight loss)
- Fasting blood glucose result of greater than or equal to 100 mg/dL demands close follow-up and repeat monitoring every 1–2 years.

Improper Results

This may occur due to:

- Dirty glucometer
- Glucometer or test strip that is not at room temperature
- Outdated test strips
- Too much or too little blood on the test strip
  Care should be taken to avoid the above.

SEEK HEALTH SERVICES

Routine Checkup

- Though health care providers try on moving the health care at the doorsteps of the people, there is no guarantee on how far people are willing to come forward for seeking health services. It is increasingly important to learn the factors that facilitate or impede the appropriate utilization of routine health care services.
- It is a well-known fact that the knowledge, health beliefs and attitudes of people predispose the use or avoidance of health care services. For example, people who disbelieve in medical care may not visit service facility or receive any routine checkup or preventive services.
- Uneducated patients very rarely seek preventive care.
- People with socially unacceptable health-related practices like alcoholics, smokers and drug addicts may not want to see the medical practitioners.
- People with (the symptoms worry them more or intolerable) real need most likely to seek routine health services.
- Some religious beliefs do not allow them use medicine or undergo surgeries.
- People with known chronic disease, postsurgeries seeks routine services.
- Poor people avoid health services due to unaffordability.
- Mothers and babies are the most seen people in the clinics and dispensaries.

Good Practices to Enhance Health Seeking in Patients

Research evidence shows the following measures to help people come for routine checkup:

- Creating awareness
- Health care providers and professionals should use friendly approach
- Health professionals should be unbiased
- Health professionals should listen patiently
- Long-wait times not appreciated. Increase the number of clinicians
- Progression should be explained
- Schedules should be announced (clinic schedule and timing).

Immunization

Vaccines are available for many of the communicable diseases in children. Some of the examples for vaccine preventable diseases are measles, poliomyelitis, tuberculosis, diphtheria, tetanus, whooping cough, mumps and rubella etc.

It is essential for all children in a community should receive full course of immunization for the mentioned diseases. When a child gets a disease, it not only affects the child but also may cause outbreak in the community. In addition, these diseases may become fatal or may cause serious consequences like blindness, partial paralysis, etc.

Barriers to Immunization

Fear of poking the small baby: Family may be afraid due to various reasons like:

○ The baby may cry whole day
○ It will be very painful
○ Reactions (fever, swelling, etc.) are dangerous
○ Bad consequences learnt from neighbors
○ Suspicious on syringes and needles due fear of transmission of HIV
○ No time to visit-clinics as the clinics generally work in the busy work time.

How to Overcome Barriers?

○ Conduct meeting with village leaders and mothers
○ Decide upon convenient time to conduct immunization clinics
○ Provide effective health education and achieve full coverage of children to avoid epidemics
○ Provide information on clinic services and outreach services for immunization
○ Disseminate the list of children due for vaccine
○ Make immunization by following all the principles of immunization
○ The community health nurse should have adequate training to administer vaccine; faulty techniques may lead to harmful effects.

Counseling

On certain occasions counseling becomes necessary as part of health services.

Counseling is a kind of talking therapy that permits a person to express their problems and feelings in a confidential and dependable environment. Counseling is suggested when a person needs help to deal with and overcome issues that are causing emotional pain.

Community health nurses refers the following clients to seek counseling:

○ Person with a relationship breakdown
○ Work-related stress
○ To explore sexual identity
○ Person with ambitions but cannot reach heights
○ Feelings of sadness or depression

○ Person who is with high level anxiety

Counseling sessions are:

○ Face-to-face
○ Individual or in a group
○ Over the phone
○ By email
○ Specialized computer program

When need arise community health nurse should refer the person to a counselor.

Diagnosis and Treatment

Early detection of health impairment is defined as "the detection of disturbances of homeostatic and compensatory mechanism while biochemical, morphological and functional changes are still reversible."   —(**WHO expert committee**)

Early detection of the disease and treatment of the problem refers to secondary level care. Primary level care tries to prevent the disease and promote health. Actually early detection and treatment are the main interventions to control disease.

At many times, patients do not attend laboratory investigations to know their disease; even diagnosed and put on treatment many may default the treatment. Most importantly is the patient has to take his treatment regularly without defaulting.

Early diagnosis and treatment is not that effective and economical as a "primary prevention mode". But it is critically important in certain communicable and noncommunicable diseases. They are:

○ Communicable diseases—Tuberculosis, STDs and leprosy
○ Noncommunicable diseases—Essential hypertension, cancer breast and cervix.

For example:

○ At many times people may not want to come for investigations to know their diagnosis. This is basically, due to the fear. Sputum coughing patient does not want his sputum to be tested.
○ Defaulting will not cure the disease. Most TB and leprosy patients are defaulters.
○ Suspected HIV persons do not want their blood to be tested. They do not want their disease to be revealed.

Various reasons for defaulting:

○ Has no money
○ Fear of the diagnosis (HIV, TB, STDs, etc.)
○ No transportation facilities
○ No one to help in the family
○ Family commitments

○ Work—no leave
○ Do not like to swallow medicine
○ Stomach burns
○ Feel healthy
○ Side effects are more.

Role of Community Health Nurse in Diagnosis and Treatment

○ Early effective therapy helps in shortening the period of communicability and reduces the mortality rates in the community. Community health nurses should be actively engaged in early diagnosis and treatment disease
○ Provide health information during home visit as well in mass campaigns
○ Periodical mass education programs
○ Causing awareness through holding meetings with the community leaders, women self-help groups and *mahila mandals*
○ Coordinate with NGOs activities that focus on secondary level interventions
○ Health educating couples at the same time
○ Teaching on breast self-examination, testicular self-examination
○ Motivating men and women to seek health care when they have some problems
○ Stress on the importance of compliance on treatment prescribed
○ Arrange specific health camps based on the need
○ Follow-up measures will help in observing and health educating the patients. Follow-up helps in continued care and surveillance.
○ Follow-up is considered for infected persons until they are no longer a threat to communicate disease to others.

Follow-up

Monitoring (or follow-up) activities are the backbone of community health nurses to empower individual, family and community to involve in the care.

An assessment of the patient's condition would help the community health nurse for planning her follow-up visits. Example—Antenatal, postnatal newborn, infant, preschooler, morbidities, etc.

Otherwise, based on certain factors the community health nurse plans her follow-up visits and the frequency with which those visits may need to be made.

○ **Current health status:** Signs of progression in health
○ Presence of any serious signs and symptoms

○ **Home environment:** *Availability of* family or friends to provide care, or he is alone
○ **Self-care abilities**
○ Level of independence
○ Patient is ambulatory or bedridden
○ **Level of nursing care needed:** The level of nursing care required
○ **Patient education needs:** The level of patient or family grasped the teaching points made
○ **Further follow-up** and retraining needed
○ **Mental status:** Alertness of the patient
○ **Level of adherence:** *P*atient and family level of compliance in following the instructions provided
○ **Help:** Help extended from family members.

MAINTENANCE OF HEALTH RECORDS FOR INDIVIDUAL AND FAMILY

Today's word of importance is quality. The health services should assure quality and should be ambitious to provide evidence based practice. Failing to assure quality, equals to fail in all further tasks. Any paid health services fall under the umbrella of "Consumer Act." Community health nurses who live in the community and learn with the community on many issues that may come to her way. She is bound to answer on care and follow-up services of the community assigned for her.

One of the most important tasks of the community health nurse is the maintenance of records and reports for the population she serves.

Salient Features

○ Records consists of health problems and needs of individual
○ Measures (preventive and promotive and rehabilitative) taken so far
○ Cultural beliefs, attitudes and practices of the individual and family that provides a platform to plan for health education
○ Records also help us to reinforce health teaching if needs felt or observed.

Purposes

○ It is first of all a legal document of service providing agency
○ Plans for immediate problem/need or long-term
○ It is a main data source to learn the individual's general health

○ Functions as a communication tool between health worker, family and other personnel

○ Helps in evaluating the services provided

○ Helps in assuring further improvement in quality of services.

Types of Records

There are different types of records available based on institutional policy of care. As a care provider the community health nurse should know about these records and each one's specified areas of use.

Cumulative and Continuing Records

This helps us know about the thorough history of an individual and to evaluate.

Family Records

Each family is given a family folder with a number. This folder holds all the individual records of the family members. This is a good source to learn about the health status of the members. Individuals of the family suffering with morbidities like tuberculosis is provided with special services in TB clinics.

Collecting Information

The CHN should be skillful in eliciting information from the family. She should consider many aspects specifically the schedule to collect information. People who are busy with their work may not show much interest in entertaining the CHN. Forcing for information will not end up with solid data. Use all polite techniques. Show interest in knowing from the family member. Appreciate and encourage. Slowly move with the actual purpose of the visit. Be friendly, be a good listener and be a good communicator. Continue to build confidence in subsequent visits.

Filing Records

It is easy to pick up the card if arranged with a system: Alphabetically, numerically, geographically and with index cards.

Registers

There are various registers. It was discussed in earlier chapters.

Reports

Reports are usually the analysis of some activities. (Like how many births took place in the year, how many deaths, how many antenatals registered and what was the outcome etc.).

The report compilation is done—weekly, monthly, quarterly, annually.

Purposes of Writing Report

○ To assess the quantity of services in a given year

○ To know how far the goals attained

○ To assess the health status of the community

○ To assess the utilization of services

○ To set a proposal for asking funds for further improvement in services

○ To provide the base for risk assessment in services.

CONTINUING MEDICAL CARE AND FOLLOW-UP IN COMMUNITY FOR VARIOUS DISEASES AND DISABILITIES

There are many patients (diagnosed and undiagnosed) with communicable and noncommunicable diseases in the community. Some may be regular in seeking treatment and following the medical guidelines. Many may be defaulters or do not have much awareness on their disease and treatment. Community health nurse plays a responsible role in helping the people to seek treatment, undergo investigations, and continue prescribed medications or any other therapy and do the follow-up in morbidity clinics and during home visits. She also visits people with chronic illnesses like diabetes, heart disease, TB, bronchial asthma, leprosy, hypertension, psychiatric and other illnesses at home.

Objectives of Continued Medical Care and Follow-up

To assist favorably the functional course of the long-term patient's disease.

To help the patient's adaptation to his chronic condition or disability and to his environment, and to enable him perform his social obligations in a better way.

Factors Interfering with Disease Control

○ Inadequate intensity of treatment

○ Failure to use evidence-based guidelines

○ Lack of family support

○ Noncompliant to treatment

○ No support for self-management

○ No access to care

○ No medical insurance

○ Differences in health beliefs and practices of people

○ Costs of the treatment

○ No transportation to reach clinic.

Chronic illness interventions in community rely on multidisciplinary teams functioning at the community level. At community level there are governmental and non-governmental teams functioning to help the community on their chronic disease management. There are many national health programs established mainly to follow on specific communicable and noncommunicable diseases. Examples include antimalaria program, filaria control program, diabetes control program, diarrhea control program, acute respiratory tract infection (ARI) control and tuberculosis and HIV/AIDS control program.

Diarrhea

Acute respiratory infections and diarrheal diseases are accountable for almost 50% of annual deaths that occur in under-five children, in the South-East Asia region.

It is evident from recent years that preventive strategies took a lead role in managing diarrheal diseases and ARI. High doses of oral amoxicillin given to uncomplicated pneumonias and low-osmolarity ORS and zinc administered to diarrheal cases were effective.

Mere handwashing can pull down the incidence of ARIs and diarrheal diseases by 30–50%. Improved the quality of water is another vital factor in preventing diarrhea.

Empowering the Mother on Diarrheal Management

- Identifying diarrhea based on signs and symptoms
- Administering oral rehydration solution
- If breastfeeding infant continue to feed
- Follow handwashing
- Sterilization of feeding bottles if bottle fed
- Assessment on dehydration
- Reporting immediately.

Benefits of self-care knowledge at family in managing the diarrheal cases:

- The family/care giver will identify the symptoms of diarrhea and well in advance reach the child to health facility at an earlier stage
- The family will provide home treatment as per the prescribed standard as a follow-up measure.

Frequency of Home Visit

Noncommunicable diseases like diabetes, cancer, heart disease. Based on the patient's condition community health nurse visits at least once a month.

Communicable diseases like TB, leprosy, sexually transmitted diseases (STD) community health nurse visits at least once a month.

Acute communicable diseases like measles, mumps, cholera, typhoid—A minimum of four visits depending upon the condition of the patient.

Educating and Assisting Patients during Home Visit

- Clearing the doubts about the disease, symptoms, management
- How to prevent others in case of communicable diseases. For example, TB
- Medication—action, dosage, route of administration, duration and side effects to be observed
- Drug compliance
- Diet for self and family
- Personal hygiene
- Healthful housing
- Environmental cleanliness
- Measures to prevent seasonal and environmental triggered diseases like asthma
- Causing awareness on diseases with social stigma like leprosy, TB and HIV
- Informing on availability of health services
- Importance of periodical master checkup.

CARRYOUT THERAPEUTIC PROCEDURES AS PRESCRIBED/REQUIRED FOR INDIVIDUAL AND FAMILY

Therapeutic procedures are carried out in the community family for the sake of individual or family. The community health nurse performs these procedures as per the instructions from the agency or as an identified need or as requested by the patient. Community health nurses either use community health nursing bags or use the disposable kit provided by the family for doing certain procedures, if agency policy permits.

Intramuscular Injection—Adult (Fig. 4)
Steps Involved

- Take out the newspaper from the outer opened flap, spread it on the flat surface, and place the bag on it. Even a plastic square can be used to place the bag.
- Explain the importance of paper bag to the family and keep the paper bag stand at one corner of the newspaper.
- Explain the procedure.
- Ask the patient for injection vial and prescription to check. Patient should also provide the distilled water to reconstitute the medicine in the vial.

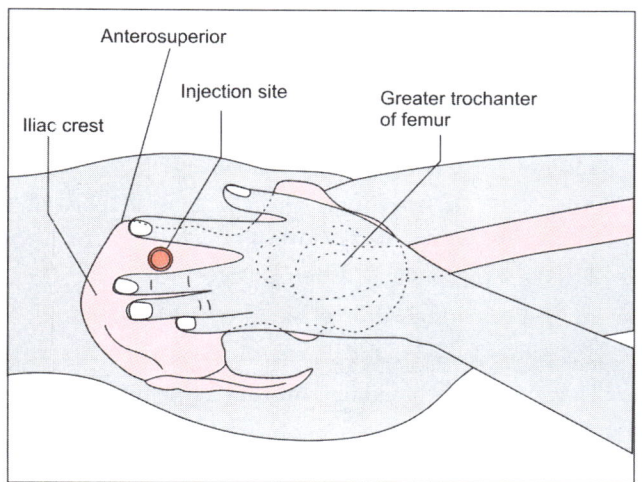

Figure 4: Intramuscular injection site in adult

- Place these on the newspaper and ask someone to take care until you return back after washing your hands.
- Remove your watch and pin it in your sari.
- Explain the procedure of catching clean urine specimen by getting a small bottle or a plastic container from the family.
- Unzip the upper compartment, do not open it.
- Unzip the side pocket and remove the soap in a soap dish and towel.
- Identify suitable washing area with the help of the family member and keep your towel and soap dish there.
- Wash your hands with soap and water and scrub for 3–5 minutes following handwashing technique. If tap water is available it is easy to wash. Otherwise you can use a mug from family and help yourself. Be economic in using the water especially in places that have water scarcity.
- Air dry or use towel to dry your hands.
- Go to working area where your bag is placed. Lift the unzipped outer covering of the upper compartment using your elbow.
- Now open the inner cardboard lining by holding the small piece of cloth attached at the center of the cardboard lining.
- Take out the spirit and two cotton swabs and disposable syringe and with needle and an extra disposable needle to withdraw, if it is a vial. Usually the pattern of practice is to receive the disposable syringe and needle from the patient to provide injection to him or her.
- Place all the articles on the newspaper and close the cardboard lining of the upper compartment.
- Wash your hands.
- Use all the rules of rights.
- Open the disposable syringe and fix the needle.
- Take distilled water and reconstitute the injection vial by wiping rubber part with spirit.

- Withdraw the correct dose and remove the needle used for withdrawing the medicine from vial and discard in the paper bag.
- Now fix another disposable sterile needle. Do not remove the cap till you reach the patient.
- Make the patient lie comfortably.
- Inject in the correct site by cleaning the area with spirit swab. Talk to the patient when you inject. Rub the site gently.
- Discard the disposable needle and cotton swab into paper bag, close it and ask the patient to burn it and discard the remains properly.
- Wash your hands thoroughly and replace the spirit by opening the inner cardboard lining and close the inner and outer lining.
- Collect the soap dish and towel and place it into the outer side pocket.
- Document the injection in the individual record, inform about your schedule for next visit, and proceed.

NOTE: Iron dextran (*Imferon*) is the major drug administered by the Z-track method: Z-track injections administered in the upper-outer quadrant of the buttocks; it should never be administered in the arm. Subsequent injections are administered alternatively in left and right buttocks.

Nasal Drops Instillation

Purpose

- To alleviate inflammation and congestion of mucous membranes
- To promote self-care in the home.

Articles

- Medication or nose drops as prescribed by the physician
- Medicine dropper
- Paper bag.

Procedure

- Place the CHN bag in suitable place
- Explain the procedure to the patient/mother/caregiver
- Make a paper bag and keep it at one corner of the paper
- Wash hands
- Place the patient with his or her head well back in a *sniffing* position
- Instill the medication directing the flow toward the floor of the nasal cavity
- Do not touch the nostril with the dropper
- Ask the patient to be in the same position for about 5 minutes to enhance the flow of medication to the lower part of the nose

o Ask patient to wipe the face and comfort him
o Discard disposable items following standard precautions
o Wash your hands
o Close the bag and clarify the doubts
o Document the procedure and reinforce teaching, if any.

Avoiding Self-Medication Errors in Patient and Family

Medication errors found to be common in elderly because many of them have multiple diseases and put on multiple medications for the same. They tend to make mistakes like taking medicines at the wrong times, taking old and out of date medicines, not taking prescribed dose or defaulting, etc. Community health nurses can help them in these conditions.

Purpose

o To provide guidelines for potential home medication errors made by the patient/caregiver
o To promote self-care in the home
o To prevent potential hazards.

Guidelines to Patient and Family

o Check the prescription and doctor's instruction
o Assess patient's compliance with the medication regimen
o Assess knowledge of family on this
o Identify if any prescribed medicine taken incorrectly or omitted
o Check the prescription and doctor's instruction
o If any medication error(s), refer the physician
o Identify the reasons for the medication error
o Teach patient and care giver about how to avoid the mistakes.

Blood-Hemoglobin Test using Sahli's Apparatus

One of the major causes of maternal mortality is anemia. As an investigative measure all the pregnant mothers should be tested for blood hemoglobin during their first antenatal visit itself. It is also essential to test adolescent girls among whom anemia is found very common. There are several methods available to test blood hemoglobin.

Articles Required

Comparator box which has brown colored two standard glass tubes on either side, a middle bi-graduated tube in the center. This central tube has two scales (percentage scale and gram per dL scale Hb pipette which is marked up to 20 mm (0.02 mL blood) glass rod dropper.

Reagents: N/10 HCL solution and distilled water.

Steps Involved

o Sahli's comparator apparatus has two standard tubes with a middle bi-graduated tube. This central tube has two scales (percentage scale and gram per dL scale). In addition there is a single mark pipette (20 µL).
o Add N/10 HCL solution into the central tube till it reaches the level of 2 in gram scale
o Clean the finger site with spirit swab
o At least get a single drop of blood
o Collect the blood in the pipette till the level of 0.02 mark
o Slowly blow the blood into the tube containing HCl
o Rinse the pipette by drawing in and blowing out the mix 3–4 times
o Mix the blood with the acid thoroughly
o Allow to stand undisturbed for 10 minutes
o Place the hemoglobin meter tube in the comparator and add distilled water to the solution drop by drop, keep stirring with the glass rod till its color matches with that of the comparator glass
o Remove the glass rod from the solution and hold vertically in the tube while matching the color
o Keep adding distilled water until it matches the color of the standard tube
o Note the reading in gram scale
o Record and show it to the patient
o Plan patient care accordingly.

Skin Suture Removal

Purpose

o To remove cutaneous sutures of surgery as per medical discharge summary (when there is no complications)
o Episiotomy sutures
o Sutures of tubectomy (Female sterilization or mini laparotomy)
o Any sutures on skin lacerations.

Equipment

o Community health bag which consists of stainless steel box with articles like thumb forceps, suture cutting scissors and stainless steel dressing cups. These articles are boiled as described in wound dressing procedure
o Sterilized cotton balls
o Sterilized gauze pieces
o Betadine or savlon as per agency's policy
o Disposable sterilized gloves (usually community health nursing bags do not have gloves). You can carry at least

few pairs of disposable gloves for meeting any routines or emergencies that needs sterile procedure

○ Paper bag to discard the soiled dressing.

Procedure

Place community health nursing bag as explained earlier in other procedures. Follow all the principles of bag technique according to the steps given below.

Steps

○ Read the discharge summary or doctor's instructions

○ Explain the procedure to the patient or a relative

○ Provide privacy in well-illuminated area

○ Make patient comfortable

○ Wash your hands and expose the site and discard the old dressing into the paper bag

○ Wash and dry you hands

○ Open the bag as per the principles and collect the articles from the bag and keep the inner lining closed

○ Wash your hands, dry and don the sterile gloves

○ Assess the wound for signs of healing. (Do not remove suture, if you feel the wound edges may separate. If any such thing observed do not proceed further and explain it to the patient).

○ Clean the sutured area with betadine (providone iodine) from dressing cup using sterile cotton

○ Hold the thumb forceps in one hand and the scissors in the other hand. Gently grasp the suture with thumb forceps

○ Slowly pull on the suture to allow entry of the scissors' blade between the suture and the skin

○ Cut the suture, and remove it by pulling smoothly with the thumb forceps

○ Repeat this until all the sutures are removed

○ Clean the incision line with antiseptic solution as per the agency policy

○ Apply a gauze dressing, if necessary or leave it open

○ Comfort the patient

○ Discard the paper bag by burning

○ Clean and replace the equipment

○ Document the healing state of the wound, any infection and discharge should be recorded

○ If any infection or malunion or gaping (episiotomy wound) found refer the patient to higher level of care.

WASTE MANAGEMENT

Basic Waste Prevention Strategies "Three –Rs"

Using various strategies "to not to waste the waste" falls in three steps like:

1. Reduce

2. Recycle

3. Reuse

The primary measure is to minimize or bring down the size or quantity of the waste that is termed as "reduce." Next is to reuse by recycling it. When there is no more possibility to prevent the waste, the volume reduction of waste is paid attention. Material is separated from the garbage for the process of recycling.

Benefits of "Three-Rs"

○ They diminish greenhouse gas discharges

○ They lessens discharge of pollutants

○ They protect and support the resources

○ They conserve energy and lessens the demand for land

○ Space and waste treatment technology.

Collection and Disposal of Waste at Home and Community

Municipal solid waste municipal solid wastes are collected by following ways:

House-to-house: Waste collectors go house to house and collect the wastes. This service is provided on payment.

Community bins: Community bins are positioned at fixed points for each area/street. Users bring and dispose their garbage in the community bin. As per schedule the assigned workers from municipality pickup the waste for disposal.

Kerbside or curbside pickup: Users places their garbage outside their homes and it is collected by the assigned workers as per the schedule.

Self-delivered: Generators deliver the waste directly to disposal sites.

Service: Municipalities often make a contract or issue license to private agencies to collect the wastes from different areas.

Treatment of Solid Waste

The main aim of treating waste is to convert the waste into a manageable form by reducing the quantity and minimizing the harmful substances so that waste disposal becomes safe.

Treatment methods are selected based on the composition, quantity and form of the waste material. Waste treatment techniques are chosen according to the volume, form and composition. Treatment methods include:

○ Thermal treatment

○ Dumps and landfills

○ Biological waste treatment

○ Integrated solid waste management.

Thermal Treatment

Using heat to treat the waste is known as the thermal method. Some methods are:

Incineration

Incineration is the most often used thermal method. In this method waste is treated by burning. Incineration converts waste into carbon dioxide, water vapor and ash. This method may be used as a means of recuperating energy to be used in the supply of electricity. There are open and closed systems of incineration. The waste is burnt in a chamber in the open system; the closed system uses a special chamber specifically planned with several parts to enable the process of incineration.

○ **Advantages**
  □ Incineration lessens the quantity of the waste
  □ Makes the waste as nonhazardous
  □ Minimizes the cost on transportation
  □ Lessens the production of the greenhouse gas, methane
  □ Requires less land for landfills
  □ The residue generated from burning is acceptable as fill material since it is free from organic matter
  □ Almost all kinds of waste can be burned
  □ Climate changes cannot affect it
  □ Flexibility is possible—no restriction for its operation
  □ Sale of waste for steam or power generates income.

○ **Disadvantages**
  □ Skilled manpower is required to operate
  □ Not easy to find the suitable site for installation
  □ Cost for construction and operation is too high.

Pyrolysis

"Pyro" means fire and "lysis" means separating. In this method burning of the waste occurs in the absence of oxygen. Organic waste is separated into gas and gaseous fractions (CO, CO_2, CH_4, tar and charred carbon). At the end of pyrolysis a mixture of combustible and noncombustible gases as well as pyroligneous liquid is produced. These end-products have very high heat energy that can be used for various purposes.

○ **Advantages**
  □ The major advantage is the conservation of energy with no air pollution.

Open burning

It is the act of burning waste materials in open air that causes smoke and other discharges directly into the air without passing through a chimney or stack.

○ **Advantages**
  □ Cheaper and easier method
  □ Disadvantages
  □ Open burning of refuse discharges many pollutants into the environment
  □ These pollutants may result in adverse effects on health
  □ The discharge of acidic gases can cause acid rain
  □ The mixture of extremely small particles and liquid droplets (particulate matter) may cause smoke leads to air pollution.

Open Dumping

In this method solid waste is dumped in low lying areas. In a course of time the dumped refuse decreases in volume and is slowly converted into humus as a result of bacterial action.

○ **Advantages**
  □ Efficient to treat all types of refuse except garbage. Selection of proper dumping site reduces the health problems
  □ Labor and supervision required is less.

○ **Disadvantages**
  □ Exposed to flies and rodents
  □ Source of annoyance from the smell and unpleasant appearance
  □ Movable refuse is spread by wind
  □ Drainage from dumps causes pollution of water and land.

Landfills

Sanitary landfills or controlled tipping

In this method a pit is dug then the refuse is filled in layers. It means the solid waste is buried in layers, pressed well and covered with layers of earth. When the trench or pit reaches its full volume or quantity, a cap or top cover is applied to close the site. Some harmful plants are planted over the site to keep away the animals.

Steps in making sanitary landfills

○ Selecting a suitable location or spot is the first step. The site should be preferably a wasteland and located away from residential areas

○ The generated waste is collected and transported to the area by using vehicles designed for these purposes

○ Laying the wastes in appropriate heap to a predetermined height

○ Compacting the layer mechanically

○ Covering the compacted layer with a thin layer of earth up to 22 cm depth at the end of each work day. The same steps are repeated for each work period.

The followings are some of the methods used for landfill:

○ **Trench method:** Refuse is dumped in a long trench measuring 2–3 m deep and 4–12 m wide, compacted and covered with excavated earth.

○ **Ramp method**: The available sloppy area is used to dump the waste. Some excavation is done to secure the covering material.

○ **Area method:** Land depressions are used for filling. The refuse is deposited, packed and consolidated in uniform layers and sealed to prevent infestation by flies and rodents and suppresses the nuisance of smell and dust. Chemical, bacteriological and physical changes occur in buried refuse leading to complete decomposition of organic matter.

○ **Advantages**
  ❑ It is easy to establish
  ❑ Many disposal areas can be used concurrently
  ❑ Terminated landfill sites can be utilized for farming
  ❑ This overcome the harmful effects that occur with open dumping
  ❑ It is possible to reclaim and use the terminated sanitary land fill areas for the benefits of community.

○ **Disadvantages**
  ❑ Finding the suitable site within easy reach is not always possible
  ❑ It needs huge areas to meet the slow processing of decomposition
  ❑ Selection of improper site for sanitary landfill may cause seepage into water streams promoting pollution and diseases
  ❑ It is not always possible to get sufficient supply of earth cover
  ❑ Requires skilled supervisors.

Bioreactor landfills

The bioreactor landfills use enhanced microbiological processes to accelerate the decomposition of waste. The main controlling factor is the constant addition of liquid to maintain optimum moisture for microbial digestion. These enhanced microbial processes have the advantage of rapidly reducing the volume of the waste creating more space for additional waste.

Biological Waste Treatment

Composting

○ Composting is natural process of recycling decomposed organic materials into a rich soil known as compost. Anything that was once living will decompose.

Composting is the controlled aerobic decomposition of organic matter by the action of microorganisms and small invertebrates. There are number of composting techniques being used today. The end result of composting is an accumulation of partially decayed organic matter called **humus**.

○ Optimum temperatures for the process are in the range of 50°–60°C with the ideal being 60°C.

○ Composting is a combined method of refuse and night-soil or sludge.

Methods of Composting

○ Bangalore method (Anaerobic method)

○ Mechanical composting (Aerobic method)

Bangalore method (anaerobic method)

○ In this method a trench measuring 3 ft deep, 15–30 ft long and 8 ft broad is used to dispose the refuse or night soil.

○ Usually, the size of the trench is based on the volume of refuse.

○ The night soil and organic residues forms the alternate layers.

○ At the end of filling, the pit is covered with a 15–20 cm layer of refuse.

○ This is permitted to remain in the pit for 3 months without turning and watering. In this period, the material settles and reduction occurs in biomass volume.

○ Second round of night soil and refuse are put in alternate layers and plastered or covered with mud or earth.

○ This helps in preventing the loss of moisture and breeding of flies.

○ Aerobic composting takes place in about 8–10 days, following which the material undergoes anaerobic decomposition at a very slow rate.

○ This takes about 6 to 8 months to obtain the finished product.

Mechanical composting (aerobic method)

○ **Manure pits**
  ❑ Manure pit is the most suitable method for collection and disposal of refuse in rural areas.
  ❑ The garbage, cattle dung, straw and leaves should be dumped into the manure pits and covered with earth after each day's dumping.
  ❑ Two such pits will be needed, when one is closed, the other will be in use. The refuse gets converted into manure within 5–6 months and can be returned to the field.

○ **Burial**
  - This method is suitable for small camps.
  - A trench of 1.5 m wide and 2 m deep is excavated, and the refuse is dumped. It is covered with 20–30 cm of earth at the end of the day.
  - When the level in the trench is 40 cm from ground, the trench is filled with earth and compacted. A new trench is dug out. The contents may be taken out after 4–6 months and used on the fields.

○ **Advantages**
  - **Profit making:** Manure is a profitable product. Compost or manure is a most purchased product by farmers, gardeners and others.
  - **Destruction of pathogens:** Pathogens are destroyed easily by maintaining the temperature above 40°C for a minimum of 2 weeks.
  - **Kills harmful plants:** Temperature of 40°C for minimum of 2 weeks destroys the viability of weed seeds.
  - **Volume reduction:** The mass and volume of the manure is reduced considerably when composted.
  - **No odors** or fly problems associated with raw manure. Composting minimizes the moisture content so that handling becomes easier.
  - **Improved transportability:** The reduction in mass and volume facilitates transportability.
  - **Soil conditioner:** Compost reduces the risk for soil erosion, and reduces the fertilizer requirements.
  - **Availability:** Odor free compost can be used as per the convenience of the farmer.
  - **No leakage:** Since nitrogen is transformed to a steady form it is less susceptible to leakage.

○ **Disadvantages**
  - Compost contains less than half the nitrogen of manure but if manure is not incorporated into the soil it loses nitrogen to the atmosphere and may retain less nitrogen than the compost.
  - To produce quality compost time commitment is essential.
  - Equipment like windrow turners are necessary but it is costly.
  - Considerable land area is necessary.
  - Money and time may be spent to sell.

Integrated Solid Waste Management

Integrated solid waste management (ISWM) focuses on formulating systems that are accessible, acceptable and affordable by the community. This system can sustain and serve the community to provide safe environment (Fig. 5).

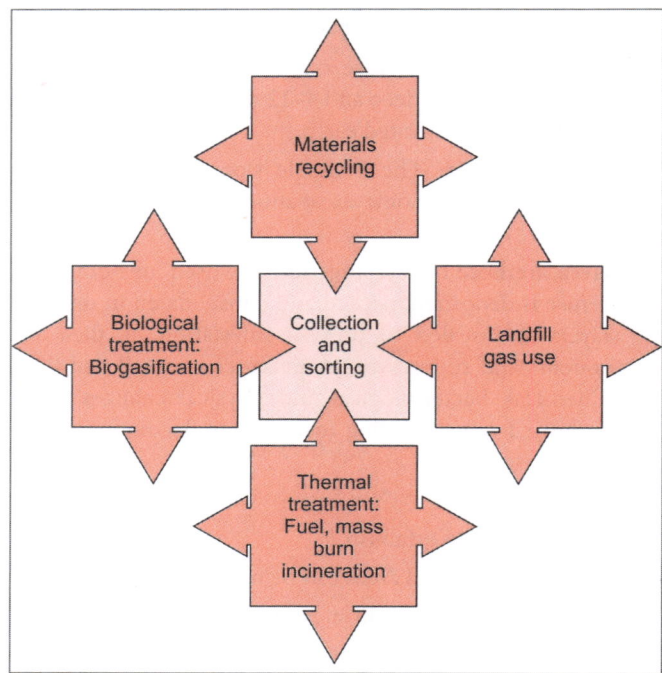

Figure 5: Integrated solid waste management (ISWM)

This ISWM method uses range of strategies and some of them are proper collection and segregation of different types of wastes.

Disposal into Sea

It is a simple and cheap method in which the solid waste is disposed under deep sea water at a remarkable distance from the coastal areas.

Source Reduction

Source reduction is the first priority in waste disposal. Source reduction helps in conserving the resources, lessening the cost of disposal by reducing the volume of waste. Source reduction is a kind of practical approach that reduces the amount of material we produce.

The basic elements of source reduction include:

○ Minimize the number of materials used in manufacturing
○ Increase the life time of the product through quality and maintenance
○ Decreased toxicity
○ Reusing the material
○ Consumer uses materials efficiently
○ High efficiency in production results in less waste.

Techniques Involved in Resource Recovery

○ Reduce the volume of solid waste mechanically by compaction
○ Use incineration to reduce the chemical volume

○ Mechanical size reduction is carried out by shredding, grinding and milling

○ Use of hand-sorting, air separation, magnetic separation and screening for component separation.

SENSITIZE AND HANDLE SOCIAL ISSUES AFFECTING HEALTH AND DEVELOPMENT FOR SELF AND FAMILY

Women Empowerment

Indian constitution honored women as legal citizens of the country and have equal rights like men. Indian women were elected and served in prestigious positions like Prime Minister, Chief Minister, Chief Justice, Governor, Collector and Police Officers. Traditionally males are dominant figures of their families and the same continued even outside. Even today, entire men do not accept the women empowerment. The very anatomy of women brand them bear children and rear them leading malnutrition and poor health in women. Patriarchal norms and values is predominantly found in our India.

Women empowerment refers to all the necessary efforts taken to improve and strengthen the women's status in various aspects of life, like social, economical, political and legal to ensure equal-right to women and enhance confidence in them to claim their rights.

Status of Women

Sex Ratio

Sex ratio is defined as the number of females to 1000 males. Sex ratio in India is 943 Females:1000 Males. Sex ratio can help in identifying the level of extent of equality between males and females in a region at a given point of time.

> **Sex Composition**
> • The small family norm and longing for a male child has changed the sex ratio. The gender discrimination is accountable for this decline in female ratio.
> • Kerala with 1084 females per 1,000 males has the highest sex ratio according to 2011 Census of India.

Nutrition and Feeding of Girl Baby

○ In many communities, girl babies treated unequally with boy babies. This discrimination starts from birth and continues until graveyard.

○ Care, obligation, and commitment of parents and society toward girl children is seeming to be less comparing to male children.

○ Girl babies are either not fed with breast milk or breastfed for only shorter duration. In addition, the girl babies are not adequately nourished.

Education

○ Increasing women education facilitates higher economic growth.

○ Worldwide increased educational attainment accounts for about 50% of economic growth. In this merely around 50% contribution comes from girls who pursue higher levels of education and achieving better equality in the number of years spent in education. However, significant number of educated women could not yield their expected translated value that equals their education.

○ Though Indian constitution assures free primary schooling to everyone up to 14 years of age, very few females attend school. But in many families girl children were not sent to school due to various reasons.

Wages for Women and Men

○ Internationally women found to get placed in work on an unequal basis in comparison to men. In 2013, the male employment-to-population ratio stood at 72.2%, while the ratio for females was 47.1%.

○ Worldwide, women are less paid than men. In most countries women get paid only 60–75% of men's wages.

○ Women are likely to be found working in low productivity areas comparing to men who work in high productive jobs.

○ If these deficits (participation and wage gap) are rectified easily women could increase their income up to 76% globally.

○ Gender gaps are also found in specific areas: Domestic cleaning, vessel washing and cooking are the household works specifically branded for women. Even if a woman is employed earning equal to her husband she needs to perform the household duties specifically designated for women.

Child Marriage

○ Child marriage is defined as marriage conducted before the age of 18 years applicable for both boys and girls. This is prevalent among young girl children.

○ United Nations Population Fund (UNFPA) stated that more than 140 million girls will become child brides between 2011 and 2020.

○ If present level of child marriages continues we can witness annually around 14.2 million girl children getting married.

○ Girls married at too young age are placed at higher risk of getting sexually abused by the partner than those who marry later.

Child marriage violates the rights of young girls

○ Terminating their education

○ Hindering any chances to get vocational and life skills

- Teen pregnancy, child bearing, and motherhood before they are physically and psychologically matured
- Intimate partner sexual violence and HIV infection.

Measures to prevent childhood marriages

- Providing equal access to education for both girls and boys
- Mobilizing girls, boys, parents and leaders to change the practices that discriminate girls from boys
- Providing girls who are already married with options for schooling, employment and livelihood skills, sexual and reproductive health information and services (including HIV prevention), and offering recourse from violence in the home
- Assess the factors for predisposing child marriage, gender inequality and discrimination and child-sexual abuse. Draw an appropriate action plan to eliminate these problems.

Dowry System

Families become cheerful and celebrate the day if boy is born; girl baby's arrival puts them sad and take away their happiness. Most families feel that the girl children are the "pain in the eyes-big burden" since they need to spend such a lot of money for her marriage.

Though the "dowry system" was banned by the Indian government in 1961 we still witness many bad consequences of unpaid dowry.

Sexual Violence

- Statistics reveal that around 120 million girls worldwide have experienced forced sexual acts at some point in their lives.
- According to statistics every day close to five women are raped and 10 women are molested in the National Capital, Delhi.

Prevention of Female Feticide

Determination of sex has been prohibited and is a punishable offence.

- No Genetic Counseling Center or Genetic Laboratory or Genetic Clinic shall conduct or cause to be conducted in its Center, Laboratory or Clinic, prenatal diagnostic techniques including ultrasonography, for the purpose of determining the sex of a fetus.
- No person shall conduct or cause to be conducted any prenatal diagnostic techniques including ultrasonography for the purpose of determining the sex of a fetus.
- No person shall, by whatever means or cause allowed to selection of sex before or after conception.

Women Abuse—Definition

Woman abuse is the intentional and systematic use of tactics to establish and maintain power and control over the thoughts, beliefs, and conduct of a woman through the inducement of fear and/or dependency. The tactics include, but are not limited to, emotional, financial, physical, and sexual abuse, as well as, intimidation, isolation, threats, using the children and using social status and privilege. Woman abuse includes the sum of all past acts of violence and the promise of future violence that achieves enhanced power and control for the perpetrator over the partner. (Reynolds and Schweitzer 1998, the London Abused Women's Center).

Preventive Measures on Women Abuse

- Enforcement of laws on violence against women
- Supporting gender sensitization by conducting public awareness programs
- Encourage the media to play a constructive role
- Provision of easily accessible 24 × 7 information services to inform any violence related to women
- Provision of legal services free of cost or at affordable cost
- Regional women related policies
- Strengthening *mahila mandals* and women's organization all over India
- Education to all women
- Family support
- Informing on helplines

Women Helplines in India: The community health nurses working in different parts of India should alert the community about the availability of telephone lines for helping the women in emergencies (Table 6).

Table 6: Women helplines in India

Women's helpline (All India)	1091/1090
National Commission for Women (NCW)	011-23219750
Delhi	
Delhi Commission for Women (DCW)	011-23378044/23378317/23370597
Outer Delhi Helpline	011-27034873/27034874
Women in distress	1091
Police Control Room	100
Child Helpline	1098
Anti-stalking/Obscene calls	1096

Contd...

Child, student and senior citizen	1291
DCP, North East Special Unit	9818099070
IGP–Nodal Officer for Northeasterners	(WhatsApp no) – 9810083486
Andhra Pradesh	
Hyderabad/Secunderabad – Women Police Station	040-27853508
Hyderabad Women Police Station	04027852400/4852
Bengaluru	
Women's Police Helpline	08022943225
Bengaluru Traffic Police	080-22868444/22868550
Chandigarh	
Women Police Exchange	1722741900
Haryana	
Women and Child Helpline	0124-2335100
Himachal Pradesh	
Women Commission	9816066421, 9418636326, 9816882491, 9418384215
Mumbai	
Railway Police	9833331111
Mumbai Police Helpline	100, 103
Navi Mumbai Police Station	0222758 0255
Punjab	
Women's Helpline	9781101091
Tamil Nadu	
Women's Helpline	044-28592750
Women Police Station, Adayar	044-24415732, 044-23452586
Tripura	
Women's Helpline Numbers	0381-2323355, 03812322912
Rajasthan	
Nirbhaya Sambhali Helpline	1800-1200020
Women Police Station Jodhpur	0291-2012112
Karnataka	
Women Police Helpline	0821-2418400
Mysore Women Police Station	0821-2418110/2418410
Kerala	
Vanitha Helpline Number of Kerala Police, Trivandrum	9995399953
State Vanitha Cell	0471-2338100
Women's Cell, Kollam	0474-2742376
Women's Cell, Kochi	0484-2396730

Women Welfare Programs in India

○ Prime Minister Modi is leading a campaign **"Save your daughters, educate your daughters"** ('*Beti Bachao Beti Padhao*'). In Haryana state 12 districts were chosen for the initial campaign, the sex ratio varies here from 775 to 837 females per 1,000 males.

○ Under this scheme, the core principles of respecting, protecting and fulfilling the rights of girls and women, and putting a full stop to gender based violence will be adopted.

Swayamsidha

○ Swayamsidha is an integrated scheme for the development and empowerment of women through self-help groups.

○ It covers services, access to micro-credit and promotes microenterprises.

Swashakti Project

○ Swashakti project aims at increasing women's access to resources for better quality of life.

○ This is achieved through time reduction devices, health education and training women on income-generating schemes.

Integrated Child Development Services Scheme (ICDS)

○ The scheme started in 1975 with the objective to give special coverage to slums in urban areas.

○ The scheme also envisages delivery of an integrated package of services consisting of immunization, health checkups, nutrition and health education and refreshment services to child and pregnant women.

Training and Employment Program for Women

○ It provides new skills and knowledge to women who do not have any income or property.

○ They are trained in areas like agriculture, animal husbandry, dairying, fisheries, handlooms, handicrafts, etc. to get employed and get income to lead their life.

Swavlamban

This scheme provides training and skills to women to enable them to obtain employment or become self-employed. Some of the areas in which training given are: computer programming, medical transcription, electronic assembling, radio and TV repairs, garment making, handloom weaving, handicrafts, secretarial practice, embroidery and community health.

Hostels for Working Women

This scheme, provides financial assistance for construction or expansion of hostel buildings for working women. The main aim is to provide safe and affordable accommodation to working women. This also includes women on training and girl students pursuing professional courses.

Swadhar

This scheme provides integrated services to women who has no support. This covers:

o Widows living alone

o Women released from prison

o Survivors of natural calamities

o Women and girls rescued from brothel area or other places

o Victims of sexual crimes

o This scheme provides food, clothing, shelters, health care, counseling and legal aid.

o This also rehabilitate them through education, skill formation and behavioral training.

Rashtriya Mahila Kosh

The National Credit Fund for Women is meant to facilitate credit support or micro-finance to poor women to start such income-generating schemes as agriculture, dairying, shop keeping, vending and handicrafts.

Childhood Abuse

India, Nigeria, Democratic Republic of Congo, Pakistan and China collectively accounted for half of the total number of under-five deaths globally. In India, around 1.7 million children died before reaching the age of 5 years in 2010, and more than half of them (52%) died in the first month of life. *Each of the major causes…can be prevented or treated with known, highly effective and widely practicable interventions such as improvements in prenatal care,* "wrote the researchers, led by the Registrar General of India. Apart from the diseases many deaths that occur as a result of various forms of child abuse that go unnoticed.

Children—The Weakest

o Children are consider as the weakest section and are at risk of many environmental hazards than adults till they have not attained complete maturity of their organs and physiological systems.

o The fetus in womb is open to a number of agents that can make their entry through placenta and may cause developmental abnormalities. The effects of severity of exposure to mother and baby are based on the developmental stage at which the infection occurred.

o The possibilities of unique pathways of exposure that may increase their risk. This is because the children play with mouth surface and objects.

o Children are potential for long-term exposures to environmental hazards.

o Children live, learn and play in different physical environments than adults.

o Children have considerably less knowledge and control over the hazards.

Various Types of Child Abuse

Children who are abused in various ways (physically, mentally, sexually) suffer with physical, psychological and social problems. They may involve in antisocial activities.

Psychological Child Abuse

Psychological abuse or maltreatment is one of the commonly found forms of child abuse.

Parents' attitude in psychological child abuse

o Acts of omission, e.g. Parents do not showing love and affection

o Acts of commission, e.g. rejection, insults and child is not allowed to enjoy socialization

o All the above acts will have negative impact on child's self-esteem and social competence. So the child is withdrawn and emotionally disengaged.

Neglect

o Neglect can be defined as 'any serious act or omission by a person having the care of a child that, within the bounds of cultural tradition, constitutes a failure to provide conditions that are essential for the healthy physical and emotional development of a child'. (CFCA Resource Sheet, 2016)

o Parent fails to adequately meet the needs of the child like provision of food, shelter, clothing, medical care, love and affection and supervision on child's activities, etc.

o Such neglected children will not have much attachment with parents he/she will lack confidence and socially isolated.

Physical Abuse

o Physical abuse is defined as, 'any nonaccidental physical act inflicted upon a child by a person having the care of a child'. It is not necessarily the "intent to hurt" but can also be a justified action to discipline the child.

o Physically abused children will have constant threat, fear with poor academic performance, depression and low self-esteem.

Domestic and Family Violence

- It occurs in intimate relationship, usually one person in a position of power over another. It may include a range of abuse like physical, sexual, emotional financial abuse, psychological, etc.
- Children are fearful, anxious and unpredictable about the threats.

Sexual Abuse

- Child sexual abuse is defined as any incident in an adult, adolescent or child uses their power and authority to engage a minor in a sexual act, or exposes the minor to inappropriate sexual behavior or material.
- Sexually abusive behaviors can include the fondling of genitals, masturbation, oral sex, vaginal or anal penetration by a penis, finger or any other object, fondling of breasts, voyeurism, exhibitionism and exposing the child to or involving the child in pornography (CFCA Resource Sheet, 2015: Bromfield, 2005; US National Research Council, 1993).
- In general, girls are more prone to be sexually abused than boys.
- Sexually abused children are withdrawn, unhappy with self-harm and suicidality.

Child Protective Measures in India

If you are concerned that a child is being abused you can speak using the phone number:

CHILDLINE stands for a friendly '*didi*' or a sympathetic '*bhaiya*' who is always there for vulnerable children 24 hours of the day, 365 days of the year

- Whether you are a concerned adult or a child, you can dial **1098 (all over India)**, the toll free number to access the services.
- They respond to emergency needs of children and link them to services for their long-term care and rehabilitation.

Indian Legal Acts on Protection of Children

- The Child Marriage Restraint Act, 1929
- The Child Labor (Prohibition and Regulation) Act, 1986. The Juvenile Justice (Care and Protection of Children) Act, 2000. The Infant Milk Substitutes, feeding bottles and Infant
- Foods (Regulation of Protection Supply and Distribution) Act, 1992
- The Pre-Conception and Prenatal Diagnostic Technique
- (Prohibition of Sex Selection) Act, 1994.

- The Immoral Traffic Act, 1956.
- The Guardian and Wards Act, 1890.
- The Young Persons (Harmful Publications) Act, 1956.
- The Commissions for Protection of Child Rights Act, 2005.

Convention on the Rights of the Child

- After series of discussions, the United Nations General Assembly came forward to accept "Convention on the Rights of the Child" (CRC) in November 1989. It is the most extensively recognized human rights organization in the world. India, possess the load of one-fifth of world's children, endorsed the CRC in 1992. India had agreed the standards specified there in on matters relating to health care, education, legal, civil and social services. CRC provides a framework on universal standards for the care, treatment and protection of all individuals below the age of 18 years. CRC comprises distinct articles and three optional protocols.

To operate CRC focuses on the following principles:

- Children should be free of discrimination
- Government policies should focus the core interests of the children
- Children should survive and develop to their full potential
- Children's views and perspectives are important and need to be heard.

The following are some of the constitutional provisions that protect children in India:

- Right to equality (Article 14)
- Right to free and compulsory elementary education for all children in the 6–14 years of age group (Article 21 A)
- Right to be protected from any hazardous employment till the age of 14 years [Article 24)]
- Right to be protected from being abused and forced by economic necessity to enter occupations unsuited to their age or strength [Article 39(e)]
- Right to equal opportunities and facilities to develop in a healthy manner and in conditions of freedom and dignity and guaranteed protection of childhood and youth against exploitation and against moral and material abandonment [Article 39 (f)]
- Right to nutrition and standard of living and improved public health (Article 47)
- Right to early childhood care and education to all children until they complete the age of six years (Article 45).

12th Five-year Plan and Child Mortality

- Twelfth five-year plan seeks to bring down infant mortality rate (IMR) to 25. Currently the decline rate is 5% per year.

o If India moves with the same rates India should project an IMR of 32 by the year 2017.

o It is a well-known fact that the underweight children are more prone to mortality and morbidity. At the current rate of decline, the prevalence of underweight children is expected to be 27% by 2017.

Life Expectancy of a Child Increased

World health data states that a girl who was born in 2012 can expect to live around 73 years, and a boy to the age of 68. This is six years longer than the average global life expectancy for a child born in 1990.

Abuse of Elders

Elderly Population

Population aging is the one of the most significant emerging problem in almost all developing and developed countries. Government of India in its national policy on older persons (January, 1999) defines "senior citizen" or "elderly" as a person who is of age 60 years or above.

Asia holds the highest proportion of world's elderly (53%), followed by Europe, 25%. This problem is an ongoing one since the life expectancy of the people is increasing day by day due to increased awareness on healthy lifestyle, access to health care and growing medical technology. This burden of increasing numbers of elderly will build-up and take giant tides in the next 50 years. By 2050, around 82% of the world's elderly population will be found in developing regions of Asia. Population aging is considered as the biggest problem of developing nations.

Myths related to growing older: There are many myths related to aging:

o Older people are unfit mentally and physically
o All older people have alike needs
o We cannot expect any creativity or contribution in older people
o Older people's experience cannot make wonders in modern society
o Older people want to be quiet and calm
o Older people takes away resources from young people
o Expenses on older people is a waste
o Older people are not suited to modern workplaces
o You cannot teach old dog new tricks
o Older people want to live in isolation
o Older people are not worth.

Elderly Abuse—Definition

The definition developed by Action on Elder-Abuse in the United Kingdom and adopted by the International Network for the Prevention of Elder Abuse: *"Elder abuse is a single or repeated act, or lack of appropriate action, occurring within any relationship where there is an expectation of trust which causes harm or distress to an older person."* Such abuse is generally divided into the following categories:

o **Physical abuse**—*the infliction of pain or injury, physical coercion, or physical or drug-induced restraint.*

o **Psychological or emotional abuse**—*the infliction of mental anguish.*

o **Financial or material abuse**—*the illegal or improper exploitation or use of funds or resources of the older person.*

o **Sexual abuse**—*non-consensual sexual contact of any kind with the older person.*

o **Neglect**—*the refusal or failure to fulfill a care giving obligation. This may or may not involve a conscious and intentional attempt to inflict physical or emotional distress on the older person.*

Elderly abuse maybe physical, sexual, psychological, and emotional. There may be financial and material abuses too. Abandonment, neglect, ill-treatment, and disrespect of elderly persons are commonly found abuse of elderly in many families.

Older Population and Challenges

Noncommunicable Diseases

In general the most frequent cause of death of older people is noncommunicable diseases like heart disease, cancer and diabetes, etc. The role of infectious and parasitic diseases is less when comparing to noncommunicable diseases. Further, older people often suffer with quite a few health problems at the same time, like diabetes, hypertension and cardiac diseases.

Life with Disability

There are many older people live with disabilities like physical (cataract, deafness, immobile and bedridden, etc.) and mental problems. For example, about 65% are visually impaired are found in the age of 50 and more. Age group of 50 years constitutes about 20% of the world's population. With an increasing elderly population in many countries, more people will be at risk of age-related visual impairment.

Maltreatment

Statistics reveals that around 4–6% of older people in developed countries experience some form of maltreatment at home. Application of physical restraints, depriving of dignity (allowing them in soiled clothes for longer periods) and deliberately providing inadequate care (less attention leading to pressure sores) are some of the examples for abusive acts in institutions.

Long-term Care Need of the Hour

The older people are unable to perform self-care needs by themselves. The increasing elderly population needs extended care centers or hospitals and adequate health care professionals.

Number of People with Dementias on Raise

The risk of dementia rises sharply with age. Around 25–30% of people aged 85 or more found to have some degree of cognitive impairment.

Older People are Vulnerable during Disasters

It is not possible for older people to escape from disasters (earthquake, heavy flood, cyclone, fire, gas leakage, etc.), since they are weak, unable to run or jump. Usually we come across many deaths occurring among older people during disasters.

Importance of Senior Citizens

- They will teach us through experience
- They can be helpful in guiding us on how to conduct us. Example self-esteem, self-respect, self-discipline
- They make our environment joyful
- We can gain practical experience
- They have learned the lessons of humility
- They are fun companions
- They know things we would never guess unless we ask
- They help us deal with our disappointment and grief and illness.

Welfare Programs for Senior Citizens

Ministry of Social Justice and Empowerment is the nodal Ministry responsible for welfare of the senior citizens. It has announced the National Policy on older persons covering all concerns pertaining to the welfare of older persons.

Maintenance and Welfare of Parents and Senior Citizens Act, 2007

The Maintenance and Welfare of Parents and Senior Citizens Act, 2007 was introduced in December 2007 to promote need-based maintenance for parents and senior citizens.

The Act provides for:

- Maintenance of parents/senior citizens by children/relatives made obligatory
- Justifiable through court reversal or transfer of property by senior citizens in case of negligence by relatives
- Penalization in case of abandonment of senior citizens
- Establishment of old age homes for senior citizens
- Facilitate adequate medical facilities and security for senior citizens.

National Program for Health Care for Elderly (NPHCE)

National program for health care for elderly (NPHCE) was implemented by the Ministry of Health and Family Welfare in the year 2010–11 with an approved amount of ₹288 crore for the period of the 11th Five-Year Plan.

The Ministry also considers senior citizens:

- Separate queues for older persons in government hospitals
- Geriatric clinic in several government hospitals.

Travel

- Reservation of two seats for senior citizens in front row of the buses of the State Road Transport undertakings.
- Some State Governments are giving fare concession to senior citizens in the state transport. Some states introduced bus models, which are convenient to the elderly.
- Indian Railways provide 30% fare concession in all mail/express for senior citizens aged 60 years and above.
- Indian Railways also have the facility of separate counters for senior citizens for purchase/booking/cancellation of tickets.
- Wheel chairs for use of older persons are available at all junctions.
- Ramps for wheel chairs are available in some important stations.
- There is a provision in coaches for wheelchair—space, hand rail and specially designed toilet for handicapped persons.
- Air India is offering discount to senior citizens of 60 plus on flights to USA, UK and Europe. Further, Air India has now decided to reduce the age of 60 plus for discount on their domestic routes as well with immediate effect.
- Under the *Antyodaya Scheme*—the Below Poverty Line (BPL) families that has older persons are issued food grains 35 kg/family/month. The food grains are issued at ₹3/- per kg for rice and ₹2/- per kg for wheat.

Income Tax Exemptions

- Tax exemptions is provided to the senior citizens by the Ministry of Finance. Income tax exemption for Senior citizens of 60 years and above up to ₹2.50 lakh per annum.
- Income tax exemption for Senior Citizens of 80 years and above up to ₹5.0 lakh per annum.

Pensions Portal

A pension portal has been set up by the department of Pensions, Government of India, to assist senior citizens to get information regarding the status of their application, the amount of pension, documents required, etc. This portal accepts grievances from older people.

Commercial Sex Workers

Commercial sex is an act of sexual intercourse in exchange for money. HIV prevalence is 12 times greater among sex workers than among the general population. Some of the key elements that had contributed to this increased prevalence are stigma and discrimination, violence and punitive legal and social environments. Law and disciplinary environments limited the availability and accessibility to HIV prevention and treatment, care and support for sex workers and their clients. There are male and female sex workers functioning all over the world. Their occupation, puts all their customers at risk of STDs and HIV infection.

"Given the role of STIs as a co-factor of HIV infection, high rates of STI among sex workers can be interpreted as a precursor to a relatively rapid spread of the epidemic" *UNAIDS*.

Types of Prostitution

Street prostitutes, bar dancers, call girls, religious prostitutes, escort girls, road side brothel, child prostitutes, etc.

Factors Influencing Increased HIV Prevalence Among Sex-workers

Discrimination

- Significant legal and institutional discrimination shown on sex workers (male and female) put them in great struggle to meet their own health and well-being needs.
- Health service providers do not want to provide services to sex workers.
- Law enforcement officials like police most often violate the human rights of sex workers.
- Lack of programs and funding.

Facilities

Only about one-third of countries are able to provide health-related programs for sex workers to reduce the risk of STDs and HIV. The quality and reach of these programs may differ. In rest of the countries the sex workers are supposing to make arrangement to obtain services through general health-care settings. Whereas the sex workers feel that these service areas do not welcome them.

Fear to Move Out for Treatment

Sex workers also have the threat of getting attacked by the public. Hence, many hide them-self and not approach health facilities for their health needs.

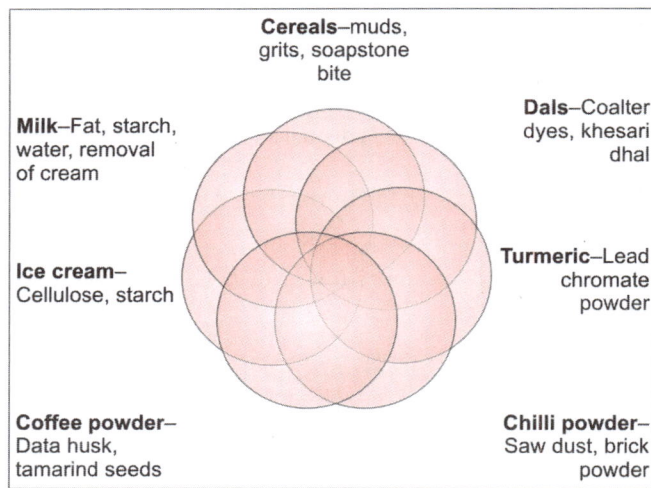

Figure 6: Adulterants added to specific food items

New WHO Guidelines

- Prevent decriminalization of sex workers
- Improve access to health services for sex workers.
- Interventions to empower sex workers
- Correct and consistent condom use.

Food Adulteration

- Food adulteration is defined as the addition of some unacceptable things to the food materials, which ruin the quality of the food for consumption (Fig. 6).
- **Adulterant:** Any material that is employed for the purposes of adulteration (Fig. 6).

Consequences of Food Adulteration

- Consumer has to pay more money for food of lower quality and quantity
- It can be harmful to health and may lead to death.

Prevention of Food Adulteration (PFA) Act, 1954

Objectives

- To provide pure and wholesome food to the consumers
- To protect them from fraudulent and deceptive trade practices
- To prevent the sale of substandard foods
- To protect the interests of the consumers by eliminating fraudulent practices.

Definition of Food

- Any article used as food or drink for human consumption other than drugs and water and includes any article which ordinarily enters into or is used in the composition or preparation of human food

❍ Any flavoring matter or condiments

❍ Any other article which the Central Government may having regard to its use, nature, substance or quality, declare, by notification in the official gazette as food for the purpose of this Act.

Adulteration

An article of food shall be deemed to be adulterated:

❍ If the article sold by vendor does not meet the nature, substance or quality demanded by the purchaser

❍ If presence of any other substance which affects the substance or its quality

❍ If any constituent of the article has been wholly or in part extracted to affect the quality thereof

❍ If the article under unsanitary conditions become injurious to health

❍ If the article consists wholly or in part of any putrefied, decomposed substance unfit for human consumption

❍ If the article is obtained from a diseased animal

❍ If the article contains any poisonous substance which renders it injurious to health

❍ If the container of the article is composed deleterious substance which renders its contents injurious to health

❍ If any coloring matter other than that prescribed present in the article

❍ If the article contains any prohibited preservative or permitted preservative in excess

❍ If the quality or purity of the Article falls below the prescribed limits

❍ If the quality or purity of the article falls below the prescribed standard which renders it injurious to health.

Sale of certain admixtures prohibited sale by himself or by his servant or agent is prohibited in case of:

❍ Cream which has not been prepared exclusively from milk or which contains less than 25% of milk fat.

❍ Milk which contains added water

❍ Ghee which contains any added matter

❍ Selling skimmed milk as whole milk

❍ Mixture of two or more edible oils as an edible oil

❍ Any article of food which contains any artificial sweetener beyond the prescribed limit

❍ Turmeric containing any foreign substance

❍ Mixture of coffee and other substance except chicory

❍ Curd not made out of milk

❍ Milk or milk products containing constituents other than of milk.

Procedure for Sampling and Analysis

❍ Where any adulterant is manufactured samples of such article or adulterant taken for analysis.

❍ Notice will be issued by the inspector to the seller indicating his intention

❍ Three samples are taken and the signature of the seller is affixed to them

❍ One sample is sent for analysis to public analyst under intimation to the local health authority

❍ The other two samples are sent to the local health authority for further reference.

Penalties

❍ Minimum 6 months imprisonment with a fine of ₹1000/-

❍ If adulteration leads to death or critical harm, punishment will be life imprisonment with fine of ₹5,000/-

❍ From 1986 amendment, consumers and NGOs are empowered to take samples of food for examination

❍ Central committee for food standards frames and revises the rules under PFA Act

❍ Any food not conforming to the standards is labeled as adulterated

❍ A chain of food laboratories are established and their report is considered final. These labs are in Kolkata, Mysore, Ghaziabad, Pune

❍ Adulteration is social evil. All are responsible for the perpetuation of the evil.

Important Miscellaneous Provisions

❍ If any extraneous additions of coloring matter is added, the same should be indicated on the labels

❍ From the labels the blending composition of ingredients should be clear to the customer

❍ Sale of kesari gram individually or as an admixture is prohibited

❍ Prohibition of use of carbide (acetylene) gas in ripening is prohibited

❍ Sale of ghee with Reichert value less than the permitted level

❍ Sale of admixture of ghee or butter is prohibited

❍ Addition of artificial sweetener should be mentioned on the label

❍ Sale of food colors without license prohibited

❍ Sale of insect damaged dry fruits and nuts prohibited

❍ Food prepared in rusted containers, chipped enamel containers and untinned copper/brass utensils are treated as unfit for human consumption

❍ Containers not made of plastic material which is not according to the standards are not to be used

○ Selling salseed fat or any other purpose except for bakery and confectionery is prohibited

○ Store of insecticides in the same premises where food articles are stored is prohibited

○ Milk powder or condensed milk can be sold only with ISI mark

○ Use of more than one type of preservative is prohibited

○ Crop contaminants beyond certain specified level is treated as adulterant

○ Naturally occurring toxic substances in the food material beyond certain level is considered as unfit for human consumption

○ No antioxidant, emulsifiers and stabilizing agent is permitted beyond the prescribed level

○ No insecticides should be sprayed on the food items

○ Oils can be manufactured only in factories licensed for such purpose.

Role of Voluntary Agencies in PFA Act

○ NGO should create awareness in the general public of the hazards of food adulteration

○ They should rise up against the cheating traders

○ They should identify the dishonest food inspectors

○ They can take samples of the food suspected to be adulterated for further evaluation.

Food Recall

○ A food recall is defined as an action taken to remove foods which may pose a safety risk. In other words, it is the action to remove food from the market at any stage of the food chain, including that possessed by consumers.

○ WHO has taken the theme food safety, from farm to plate (and everywhere in between) on World Health Day, 7 April 2015. The World Health Day 2015 slogan is: "From farm to plate, make food safe".

The FDA categorizes all recalls based on the level of hazards involved:

Class I recall is a condition in which there is a reasonable chance that the use of or exposure to a violate product will cause serious adverse health consequences or death.

Class II recall is a condition in which use of or exposure to a violate product may cause temporary or medically reversible adverse health consequences.

Class III recall is a condition in which use of or exposure to a violate product is not likely to cause adverse health consequences.

Food Standards

The codex alimentarius: This provides international food standards, guidelines and codes of practice to maintain safety and quality in international food trade. Consumers and importers can trust the safety and quality of the food products.

Agmark Standards

Agmark's expansion is agricultural marketing. Agmark is a quality certification mark provided by the Government of India.

This certification confirms

○ The product is in better term

○ The quality control and hygienic condition of the food.

○ This certification provides benefits to the producer and the consumer. The seller can sell their products easily. It satisfies the buyers.

Bureau of Indian Standards (BIS)

It is a national statutory body. The main functions of BIS are:

○ Preparation and implementation of standards

○ Implementation of certification schemes for products and systems

○ Management of testing laboratories

○ Creating consumer awareness

○ Maintaining close liaison with international standards bodies.

○ BIS product certification scheme is basically voluntary in nature. But, to assure health and safety of the consumer, 68 items are made mandatory by the government through various legislative measures such as Prevention of Food Adulteration Act, Coal Mines Regulations and Indian Gas Cylinders Rules besides BIS Act.

○ Some of the items brought under mandatory certification on consideration of health and safety are milk powder, packaged drinking water, LPG cylinders, oil pressure stoves, clinical thermometers, etc.

Food Safety and Standards Act, 2006

The Indian Parliament has passed the *Food Safety and Standards Act, in year 2006* that overrides all other food related laws:

○ Prevention of Food Adulteration Act, 1954

○ Fruit Products Order, 1955

○ Meat Food Products Order, 1973

○ Vegetable Oil Products (Control) Order, 1947

○ Edible Oils Packaging (Regulation) Order, 1988

○ Milk and Milk Products Order, 1992 etc. are repealed after commencement of FSS Act, 2006.

Food Safety and Standards Authority of India

○ The (FSSAI) has been established under Food Safety and Standards Act, 2006 which consolidates various acts and orders that have until now handled food related issues.

○ FSSAI has been created mainly for laying down scientific standards for articles of food to ensure availability of safe and wholesome food for human consumption. To achieve this it regulates food manufacture, storage, distribution, sale and import.

Functions of FSSAI

○ Formulating the regulations to set norms and procedures in relation to article of food

○ Formulating policies, procedures and guidelines to assess and provide accreditation for food businesses

○ Laying down procedure and guidelines for accreditation of laboratories

○ Supports central and state governments to formulate the policies and rules in relation to food safety and nutrition.

○ Data collection regarding food consumption, incidence and prevalence of biological risk, contaminants in food and foods products, early identification of up coming risks and introduction of rapid alert system

○ Creating an information network with public, consumers and local administrative bodies to provide fast information about food safety and related issues

○ Provide training programs for persons who are involved or intend to get involved in food businesses

○ Assist with the development of international technical standards for food, sanitary and sanitary standards

○ To promote general awareness about food safety and food standards.

Substance Abuse

The abuse of alcohol and other psychoactive substances has become widely prevalent in all levels of society. Substance abuse is the misuse of specific substances to alter mood or behavior; drug and alcohol abuse are two examples of substance abuse. A substance can be defined as a prescribed drug, an illegal drug, or a substance used in an unintended manner to produce mood or mind-altering effect (e.g. inhalants, glues, or steroids). A number of disorders can be induced through the use of a particular substance.

Drug users most often consume different drugs at a time like alcohol, barbiturates, opioids and tranquilizers, etc. IV/injecting users are at for developing HIV infection, acquired immunodeficiency syndrome (AIDS), and hepatitis B.

Family Education by Community Health Nurse

○ Instruct patient and family about adverse physiologic and psychological effects of substance use.

○ Discuss health maintenance practices to minimize potential effects of substance use (e.g. vitamin use, proper diet).

○ Explain the potential for injury from risk-taking behaviors.

○ Reinforce the need for aftercare groups and activities.

○ For general information and support, consult some agencies that run related rehabilitation programs.

UTILIZE COMMUNITY RESOURCES FOR SELF AND FAMILY

Trauma Services

Trauma refers to the services provided to people who are the victims of road traffic accidents.

Main Strategies in India

○ Ensure definitive treatment for the victim within the golden hour

○ Basic life support ambulances should be available at every 50 km along the highways

○ Designated trauma care facilities

○ Facilities at every 100 km on the highways by upgrading the existing government health care facilities. Integrated communication network to enable the public to reach the trauma care system appropriate skill training to various health professionals like—doctors, nurses and paramedics

○ Launch National injury surveillance system and trauma registry

○ To spread awareness regarding injury prevention and road safety.

Trauma System Design

No trauma victim has to be transported for more than 50 kilometers and trauma care facility is available at every 100 km.

Categories of Trauma Care Facilities

Level IV Trauma Care

Appropriately equipped and manned mobile hospital/ambulances are recognized to provide level IV trauma care.

Level III Trauma Care

○ This provides initial evaluation and stabilization (surgically if appropriate) to the trauma patient.

○ The district/tehsil hospitals with a bed capacity of 100–200 beds serve in level III.

Level II Trauma Care

○ This provides definitive care for severe trauma patients.

○ Emergency health care professionals are available to the trauma patients immediately on arrival.

○ The existing medical college hospitals or hospitals with bed strength of 300–500 should be identified as Level II Trauma Center.

Level I Trauma Care

○ This provides the highest level of definitive and comprehensive care for patient with complex injuries.

○ Mostly medical college hospitals are selected to provide this level of care since it needs specialist skill.

○ Ministry of Health and Family Welfare, Government of India is established a National Trauma Registry and Injury Surveillance System. All Trauma Care Facilities have to provide all relevant information to the said Registry in the prescribed format from time to time.

Ambulance Services

Under National health mission

○ Dial 108 for ambulance to transport patients of critical care, trauma and accident victims, etc.

○ Dial 102 for ambulance to primarily to transport pregnant women for institutional delivery and also sick infants.

Old Age Homes

The senior citizens who do not have family support, not accommodated by relatives, not wanting to stay with the family due to various reasons, look for old age homes. Some of the states like Delhi, Kerala, Maharashtra and West Bengal have developed good quality homes for aged. These homes are equipped with medical facilities, ambulances, health care professionals and provision of well-balanced meals.

There are many old age homes function in India by NGOs. Some of them provide free services and others for payment. In general all of them provide food, shelter and medical amenities to the inmates. In paid homes there is a provision for telephone, internet, etc.

Some old age homes function as "day care centers."

These homes provides a conducive atmosphere for the residents. The elderly people forget their worries by sharing their joy and sorrows with each other.

Help Age India

Help Age India established in 1978 is a leading charity voluntary organization in India working for cause of uplifting disadvantaged elderly. Through it committed services, it has become the representative voice for India's elderly. It provides medical services, poverty alleviation and income generation schemes in urban and rural India.

Help Age India provided a list of 484 homes for the aged in 16 cities of the country with information about basic facilities, key features and contact details of these homes, available on help age India's website.

Tamaraikulam Elders Village (TEV)

The TEV is the first home for the aged in Cuddalore, about 20 km from Puducherry constructed by Help Age India, by the generous donations from viewers of NDTV.

Facilities

○ Free stay facility for rural poor

○ This can provide facility for 100 inmates

○ Self-sufficient in terms of energy and food: Active people of the home raise livestock, look after a fish pond, a vegetable plot, a greenhouse and a rice paddy field.

○ They produce toiletries, banana-leaf rope, straw bags and pickles for sale.

○ Healthcare facilities available

○ They practice active ageing techniques

○ Enjoys festivals and recreational activities.

Kalyan Ashram, Kolkata

A two-storey building, model age care home for elderly women at Chetla. This can accommodate 10 persons.

Apart the other services of Help Age India include: Mobile health care, cataract surgeries, physiocare, cancer care, health camps, disaster management, etc.

Orphanages

Global estimation reveals that there are approximately 153 million children who have lost a mother or a father; 17.8 millions of them have lost both parents.

An orphan is defined as a child that has lost one or both parents. The loss of one parent classifies a child as a "single orphan" and the loss of both parents as a "double orphan."

Factors that influence separation of child from parents: Poverty, no access basic needs, childhood abuse-physical, psychological or any other, neglect by parents, disease, disabilities, emergencies—disasters like flood, storm etc, kidnapped child and bad friends, etc.

Orphanages may provide shelter and food but it is difficult to observe and care for their needs when there are big numbers of children under the care. There is less opportunity for the child to experience the love, affection, and warmth of the parents. Hence, in such centers it is a question mark on how far the child would get opportunity to get emotional security and feel of being in a family.

Adoption: Some orphan children are legally adopted and the parents who adopted hold all responsibilities for caring the child just like real parents. Many orphans indulge themselves in violence and antisocial activities since they do not have any family to teach right or wrong. Ultimately they are going to Borstals and remand homes.

Borstals

This facility falls between a certified school and adult prison. The boys of the age above 16 years are placed in Borstals when it is difficult to maintain them in a certified schools or they have misbehaved there. The prison sentence is for 3 years. This is identified as a method of training and reformation.

Remand Homes

The main objective is to improve the mental and physical well being of the child. The child is cared by doctors, psychiatrists and other trained personnel. The children here are given elementary schooling. Apart from this they are provided with art and craft work and recreational activities.

Homes for Physically and Mentally Challenged Individuals

There are many homes established for physically and mentally challenged individuals in India. There are paid home and unpaid homes providing 24 × 7 care and training activities. Apart, there are day care centers where parents/care taker accompany them and bring them back in the evening. These homes empowers and assists the differently challenged individuals to reach their full potential by providing education, training and employment.

The activities in such centers may include but not limited to:

- Screening of newborn babies
- Services to parents of disabled children
- Job-orientated training programs
- Promotion of self-help groups
- Parents support groups (PSGs)
- Physiotheraphy
- Speech therapy
- Occupational therapy
- Hydrotherapy
- Medical care, etc.

National Institute for Empowerment of Persons with Multiple Disabilities (NIEPMD)

Established in the year 2005, on East Coast Road, Muttukadu, Chennai, Tamil Nadu.

Services provided include: Rehabilitation medicine, physical therapy, occupational therapy, sensory integration, early intervention services, prosthetics and orthotics, special education, psychological assessments and interventions, etc.

Community health nurses should inform them about the availability services to mothers of differently challenged individuals.

Indira Awaas Yojana (IAY)

This is a centrally sponsored housing scheme. This provides dwelling units free of cost to the rural poor living below the poverty line at a unit cost of ₹20,000/- in plain areas and ₹22,000/- in the hilly/difficult areas.

Three percent of its funds are reserved for the benefit of disabled persons living below the poverty line in rural areas.

Adhar

Adhar is an institution by the parents, of the parents and for the parents of special children. Started in 1990 as "Association of Parents of Mentally Retarded Children."

Activities

Children are trained to make chalk sticks, candles, paper bags, agarbatties, dusters, mats, decorated earthen lamps (*diyas*) for Diwali, wall hangings, etc. as per their physical and mental abilities. The children work from 9.30 am to 4.30 pm.

Banyan

The Banyan has been an integral part of the chain of care for people with mental illness in Chennai. It also have a branch in Maharashtra. It is a nongovernmental organization.

Karuna Home

It is a rehabilitation and residential center serving the young, physically and/or mentally disabled, of Tibetan refugee parents in India.

This home is in South India near large Tibetan refugee settlements and major Tibetan monasteries. The majority of the disabled residents are from South India. Few were from North India the remaining are Indian origin from the surrounding neighborhood. The range of disabilities, impairments or handicaps arise from autism, dyslexia, epilepsy, polio, Down syndrome and cerebral palsy.

Home for Destitute

These are homes for people who do not have anybody to care. These homes mostly provide shelter and food. This may include men, women, aged and children who do have family or relatives to take care of them. In general the activities of these homes are:

- Provision of psychological support
- Empowering sick and poor and abandoned
- Providing shelter, food and clothes
- Attention on their health and well-being
- Continuing support and care and he/she perform activities of daily living independently
- Join them to their families if they have one and wish to join
- Provide social, economic and physical security
- Improve the quality of life and self-fulfillment
- Restore self-esteem and dignity.

Summary

Empowerment—"A stage of health development, whereby everyone has access to quality health care or practices self-care protected by financial security so that no individual or family experiences catastrophic expenditure that may bring about impoverishment". There need to be well-developed policies for promoting self-care activities that include self, families, groups and communities.

Self-care is everyone's responsibility. However, it is government's responsibility to provide necessary framework to promote self-care at various levels. **Growth** is an increase in physical size of the whole body or any of its parts. **Development** refers to a progressive increase in skill and capacity of function. The factors affecting growth and development are genetic inheritance, prenatal environment, under nutrition of mother etc. Growth monitoring may include: (1) Growth charting and (2) anthropometric measurements—height for age, weight for height and mid-arm circumference. Reference standards methods are (1) Mean or median, (2) Percentile or centiles, (3) Weight for age and weight for height.

Mid-arm circumference (MAC): Mid-arm circumference is considered as the reliable estimation of body's muscle mass. Any reduction in this tells that the body is adjusting the inadequate energy intakes. There are many classifications available to grade malnutrition. Some of them are: Gomez Classification, *Waterlow's Classification and Indian Academy of Paediatrics (IAP).*

Moderate acute malnutrition (MAM) is defined by WHO/ UNICEF: Many health concerns in women are closely related to normal changes or abnormalities of the menstrual cycle.

Menstrual cycle: Many of these problems occur as a result of lack of awareness on (1) menstrual cycle, (2) developmental changes, and other factors that may have an impact on the pattern of the menstrual cycle. *Advise by community health nurse:* Regular exercise, low-fat vegetarian diet, Heating pads may be very effective for cramps, Non-steroidal anti-inflammatory drugs (NSAIDs). Any woman with excessive cramping or dysmenorrhea is refer to hospital to get consultation from gynecologist. *Hygiene:* Advise all ladies to keep self and her genitals clean, use clean cotton cloth pieces or cotton pads for better absorption of the blood and to maintain hygiene. Take bath at least twice a day.

Breast self-examination (BSE): Ideally it is advisable to perform a BSE between 7 and 10 days after the first day of menstrual period. *For women with no unusual risk factors or breast problems:* For women age 20 to 39: A monthly breast self-examination. A clinical breast examination every 1–3 years by a trained health professional. *For women age 40 and older:* A monthly breast self-examination. A yearly clinical breast examination by a trained health professional and a yearly screening mammogram starting at age of 40 years.

Testicular self-examination (TSE): Testicular examination plays a major role in the early detection of testicular cancer. Perform testicular self-examination (TSE) once a month. The test is neither difficult nor time consuming.

Warning signs of breast cancer: Lump, hard knot or thickening, swelling, warmth, redness or darkening, change in the size or shape, dimpling or puckering of the skin, itchy, scaly sore or rash on the nipple, pulling in of your nipple or other parts, nipple discharge that starts suddenly and pain in one spot that does not go away.

In more recent years self-care management of **diabetes** became comparatively easy because of improved technology, various campaigns on diabetes, interest from governmental and non-governmental organizations, and involvement of community health nurses in causing awareness and promoting self-care abilities of people in the community.

Blood glucose levels interpretation—FBS greater than or equal to 126 mg/dL on two occasions, random blood sugar greater than or equal to 200 mg/dL and presence of classic symptoms of diabetes (polyuria, polydipsia, polyphagia, and weight loss), and fasting blood glucose result of greater than or equal to 100 mg/dL demands close follow-up and repeat monitoring every 1–2 years.

Vaccines are available for many of the communicable diseases in children. Some of the examples for vaccine preventable diseases are measles, poliomyelitis, tuberculosis, diphtheria, tetanus, whooping cough, mumps and rubella, etc. On certain occasions counseling becomes necessary as part of health services. Counseling is a kind of talking therapy that permits a person to express their problems and feelings in a confidential and dependable environment.

Early detection of the disease and treatment of the problem refers to secondary level care. Primary level care tries to prevent the disease and promotes health. At many times patients do not continue the treatment appropriately. The health services offered should assure quality and should be ambitious to provide evidence based practice. Failing to assure quality, equals planning to fail in all further tasks. One of the most important tasks of the community health nurse is the maintenance of records and reports for the population she serves.

There are many patients (diagnosed and undiagnosed) with communicable and noncommunicable diseases in the community. Some may be regular in seeking treatment and following the medical guidelines. Community health nurse plays a responsible role in helping the people to seek treatment, undergo investigations, and continue prescribed medications or any other therapy and do the follow-up in morbidity clinics and during home visits.

Basic waste prevention strategies "Three—Rs"-Using various strategies "to not to waste the waste" falls in three steps like: Reduce, Reuse and Recycle. **Dumps**—In this method solid waste is dumped in low lying areas. In a course of time the dumped refuse decreases in volume and is slowly converted into humus as a result of bacterial action. *Sanitary Landfills or Controlled Tipping*—In this method a pit is dug then the refuse is filled in layers; means the solid waste is buried in layers, pressed well and covered with layers of earth. When the trench or pit reaches its full volume or quantity, a cap or top cover is applied to close the site. Some harmful plants are planted over the site to keep away the animals.

Integrated solid waste management (ISWM) focuses on formulating systems that are accessible, acceptable and affordable by the community. This system can sustain and serve the community to provide safe environment. Indian constitution honored women as legal citizens of the country and have equal rights like men. Traditionally males are dominant figures of their families and the same continued even outside. *Woman abuse is the intentional and systematic use of tactics to establish and maintain power and control over the thoughts, beliefs, and conduct of a woman through the inducement of fear and/or dependency.*

The community health nurses working in different parts of India should alert the community about the availability of **telephone lines** for helping the women in emergencies. In India, around 1.7 million children died before reaching the age of 5 years in 2010, and more than half of them (52%) died in the first month of life. Apart from the diseases many deaths that occur as a result of various forms of child abuse go unnoticed.

Old age homes: The senior citizens who do not have family support, not accommodated by relatives, not wanting to stay with the family due to various reasons, look for old age homes.

There are many old age homes function in India by NGOs. Some of them provide free services and others for payment. In general, all of them provide food, shelter and medical amenities to the inmates. In paid homes there is a provision for telephone, internet, etc.

Help age India: Help Age India established in 1978 is a leading charity voluntary organization in India working for cause of uplifting disadvantaged elderly.

There are many homes established for **physically and mentally** challenged individuals in India. There are paid homes and unpaid homes providing 24/7 care and training activities. Apart there are day care centers where parents/care taker accompany them and bring them back in the evening.

Assess Yourself

I. Multiple Choice Questions (Choose the Correct Answer)

1. Which of these following "laws" overrides all the other "food related laws"?
   a. Food Safety and Standards Act, 2006
   b. Prevention of Food Adulteration Act, 1954
   c. Fruit Products Order, 1955
   d. Meat Food Products Order, 1973

2. Cephalocaudal refers to the direction of development occurring in:
   a. Head-to-toe direction
   b. Transverse direction
   c. Vertical
   d. Horizontal

3. Proximodistal refers to the direction of development occurring in:
   a. Head-to-toe direction
   b. Longitudinal direction
   c. Inward to outward pattern
   d. Linear vertical

4. In which of these methods solid waste is buried in layers?
   a. Pyrolysis
   b. Dumping
   c. Controlled tripping
   d. All of the above

5. Which of these following refers to "anaerobic method" of composting?
   a. Bangalore method
   b. Mechanical composting
   c. Manure pits
   d. Burial

II. Short Answer Questions

1. Define growth and development.
2. Write four principles of growth and development.
3. Define self-care.
4. Self-care promotion at various levels.
5. Write four factors that affect growth and development.
6. Write four parental guidance of one month old infant.
7. Write four basic features of a growth chart.
8. Define level I and II trauma care.
9. Write four functions of Bureau of Indian Standards (BIS).
10. What are Codex Alimentarius and *Agmark Standards*.
11. Write four roles of Voluntary Agencies in PFA Act.
12. List four methods of composting.
13. List four disadvantages of open dumping.
14. Mention about "Ambulance Services" under national health mission.
15. Write four advantages of sanitary landfill method.

III. Short Notes

1. Growth monitoring
2. Growth and development
3. Breast self-examination
4. Testicular self-examination
5. Solid waste management
6. Incineration
7. Warning signs of specific diseases
8. Maintenance of health records for family
9. Women empowerment
10. Child abuse
11. Women abuse
12. Commercial sex workers
13. Old age homes
14. Trauma services
15. Food Adulteration Act
16. Substance abuse
17. FSSAI
18. Self-care promotion at various levels
19. Trauma care
20. Bureau of Indian Standards (BIS)

IV. Write Essay on:

1. State the different types of solid waste disposal. Write the role of community health nurse in solid waste disposal.
2. What is women empowerment? Discuss the status of women and women welfare programs available in India.

ANSWERS

I. 1. a **2.** a **3.** c **4.** c **5.** a

National Health and Family Welfare Programs and the Role of Community Health Nurses

6
Unit

Learning Objectives

At the end of this unit the learners will be able to:

- List various national health programs in India
- List the objectives for each specific program
- State the historical mile stones of reproductive and child health program
- List various programs that are incorporated into reproductive and child health program (RCH)
- Describe the role of community health nurse in RCH program
- Describe revised national tuberculosis control program
- Describe National Vector Borne Disease Control Program (NVBDCP)
- Explain the role of community health nurse in NVBDCP
- Describe malaria control program
- Describe national leprosy eradication program
- Describe STDs control program
- Describe AIDS control program
- Describe expanded immunization program
- Describe Pulse polio eradication program
- Describe ICDS program
- Describe ESI scheme
- State the national health insurance schemes in India

KEY TERMS

- Acute Respiratory Infection (ARI) program
- Reproductive and Child Health (RCH) Programs Phase-I and II
- Essential obstetric care
- Emergency obstetrical care
- Essential newborn care
- Diarrheal Disease Control and control of vitamin A deficiency
- Prevention and control of anemia in children
- Revised National Tuberculosis Control Program (RNTCP)
- National Vector Borne Disease Control Program (NVBDCP)
- Malaria control program
- National Filaria Control Program (NFCP)
- Role of community health nurse in elimination of filariasis
- Japanese encephalitis, dengue fever, chikungunya

KEY TERMS

- National Leprosy Eradication Program (NLEP)
- National AIDS Control Program (NACP)
- HIV Testing and Counseling
- Sexually Transmitted Disease (STD) Control Program
- Surakhsha clinics
- National program for control of blindness (NPCB)
- Iodine deficiency disorder program (IDD)
- Expanded program on immunization
- National water supply and sanitation program
- Swajaldhara
- Bharat Nirman
- Rural Sanitation Program
- Swachh Bharat Mission (SBM)
- Nirmal Bharat Abhiyan (NBA)
- Minimum need program
- 20-Point Program
- Polio Eradication: Pulse Polio Program
- Acute Flaccid Paralysis Surveillance
- National Program for Prevention and Control of Cancer, Diabetes, Cardiovascular Disease and Stroke (NPCDCS)
- Cancer Prevention and control Components under NPCDCS
- Tobacco Control Legislation
- National Mental Health Program (NMHP)
- Yaws Eradication Program
- National nutritional programs
- Vitamin A prophylaxis program
- Integrated Child Development Services (ICDS) Scheme
- Kishori shakti yojana
- Nutrition Program for Adolescent Girls
- Anganwadi worker (AWW)
- Employees state Insurance Scheme (ESI Act, 1948)
- Rajiv Gandhi Shramik Kalyan Yojna
- The Central Government Health Scheme in India
- Rashtriya Swasthya Bima Yojana (RSBY)
- Aam Aadmi Bima Yojana (AABY)

It is a herculean task if any government plans to meet all health care needs of the people in solo. National health programs were launched time to time to prevent, control, eliminate or eradicate certain communicable and noncommunicable diseases. National health programs either find its place in five-year plans to control or eradicate a specific disease based on the national priority. Currently, our country has health program against almost all diseases of public health importance. Some of these are centrally sponsored; some state sponsored and the others by state and center. Apart from the above, other health programs get assistance from international agencies.

Contd…

NATIONAL VECTOR-BORNE DISEASES

NATIONAL VECTOR-BORNE DISEASE CONTROL PROGRAM (NVBDCP)

In India, the Directorate of National Vector Borne Disease Control Program (NVBDCP) is the central agency for the prevention and control of the six most common VBDs in the country. They are: malaria, dengue, lymphatic filariasis, kala-azar, japanese encephalitis (JE) and chikungunya.

The NVBDCP takes care of planning, policy making, technical guidance and evaluation of the program implementation.

All the above mentioned diseases are transmitted by mosquitoes except Kala-azar which is transmitted by sand flies.

Prevention and Control Strategies for VBD Under NVBDCP

There are important strategies listed under three broad headings to tackle the problem of vector-borne diseases (Fig. 1).

Objectives

○ Integrated accelerated action toward reducing mortality of malaria, dengue and JE by half
○ Elimination of kala-azar by 2010
○ Elimination of lymphatic filariasis by the year 2015

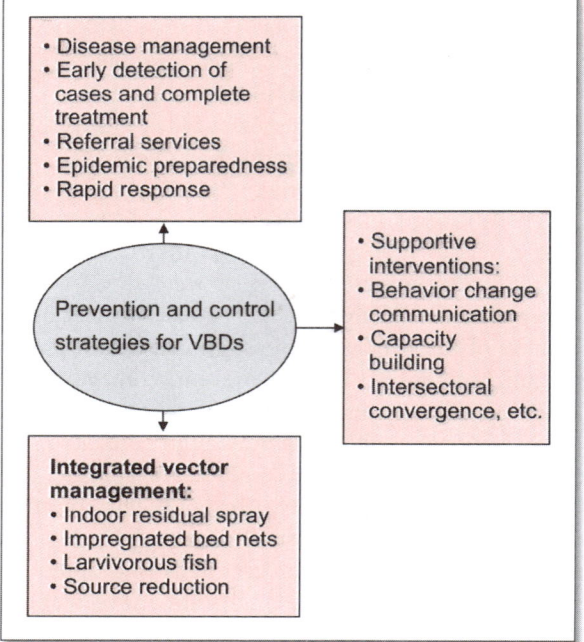

Figure 1: Vector-borne disease: Prevention and control

MALARIA CONTROL PROGRAM (TABLE 1)

Malaria control program was launched during first five-year plan, in 1953. The increased success rates motivated India to convert the program into eradication program. Following which, the program had gone through many changes.

Table 1: Historical events in malaria control activities in india

Years	Activities
Before 1940	There was no organized malaria control program in India
Scenario before 1953	Estimated number of malaria cases and deaths in India were 75 million and 1 million respectively
1953	National malaria control program launched
1958	National malaria eradication program launched
1966	Malaria cases reduced to 0.1 million
Early 1970s	Resurgence of malaria
1971	Urban malaria scheme launched
1976	Malaria cases—6.46 million highest in post DDT period
1977	Modified plan of operations (MPO) implemented
1984–1998	Annual reported incidence of malaria within 2–3 million cases
1995	Modified action plan for malaria control implemented
1997	World Bank assisted enhanced malaria control project (EMCP) started
1999	Renaming of program to national antimalaria program
2002	Integration of malaria control progamme into the national Vector-borne disease control program
2005	○ Global fund assisted intensified malaria control project (IMCP) ○ Launched in 94 districts of 10 states (2005–2010) ○ Introduction of RDTs in the program
2008	Revision of drug policy with ACT (Artemisinin—based combination therapy) use extended to high-risk P. falciparum districts covering about 95% of P. falciparum infections
2009	○ World Bank assisted National Vector borne diseases control project; covering 185 million population 93 districts in 8 states. ○ Introduction of Long lasting insecticidal nets (LLINs)
2010	Revised National Drug Policy 2010. ACT for all *P. falciparum* cases in the country; Global Fund (Rd 9) assisted intensified malaria control project (IMCP-II) –Oct. 2010 to Sept. 2015
2012	Introduction of bivalent RDT
2013	New drug policy 2013

Main Activities

- Formulating policies and guidelines
- Technical guidance
- Planning
- Logistics
- Monitoring and evaluation
- Coordination of activities through state/UTs and in consultation with National Center for disease control (NCDC), National Institute of Malarial Research (NIMR)
- Collaboration with international organizations like the WHO, World Bank, GFATM and other donor agencies
- Training
- Facilitating research through NCDC, NIMR, Regional medical research centers
- Coordinating control activities in the inter-state and inter-country border areas.

Strategic Action Plan for Malaria Control in India (2012–2017)

Vision

Substantial and sustained reduction in the burden of malaria in the near and mid-term, and elimination of malaria in the long-term, when new tools in combination with strengthening of health systems will make national elimination possible.

Malaria control is incorporated under the umbrella of NRHM.

Objective

To achieve Annual Parasite Index <1 per 1000 population by the end of 2017.

Goals

- Screening all fever cases suspected to malaria (60% through quality microscopy and 40% by rapid diagnostic test).
- Testing all *P. falciparum* cases with full course of effective ACT and primaquine and all *P. vivax* cases with 3 days chloroquine and 14 days primaquine.
- Equipping all health institutions especially in high-risk areas.
- Strengthening all district and sub-district hospitals in malaria endemic areas.

Outcome Indicators

- At least 80% suffering from malaria get correct, affordable, appropriate and complete treatment within 24 hours of reporting

- At least 80% of those at high-risk of malaria get protected
- At least 10% of population in high-risk areas is surveyed annually.

Malaria Control Strategies

Surveillance and Case Management

- Case detection (passive and active)
- Early diagnosis and complete treatment
- Sentinel surveillance.

Integrated Vector Management

- Indoor residual sprays (IRS)
- Insecticide treated bed-nets (ITNs) long-lasting insecticide nets (LLINs)
- Antilarval measures including source reduction.

Epidemic Preparedness and Early Response Supportive Interventions

- Capacity building
- Behavior change communication
- Intersectoral coordination
- Monitoring and evaluation
- Operational research and applied field research.

Mosquito Control Measures

Preventive measures include:

Antilarval measures: This includes treating stagnant water with larvicides. The larvicides used are:

- Oil
- Paris green
- Temphos

Antiadult measures:

- Residual spraying of DDT, malathion, fenitrothion against adult mosquitos
- Space application of pesticides in the form of fog or mist.

Protection against Mosquito Bite

The followings are used to protect people from mosquito bites:

- Protective clothing
- Repellents
- Mosquito nets
- Mosquito coils
- Screening of the houses
- Mosquito mesh to windows and doors

Reduction of Mosquito Breeding Sites

○ Promotion of proper drainage system
○ Thorough drainage or filling measures
○ Management of water level
○ Changing the salt content of water
○ Keeping water coolers clean
○ Maintain clean surroundings with no stagnation of water.

Health Education

Community must be educated on cause, spread, prevention, and management of malaria. Individual, group, and mass educational approaches have to be used to educate the community.

Integrated Approach

In present day's world attempts are being paid on bioenvironmental and personal protective measures known as integrated vector control methodology.

NATIONAL MALARIA CONTROL PROGRAM UNDER NVBDCP

○ This plays the most important role in controlling malaria.
○ This functions according to the strategies and goals set in the program.
○ Diagnosis and treatment of malaria (Flowchart 1)

Role of Community Health Nurse in Caring Malaria

○ Monitoring of vital signs for all cases attending the subcenter/primary health center
○ No single fever case should be ignored
○ Thin and thick blood smears should be done and dispatched to lab
○ While waiting for the report start the person on presumptive treatment

Flowchart 1: Diagnosis and treatment of malaria

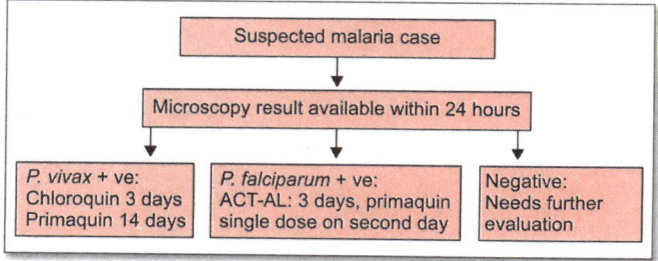

○ Avoid starting treatment on an empty stomach
○ The first dose should be given under observation
○ Provide health education to the individual and family about malarial fever
○ Advise to drink plenty of water
○ After administration of the oral antimalarial drugs observe for vomiting; repeat the dose if vomiting occurs within half an hour of intake antimalarial tablets
○ Intravenous fluids should be started for those who are unable to tolerate anything orally
○ Any patient complains of drowsiness immediate referral to hospital is necessary for further diagnosis management.
○ Follow-up of the family is important.

LYMPHATIC FILARIASIS ELIMINATION PROGRAM

○ Lymphatic filariasis, popularly known as elephantiasis, is a much ignored tropical disease. Health statistics reveals that worldwide over 120 million people are infected which about 40 million disfigured and incapacitated by the disease. There are 600 million people exposed since 1955, National Filarial Control Program in operation (NFCP). In June 1978, NFCP was merged with Urban Malarial scheme. In 2003 it was included in NVBDCP.
○ Director of National Institute of Communicable disease, Delhi continue to take of training and research related to NFCP.
○ Three Training Research Centers in filariology located in: (i) Kerala (ii) Rajahamundry Andhra Pradesh (iii) Varanasi Uttar Pradesh Under National Institute of Communicable disease, Delhi.
○ Twelve headquarters bureau are functioning at state level.

Definition

Elimination is defined as "lymphatic filariasis ceases to be the public health problem, when the number of microfilaria carriers is less than 1% and the children born after initiation of elimination of lymphatic filariasis (ELF) are free from circulating antigenemia (presence of anti filarial worm in human body).

Major Activities

National Health Policy 2002 set the goal to eliminate lymphatic filariasis by 2015.

○ Antilarval and antimosquito measures in endemic area
○ Filaria clinics established for the early detection and treatment of positive cases
○ Underground drainage facilities in hyperendemic cities and towns.

- As a measure to achieve elimination of lymphatic filariasis in 2004, India initiated mas drug administration (MDA) with single dose of DEC tablet and other measures like home-based foot care and hydrocelectomy surgeries. DEC and Albendazole tablets were upscaled since 2007.

- In 2012, as a part of validation process, India stopped MDA in 16 districts of Tamil Nadu and in some union territories. Microfilarial survey through night blood smear before MDA is done in implementation units.

Lymphatic Filariasis-Elimination Strategies

- Annual mass drug administration
  - Single dose of antifilarial drug for 5 years or more to the eligible population
  - People excluded under mass drug administration are pregnant women, children below the age of 2 years and people who are seriously ill, to interrupt transmission of the disease.
- Home-based management of foot care for lymphedema
- For men—up scaling of hydrocele operations in identified CHCs/district hospitals/medical colleges.
- Application of insect repellant creams over the body
- Using insecticide impregnated bed nets
- Prevent access to mosquito by putting mosquito mesh to windows and doors.
- Health educate on environmental sanitation
  - Avoid water stagnation in and around the house
  - Filling up of ditches and cesspools
  - Routine maintenance of septic tanks soakage pits
- Treatment:
  - Create awareness on treatment availability
  - Motivate to have treatment on regular basis
- Information
  - Inform to report complications related to filariasis like excessive lymphedema and hydrocele etc.
- Assistance
  - Assist in home care management
- Survey and MDA
  - Involve in mass microfilarial survey and MDA.

KALA-AZAR CONTROL PROGRAM

Kala-azar control program is a centrally sponsored program, launched in 1990–91. Prior to introduction of DDT, Kala-azar was highly endemic in India and had disturbed the economic growth of country due to its high morbidity and mortality rates. This has brought down the incidence from 77,102 cases in 1992 to 13,869 cases in 2013.

Elimination Strategies for Kala-azar

- Enhanced case detection and complete treatment.
- The introduction of PK39 rapid diagnostic kits and oral drug "Miltefosine" in treatment.
- Interruption of transmission through vector control-Fogging with pyrethroid in place of DDT to eliminate sandfly.
- Communication for behavioral impact and intersectoral convergence.
- Capacity building.
- Supervision, monitoring and evaluation.
- Dissemination of formulated research guidelines to all states on prevention and control of Kala-azar.

Case Search for Kala-azar

- Quarterly case searches in place of annual search: The active case searches carried during a fortnight referred to "Kala-azar fortnight survey" where door-to-door survey conducted
- Accredited social health activist (ASHA) gets ₹300/far each case identification and ₹100/ for ensuring community support during insecticide sprays
- Patient is paid ₹500/ during his hospitalization to compensate his wages
- The above "Revised strategy of eradication of Kala-azar" was launched on 2nd December 2014.
- The new strategy also includes: Introduction of RDT developed by ICMR; Treatment with Liposomal Amphotericin B, (IV 10 mg—single dose) which is supplied free of cost by World Health Organization.

JAPANESE ENCEPHALITIS CONTROL

Recent literature maintains that there are nearly 68,000 clinical cases of Japanese Encephalitis (JE) occurs each year, with up to 20,400 deaths, globally. (Bulletin-WHO, October 2011).

And again among survivors 20–30% suffer with permanent intellectual, behavioral, or neurological problems such as paralysis, recurrent seizures or the inability to speak. The disease is mostly found in rural and peri-urban areas, where people live in closely with vertebrate hosts. Maximum number of cases reported from Andra Pradesh, West Bengal, Assam, Tamil Nadu, Karnataka, Kerala, Bihar, Maharashtra, Manipur, Haryana and Uttar Pradesh.

Vector Control Intervention Strategies

Alternate wet and dry irrigation (AWDI): As recognized, flooded rice fields have been the ideal breeding place for several mosquito species including those that transmit JE.

The alternate wetting and drying of paddy fields, helps in interfering with the development of the mosquito from larvae and pupae to adult which in turn helps as a technique to control the mosquitos of JE.

Biological Control Strategies

Natural fishes like *Gambusia affinis*, *Tilapia* spp, *Poecilia reticulata* or Cyprinidae, *Killifish*, *Nematodes* and *Crustaceans* are used in biological control.

Chemical Control

Deltamethrin, organophosphates and carbamates are used to control vectors.

Health Education

- Educate community on cause, spread, prevention and management of JE
- Involve community members to keep the surroundings clean
- Engage community in the activities like filling pools, draining of accumulated water weekly, lowering water levels in rice fields, etc. that would cut down the mosquito breeding places.

Personal Protective Measures

- Wear full sleeved clothes
- Use of mosquito coils
- Burn neem leaves around the house
- Avoid water stagnation
- Avoid sleeping outdoors
- Insecticide treated mosquito nets
- Apply repellents to avoid mosquito bites
- Eliminate pig farming

Management

- There is no specific treatment available. Most often hospitalized patients are managed with feeding, airway management, and anticonvulsants for seizure control
- These patients may require long-term care and rehabilitation.

Surveillance

The component of JE surveillance consists of three major areas:

- Clinical surveillance through early diagnosis and management of JE patients at primary health centers.
- Vector surveillance in risk areas of JE to assess the vector behavior and strengthen the system accordingly.

- Sero-surveillance to monitor JE specific antibodies in sentinel animals or birds as well to recognize high-risk areas.

DENGUE CONTROL

Dengue mostly occurs in tropical and subtropical climates, globally. Severe dengue is a major cause of death among children in some of the Asian and Latin American countries. An outbreak of dengue was reported in Delhi in the year 1996. Government in consultation with states identified 311 hospitals to provide support for laboratory investigations in endemic areas. In addition 14 Apex Referral Laboratories linked with the hospitals.

Eight Key Elements for Prevention and Control of Dengue

Surveillance

- Surveillance is indicated in all endemic areas of *Aedes aegypti* and *A. albopictus*.
- Sentinel clinics should report to public health authority the number of cases reported with temperature above 38°C. This would assist for further identification of the cases by blood tests.

Case Management

Laboratory diagnosis and clinical management.

Vector Management

- Source reduction
- Chemical control
- Personal protection
- Legal measures.

Outbreak Response

- Epidemic preparedness
- Media management.

Capacity Building

- Training
- Infrastructure development
- Operational research.

Behavioral Change Communication

- Social mobilization
- IEC.

Inter-sectoral Coordination

Coordination with health and nonhealth sectors.

Monitoring and Supervision

- Review, field visit, analysis of reports
- Feedback

CHIKUNGUNYA

The name "chikungunya" originated from a word in the Kimakonde language, meaning "to become contorted", that describes the sufferer with stooped appearance and joint pain. Chikungunya has been found in more than 60 countries in Asia, National Filaria Control Program (NFCP).

The same prevention, control and surveillance strategy of Dengue is applied in chikungunya too.

Role of Community Health Nurse

Educate on environmental control: Actually prevention and control relies profoundly on reducing the number of natural and artificial water filled containers that largely support mosquito-breeding.

Educate on personal protective measures

- Clothing which minimizes skin exposure to the day biting vectors
- Where possible, clothes can be treated with permethrin to repel mosquitoes
- Application of repellents to exposed skin; repellents should contain DEET
- Use of insecticide-treated mosquito nets for protection.
- Mosquito coils or other insecticide vaporizers to prevent indoor biting
- Living rooms should be fitted with insect screens on windows and on doors.

NATIONAL GUINEA WORM DISEASE (ERADICATION PROGRAM)

- Guinea worm disease is a disabling parasitic disease. This disease was popular in rural areas where step-wells were common. The World Health Organization (WHO) officially declared countries of South East Asian region as free of guinea worm disease (dracunculiasis).
- Last case of guinea worm disease in India was identified in 1996 (Box 1).

Box 1: Last case of Guinea worm in India

- 6 July 1996
- Mr Bhanwara Ram, 25 years
- Village: Aau, PHC: Peelwa
- District: Jodhpur, Rajasthan
- Father had guinea worm in 1995
- Brother and sister had guinea worm in 1996

- The International certification team (ICT), presented its report on guinea worm disease status in India to the ICCDE in the meeting held in February 2000 in Geneva. On the basis of ICT report, India was declared as Guinea Worm disease free country by International Commission for Certification of Dracunculiasis Eradication (ICCDE).

Activities continued as per the guidelines of international team:

- Health education specifically to rural women and children
- Rumor registration and rumor investigations
- Maintaining guinea worm disease in the notified list of disease and continuation of surveillance in previously infected areas
- Close watch on functioning of hand pumps and other sources of safe drinking water.

MATERNAL AND CHILD HEALTH RELATED PROGRAMS

JOURNEY OF MOTHER AND CHILD RELATED PROGRAMS

- 1951—India initiated family planning program to reduce birth rate and control population growth
- 1966—Separate department of family planning established
- 1974–79—During 5th five-year plan the aim was to reduce birth rate to 30 per thousand by the end of 1978–1979. This was tried by integrating family planning services with maternal and child health, and nutrition. The program became readily acceptable. But the program had to face a set-back during 1977–78 due to rigid enforcement of law on people.

1977–1978—Subsequent to great learning from pros and cons of "Family planning program"

India changed its name as, "Family welfare program." The approach used thereafter was motivation and health education. Family welfare program emphasized on voluntary approach.

- **1992—Child survival and safe motherhood (CSSM).** Mother and Child related programs like universal immunization program (UIP), oral rehydration therapy (ORT) and prophylaxis programs for mother and child to control anemia and vitamin "A" deficiency respectively were incorporated under CSSM in 1992.

○ **In 1992, all the other programs including "Family welfare program" were brought under CSSM project.** Acute respiratory infection (ARI) control program (ARI), first referral units (FRUs) and "Disposable delivery kit" to pregnant ladies were also became the components of CSSM project. CSSM project continued until 1997.

REPRODUCTIVE AND CHILD HEALTH (RCH) PROGRAMS

Definition—Reproductive and Child Health Approach

Reproductive and child health approach is defined as "people have ability to reproduce and regulate their fertility, women are able to go through pregnancy and their birth safely, the outcome of pregnancy is successful in terms of maternal and infant survival and well-being, and couples are able to have sexual relations free of fear of pregnancy and of contracting disease". **—WHO**

Historical Development

Indian government put constant efforts in improving maternal and newborn health by introducing series of health programs time to time.

Now many programs relating to mother and child are placed under RCH program.

Major mile stones are:

○ 1992—Child survival and safe motherhood program
○ 1997—Reproductive and child health Phase-I
○ 1997—Reproductive and child health Phase-II
○ 2005—National rural health mission
○ 2013—RMNCH+A strategy
○ 2013—National rural health mission
○ 2014—India newborn action plan

Reproductive and child health program is an integrated approach aimed to concentrate on health status of young women, young children which has been fragmented under the names of various programs. The programs previously run independently and now incorporated into RCH are:

○ The components of family welfare program
○ Universal immunization program
○ Oral rehydration therapy

○ Child survival and safe motherhood program
○ Acute respiratory infection (ARI) control program

Care of mother and child takes an important place in our health care delivery system. India showed keen interest in improving the maternal and child health. It was reflected from the fact that 9 out of 17 goals of National Health Policy (1983) were specifically on maternal and child health.

Reproductive and Child Health Program Phase-I

This program was incorporated family planning, CSSM, prevention and management of reproductive tract infections (RTIs), sexually transmitted diseases (STDs), and acquired immunodeficiency syndrome (AIDs). On the above it had used client approach to health care (Fig. 2). This program was formally launched on October 15 1997.

Major Interventions under RCH-I

This program integrates all interventions of fertility regulation, maternal and child health and reproductive health for men and women.

○ Provides client-oriented services
○ Upgrading of the health facilities at all levels to assure quality care
○ Establishment of first referral units (FRUs) at sub-district level to provide comprehensive emergency obstetric and newborn care

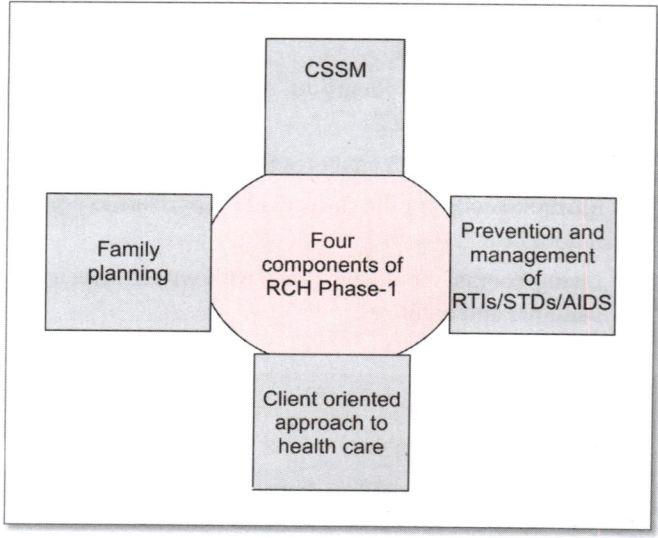

Figure 2: Four components of RCH phase-1

Abbreviations: AIDS, acquired immunodeficiency syndromes CSSM, child survival and safe motherhood; RCH, reproductive and child health; RTIs, reproductive tract-infections; STDs; sexually transmitted disease

- Provision of facilities for obstetric care, medical termination of pregnancy and for insertion of intrauterine devices in PHC
- Provision of IUD facilities at sub-centers
- Provision of specialist facilities in all district hospitals and sub-district level hospitals to treat RTIs and STDs
- To Improve outreach services for the vulnerable population.

Essential Obstetric Care

Basic maternity services to all women through:

- Early registration of antenatals
- Minimum three antenatal checkups
- Provision for safe home delivery or institutional delivery
- Provision of three postnatal visits to assess recovery and detect complications.

Emergency Obstetrical Care

- Emergency obstetric care is very vital to reduce maternal neonatal mortalities. Under CSSM project 1748 FRUs were supplied with disposable kits. However, due to poor staffing and infrastructure this was not in full-fledged operation.
- After the inception of RCH-I, infrastructure and staffing have been improved. Traditional birth attendants play their role with enhanced skills through training.

24-hour Delivery Services at PHCS/CHCS

Additional honorarium to staff to promote 24-hour delivery services.

Medical Termination of Pregnancy Act 1971

Medical termination of pregnancy (MTP) Act helps to reduce deaths occurring due to unsafe abortions. Central government provides financial assistance to this program.

Control of Reproductive Tract Infections and Sexually Transmitted Diseases

- The components of STDs and RTIs are linked with National Aids Control Organization (NACO)
- NACO provides assistance to setup RTI and STD clinics
- Central government provides assistance in training staff and provision of drug kit
- Two lab technicians posted in each district.

Immunization

- Universal immunization program (UIP) became a component of CSSM in 1992 and part of RCH since 1997.

- It will continue to take care of vaccine needs like polio, tetanus, DPT, DT, TB and measles.
- Extend help for cold chain maintenance.

Essential Newborn Care

- To reduce perinatal and neonatal mortality
- Provision of basic facilities in FRUs
- The vital strategies are to train medical and other health personnel in essential newborn care
- The main components of care include prevention of hypothermia and infection, exclusive breastfeeding and timely referral of sick newborn.

Diarrheal Disease Control

- Diarrheal disease control program will continue in the areas where integrated management in not established
- India is the first nation to introduce low osmolarity oral rehydration solution
- Addition of zinc helps in reducing the severity of diarrhea
- Provision of deworming guidelines
- Provision of safe drinking water to reduce the incidence of diarrhea.

Prevention and Control of Vitamin A Deficiency in Children

Administration of vitamin A solution to all children:

- 1 lakh international units of vitamin A solution at the age of 9 months—First dose
- 2 lakh international units of vitamin A solution given after 9 months—Second dose
- 2 lakhs international units of vitamin A solution— subsequent doses at 6 months intervals up to 5 years of age.

Prevention and Control of Anemia in Children

- *From 6 months to 5 years*: Liquid formulation of 20 mg of elemental iron and 100 mcg of folic acid per day per 100 days in a year
- *From 6 years to 10 years*: Liquid formulation of 30 mg of elemental iron and 250 mcg folic acid per day for 100 days in a year
- *Children above 10 years*: Adult dose will be given

Introduction of Hepatitis B Vaccine

Hepatitis B vaccine will be administered along with primary doses of DPT.

Training of Dais

○ *Dais'* training was introduced in 2001–2002. This was implemented in 156 districts in 18 states/union territories that had safe delivery rates of less than 30%

○ The scheme was activated in all empowered action group (EAG) states with the aim of training at least one *dai* in each village to promote safe delivery.

Reproductive and Child Health Program-Phase-II

This RCH phase-II was launched on April 1 2005 with the aim to reduce maternal and child mortality and morbidity while concentrating on rural health care. The major strategies are:

○ Essential obstetric care
  ❑ Institutional delivery
  ❑ Skilled attendance at delivery
○ Emergency obstetric care
  ❑ Operationalizing first referral units
  ❑ Operationalizing primary health centers (PHCs) and community health centers (CHCs) to provide round the clock delivery services
○ Strengthening referral system India has formulated certain guidelines to reduce maternal and infant mortality rates. The main initiatives are:

> **Three critical determinants to declare a facility as first referral unit (FRU):**
> • *Surgical interventions*
> • *Newborn care*
> • *Blood storage facility*
> • *(All these must be available on a 24 hours basis)*

Essential Obstetrical Care

To Promote Institutional Delivery

○ Fifty percent of PHCs and all CHCs would be made operational as 24-hours delivery centers in a phased manner by the year 2010

○ Responsible to provide basic obstetrical and essential newborn care and basic newborn services round the clock

○ Staff PHCs with 3–4 staff nurses/ANM to provide round the clock services.

Skilled Attendance to Conduct Delivery

○ Delivery conduction by skilled people reduces maternal mortality

○ Appropriate referral services

○ Formulated guidelines for normal delivery and management of complications for medical officers at primary health centers and community health centers

○ Formulated guidelines on antenatal care and skilled birth attendance for ANMs and LHVs (Lady health visitor or female health assistant)

○ Policy decisions

○ ANMs/LHVs/Sector health nurses are permitted to use some interventions in specific emergency conditions when life of the mother is at risk.

Emergency Obstetric Care

○ Operationalizing FRUs and skilled attendance at birth

○ Services at FRUs

○ Twenty-four hour delivery services including normal and assisted deliveries

○ Emergency obstetrical care that includes surgical interventions like cesarean section

○ Newborn care

○ Emergency care of sick children

○ Family planning services that include laproscopic services

○ Safe abortion services

○ Treatment of STI/RTI

○ Blood storage facility

○ Essential laboratory services

○ Referral services.

Criteria to Function as Full-Fledged

○ A minimum bed strength of 20–30

○ North east states and underserved areas of EAG states bed strength of 10–12

○ A fully functional operation theater

○ A fully functional labor room

○ An area earmarked and equipped for newborn care in the labor room and in the ward

○ A functional laboratory

○ Blood storage facility

○ 24-hour electricity and water supply

○ Waste disposal facilities

○ Ambulance facility.

Strengthening Referral System

○ Phase of RCH provided funds to panchayat for helping poor people in obstetrical emergencies. Since this did not work well some of the suggestions were provided for strengthening the RCH referral link. They are self-help groups, NGOs and women groups and outsourcing

- New initiatives under RCH phase II
- Training of MBBS doctors to handle obstetrical emergencies
- Operationalizing FRUs in sub-district level
- Training to MBBS doctors in obstetric management skills including cesarean section
- Federation of Obstetrics and Gynecology Society prepared a training plan for 16 weeks for the same
- Setting blood storage centers in FRUs as per government guidelines.

Recent Initiatives under RCH Phase-II

- Rashtriya Bal Swasthya Karyakram (RBSK)
- Rashtriya Kishore Swasthya Karyakram (RKSK)
- Weekly Iron Folic Acid Supplementation (WIFS) program.

Role of Community Health Nurse in RCH Program

Community health nurses play various roles in planning, implementing and providing feedback received from the community on the program.

In Caring Antenatal Mothers

- She actively participates and supervises the early registration of antenatal mothers
- She is responsible for all the care activities that may happen in antenatal period. This starts from the identification and registration of antenatal (AN) mothers. Following which:
  - Regular antenatal checkup
  - Nutrition during pregnancy
  - Regular watch on weight gain, pedal edema, blood pressure, urine albumin, urine sugar and fetal growth
- Administration of injection. Tetanus toxoid as prescribed
- Supplementation of iron and folic acid as per the guidelines
- Screening for high risk pregnancies and referral
- Follow-up on investigation
- Preparation of mother to breastfeed the baby after delivery
- Identification of any complications and referral for the same
- Supervision of the schemes like *Janani Suraksha Yojana* and any other

- Preparation for delivery—home/institutional
- Maintenance of health cards for child
- Training and supervision of *dais*
- Advice on available of facility for safe abortion in recommended cases
- Assessment and follow-up on reproductive infections and sexually transmitted infections.

Care for Postnatal Period

- Postnatal visits during postpartum period—Assessment on involution process, umbilical cord stump of the baby for any infection, breastfeeding, nutrition of the mother and temporary/permanent contraceptive advice to mothers
- Supervision of utilization of disposable delivery kit by *dais*.

Caring for Child

- Newborn care
- Maintenance of health cards for child
- Appropriate management of diarrhea
- Appropriate management of ARI—Assessment on respiratory infections and administration of oral amoxicillin as per guidelines
- Administration of vitamin A solution to children as per the guidelines
- Supervision on cold chain maintenance and immunization to children (All vaccines under universal immunization program)
- Assessment on growth and development and nutrition.

RMNCH

RMCH+A approach was launched in to 2013 address the major causes of mortality among women and children as well as the delay in accessing and utilizing health care and services. The RMNCH+A strategic approach has been developed to provide an understanding of 'continuum of care' to ensure equal focus on various life stages. Priority interventions for each thematic area have been included in this to ensure that the linkages between them are contextualized to the same and consecutive life stage. It also introduces new initiatives like the use of Score Card to track the performance, National Iron + Initiative to address the issue of anaemia across all age groups and the Comprehensive Screening and Early interventions for defects at birth, diseases and deficiencies among children and adolescents. The RMNCH+A appropriately directs the States to focus their efforts on the most vulnerable population and disadvantaged groups in the country. It also emphasizes on the need to reinforce efforts in those poor performing districts that have already been identified as the high focus districts.

Objectives

The 12th Five Year Plan has defined the national health outcomes and the three goals that are relevant to RMNCH+A strategic approach as follows:

Health Outcome Goals established in the 12th Fiver Year Plan

- Reduction of infant mortality rate (IMR) to 25 per 1,000 live births by 2017
- Reduction in maternal mortality ratio (MMR) to 100 per 100,000 live births by 2017
- Reduction in Total Fertility Rate (TFR) to 2.1 by 2017

Coverage Targets for key RMNCH+A Interventions for 2017

- Increase facilities equipped for perinatal care (designated as 'delivery points') by 100%
- Increase proportion of all births in government and accredited private institutions at annual rate of 5.6 % from the baseline of 61% (SRS 2010)
- Increase proportion of pregnant women receiving antenatal care at annual rate of 6% from the baseline of 53% (CES 2009)
- Increase proportion of mothers and newborns receiving postnatal care at annual rate of 7.5% from the baseline of 45% (CES 2009)
- Increase proportion of deliveries conducted by skilled birth attendants at annual rate of 2% from the baseline of 76% (CES 2009)
- Increase exclusive breastfeeding rates at annual rate of 9.6% from the baseline of 36% (CES 2009)
- Reduce prevalence of under-five children who are underweight at annual rate of 5.5% from the baseline of 45% (NFHS 3)
- Increase coverage of three doses DTP (12–23 months) at annual rate of 3.5% from the baseline of 7% (CES 2009)
- Increase ORS use in under-five children with diarrhoea at annual rate of 7.2% from the baseline of 43% (CES 2009)
- Reduce anaemia in adolescent girls and boys (15–19 years) at annual rate of 6% from the baseline of 56% and 30%, respectively (NFHS 3).
- Decrease the proportion of total fertility contributed by adolescents (15–19 years) at annual rate of 3.8% per year from the baseline of 16% (NFHS 3).

Rational of RMNCH A+ strategies

- In order to bring greater impact through RCH program, it is important to recognise that reproductive, maternal and child health cannot be addressed in isolation

- RMNCH+A strategic approach focuses on what the health delivery system can do to help achieve maternal and child health goals
- Purpose RMNCHA +A approach is to provide an understanding of comprehensive approach to improve child survival and safe motherhood

Why '**Plus**' in RMNCHA

The '**Plus**' in the strategic approach of RMNCH+A denotes:

- Inclusion of **adolescence** as a distinct '**life stage**' in the overall strategy
- **Linking** of maternal and child health to reproductive health and **other components** like family planning, adolescent health, HIV, and preconception and prenatal diagnostic techniques (PC and PNDT)
- **Linking** of community and facility-based care as well as referrals between various levels of health care system to create a continuous care pathway, and to bring an additive/synergistic effect in terms of overall outcomes and impact.

Janani Suraksha Yojana

Introduction

Janani Suraksha Yojana (JSY) is a safe motherhood intervention under the National Rural Health Mission (NRHM). It is being implemented with the objective of reducing maternal and neonatal mortality by promoting institutional delivery among poor pregnant women. The scheme is under implementation in all States and Union Territories (UTs), with a special focus on low performing states (LPS). JSY was launched in April 2005 by modifying the National Maternity Benefit Scheme (NMBS). The NMBS came into effect in August 1995 as one of the components of the National Social Assistance Programme (NSAP). The scheme was transferred from the Ministry of Rural Development to the Department of Health and Family Welfare during the year 2001–02. The NMBS provides for financial assistance of ₹ 500/- per birth up to two live births to the pregnant women who have attained 19 years of age and belong to the below poverty line (BPL) households. When JSY was launched the financial assistance of ₹ 500/-, which was available uniformly throughout the country to BPL pregnant women under NMBS, was replaced by graded scale of assistance based on the categorization of States as well as whether beneficiary was from rural/urban area. States were classified into low performing states (LPS) and high performing states (HPS) on the basis of institutional delivery rate, i.e. states having institutional delivery 25% or less were termed as LPS and those which have institutional delivery rate more than 25% were classified as HPS. Accordingly, eight erstwhile EAG States namely Uttar Pradesh, Uttarakhand, Madhya Pradesh, Chhattisgarh, Bihar, Jharkhand, Rajasthan, Odisha and the States of Assam and Jammu and Kashmir were classified as Low Performing States. The remaining States were grouped into High Performing States.

Goals

To reduce maternal and infant mortality through increasing institutional delivery

○ Access to quality antenatal and postpartum health care the program provides a continuum of care package that includes ANC, institutional delivery, postpartum care, and family planning coordinated by the ASHA.

Vision

○ To promote institutional deliveries
○ To reduce overall maternal mortality ratio and infant mortality rate.

Beneficiaries

○ Pregnant women of all section of the society. Pregnant women of all section of the society.
○ No age bar.
○ Irrespective of birth order irrespective of birth order.
❑ In rural and urban areas.

Important Features of Janani Suraksha Yojana

The scheme focuses on the poor pregnant woman with special dispensation for states having low institutional delivery rates namely the States of Uttar Pradesh, Uttaranchal, Bihar, Jharkhand, Madhya Pradesh, Chhattisgarh, Assam, Rajasthan, Odisha and Jammu and Kashmir. While these states have been named as Low Performing States (LPS), the remaining states have been named as High Performing States (HPS).

Tracking Each Pregnancy: Each beneficiary registered under this yojana should have a JSY card along with a MCH card. ASHA/AWW/any other identified link worker under the overall supervision of the ANM and the MO, PHC should mandatorily prepare a micro-birth plan. This will effectively help in monitoring antenatal check-up, and the post delivery care.

Eligibility for Cash Assistance: BPL Certification—This is required in all HPS. However, where BPL cards have not yet been issued or have not been updated, States/UTs would formulate a simple criterion for certification of poor and needy status of the expectant mother's family by empowering the gram pradhan or ward member (Table 2).

Cash Assistance for Home Delivery

The BPL pregnant women, who prefer to deliver at home, are entitled to a cash assistance of Rs. 500 per delivery regardless of the age of pregnant women and number of children.

Table 2: Cash assistance for institutional delivery (in ₹)

Category	Rural area		Urban area	
	Mother's package	ASHA's package*	Mother's package	ASHA's package**
LPS	1400	600	1000	400
HPS	700	600	600	400

*ASHA package of Rs. 600 in rural areas include Rs. 300 for ANC component and Rs. 300 for facilitating institutional delivery
**ASHA package of Rs. 400 in urban areas include Rs. 200 for ANC component and Rs. 200 for facilitating institutional delivery

Direct Benefit Transfer Under Janani Suraksha Yojana

Direct benefit transfer (DBT) mode of payment has been rolled out in 43 districts with effect from January 1, 2013 and in 78 districts from July 1, 2013. Recently, instructions have been issued to all States/UTs regarding extension of DBT mode of payment throughout the country in all districts. Under this initiative, eligible pregnant women are entitled to get JSY benefit directly into their bank accounts.

Janani Shishu Suraksha Karyakaram (JSSK)

Introduction

In view of the difficulty being faced by the pregnant women and parents of sick new-born along-with high expenditure on delivery and treatment of sick-newborn, Ministry of health and Family Welfare (MoHFW) has taken a major initiative to ensure better facilities for women and child health services. It is an initiative to provide completely free and cashless services to pregnant women including normal deliveries and caesarean operations and sick newborn (up to 30 days after birth) in Government health institutions in both rural and urban areas.

Government of India has launched Janani Shishu Suraksha Karyakaram (JSSK) on 1st June, 2011.

The scheme is estimated to benefit more than 12 million pregnant women who access Government health facilities for their delivery. Moreover it will motivate those who still choose to deliver at their homes to opt for institutional deliveries. . It is an initiative with a hope that states would come forward and ensure that benefits under JSSK would reach every needy pregnant woman coming to government institutional facility. All the States and UTs have initiated implementation of the scheme.

The following are the Free Entitlements for pregnant women:

○ Free and cashless delivery
○ Free C-Section

○ Free drugs and consumables

○ Free diagnostics

○ Free diet during stay in the health institutions

○ Free provision of blood

○ Exemption from user charges

○ Free transport from home to health institutions

○ Free transport between facilities in case of referral

○ Free drop back from Institutions to home after 48 hrs stay

The following are the Free Entitlements for Sick newborns till 30 days after birth. This has now been expanded to cover sick infants:

○ Free treatment

○ Free drugs and consumables

○ Free diagnostics

○ Free provision of blood

○ Exemption from user charges

○ Free transport from home to health institutions

○ Free transport between facilities in case of referral

○ Free drop back from institutions to home

Mother and Child Tracking System

Mother and Child Tracking System (MCTS) is an initiative of Ministry of Health & Family Welfare to leverage information technology for ensuring delivery of full spectrum of healthcare and immunization services to pregnant women and children up to 5 years of age. It is an innovative, web-based application, developed by NIC, to facilitate and monitor service delivery as well as to establish a two-way communication between the service providers and beneficiaries. Generation of work plans of ANMs, sending regular alerts to the service providers as well as beneficiaries about the services due and a user-friendly dash board for health managers at various levels to monitor delivery of services will go a long way in ensuring quality service delivery, micro birth planning, ensuring universal immunization and will have positive impact on important health indicators like Infant Mortality Rate and Maternal Mortality Ratio. It will also help in evidence based planning and continuous assessment of service delivery to pregnant women and children.

India Newborn Action Plan

The India Newborn Action Plan (INAP) is India's committed response to the Global Every Newborn Action Plan (ENAP), launched in June 2014 at the 67th World Health Assembly, to advance the global strategy for women's and children's health. The ENAP sets forth a vision of a world that has eliminated preventable newborn deaths and stillbirths. INAP lays out a vision and a plan for India to end preventable newborn deaths, accelerate progress, and scale up high-impact yet costeffective interventions. INAP has a clear vision supported by goals, strategic intervention packages, priority actions, and a monitoring framework. For the first time, INAP also articulates the Government of India's specific attention on preventing stillbirths. INAP was launched in September 2014, for accelerating the reduction of preventable newborn deaths and stillbirths in the country with the goal of attaining 'Single Digit Neonatal Mortality Rate (NMR) by 2030' and 'Single Digit Still Birth Rate (SBR) by 2030'. Currently, there are estimated 7.47 lakh neonatal deaths annually. The neonatal deaths are expected to reduce to below 2.28 lakh annually by 2030, once the goal is achieved. The INAP is a concerted effort towards translating commitments into meaningful change for newborns. INAP will serve as a framework for the states to develop their area-specific action plans.

Milestones in Child Survival Programmes in India

○ 1992 – Child Survival and Safe Motherhood Programme (CSSM)

○ 1997 – RCH I

○ 2005 – RCH II

○ 2005 – National Rural Health Mission

○ 2013 – RMNCH+A Strategy

○ 2013 – National Health Mission

○ 2014 – INAP

India Newborn Action Plan

○ Builds on existing commitments under the National Health Mission and 'Call to Action' for child survival and development

○ Aligns with the ENAP; defines commitments based on specific contextual needs of the country

○ Aims at attaining single digit NMR by 2030, five years ahead of the global plan

○ Emphasizes strengthened surveillance mechanism for tracking stillbirths

○ Focuses on ending preventable newborn deaths, improving quality of care and care beyond survival

○ Prioritizes those babies that are born too soon, too small, or sick—as they account for majority of all newborn deaths

○ Aspires towards ensuring equitable progress for girls and boys, rural and urban, rich and poor, and between districts and states

○ Identifies major guiding principles under the overarching principle of integration: equity, gender, quality of care, convergence, accountability, and partnerships

○ Defines six pillars of interventions: pre-conception and antenatal care; care during labour and child birth; immediate newborn care; care of healthy newborn; care of small and sick newborn; and care beyond newborn survival

○ Serves as a framework for states/districts to develop their own action plan with measurable indicators.

Goals

The two specific goals of INAP are as follows:

Goal 1: Ending preventable newborn deaths to achieve "Single Digit NMR" by 2030, with all the states to individually achieve this target by 2035

Goal 2: Ending preventable stillbirths to achieve "Single Digit SBR" by 2030, with all the states to individually achieve this target by 2035

Under INAP, the newborn care/postnatal care component of the RMNCH+A continuum (for high impact interventions and commodities) has been further delineated into four distinct categories: immediate newborn care, Care of Healthy Newborn, Care of Small and Sick Newborn, and Care of Newborn Beyond Survival. Further, pre-conception and Antenatal care and care during labour and childbirth—the two stages impacting newborn outcomes including stillbirths have been included.

As a result, six pillars of intervention packages have been identified. The interventions under each of the six pillars have been described below in detail including the strategic/priority actions required to deliver high-impact interventions for achieving effective coverage. As such, the interventions have been categorized as:

○ Essential (E), to be implemented universally

○ Situational (S), implementation dependent on epidemiological context

○ Advanced (A), implementation based on health-system capacity of the state/district.

○ The states are urged to develop their action plan based on the **Six Packages** described below in Table 3.

Table 3: Action plan based on six packages develop by state

Package 1	Preconception and antenatal care
Package 2	Care during labor and childbirth
Package 3	Immediate newborn care
Package 4	Care of healthy newborn
Package 5	Care of small and sick newborn
Package 6	Care beyond newborn survival

Package 1: Preconception and Antenatal Care

Priority actions

○ Prioritize actions for delaying age at 1st pregnancy in convergence with stakeholders and other departments with special focus on teenage pregnancy

○ Train an adequate number of service providers for Family Planning Services and ensure availability of commodities, as per FP 2020

○ Saturate high case-load facilities to provide PPIUCD

○ Train an adequate numbers of ANMs in SBA (including ANC component)

○ Scale up nutritional interventions of peri-conceptional folic acid, maternal calcium supplementation, and iron folic acid supplementation (NIPI/WIFS)

○ Strengthen convergence with related departments for nutrition counselling

○ Screening of high-risk pregnancies and their management as per protocols

○ Accelerate implementation of preventive measures against malaria for pregnant women in endemic area

○ Promote counselling and birth preparedness.

Package 2: Care during Labour and Childbirth

Priority actions

○ Prioritize and strengthen public health facilities at all levels (L1, L2, L3) for conducting safe delivery, including provision of emergency obstetric care as per the norms of MNH Toolkit.

○ Provision of dedicated MCH wings in facilities with high caseload, including functional WASH facilities.

○ All delivery points to be saturated with adequately trained health workers: Ensure trained and skilled staff at all designated delivery points: L1 delivery point should have SBA trained ANMs/SNs, L2 delivery point to have at least one BEmOC trained MO, and L3 delivery point must have at least four obstetrician and gynaecologist /CEmOC trained MOs and four Anaesthetist/LSAS trained MOs.

○ Expand the availability of SBA-trained birth attendants. In addition to ANM, SBA training to be rolled out for AYUSH doctors (as per state-specific need).

○ Establish Quality Assurance mechanism at each level, like—use of safe birth checklist and regular quality audits including perinatal death audits.

○ Institutionalize referral mechanism to ensure to-and-fro referral, including inter-facility referral, as and where required.

- Accelerate scale-up of new policy decisions on management of preterm labour through use of antenatal corticosteroids and antibiotics for premature rupture of membranes.
- Develop a mechanism of supportive supervision through existing systems or through partnerships (with professional organizations, medical colleges, and private hospitals) at the regional and state level.
- Generate awareness on JSSK entitlements, promote community participation, and demand for safe institutional delivery.
- Establish a sound surveillance system for tracking stillbirths.

Package 3: Immediate Newborn Care

Priority actions

- Establish fully functional NBCCs at all facilities conducting deliveries, according to the norms prescribed in the MNH toolkit
- Saturate all facilities conducting deliveries with NSSK-trained staff
- Implement standardized clinical protocols for essential newborn care, including resuscitation
- Develop quality assurance mechanisms/cells to monitor training quality and adherence to standard protocols
- Regular quality audits of facilities, including death audits
- Ensure availability of injection vitamin K at all delivery points and its inclusion in the State's Essential Drugs List
- Develop a mechanism of ongoing supportive supervision at the facility level
- Strengthen counselling for breastfeeding, postnatal care, and community and home care practices
- Focus on community strategies to promote demand for essential newborn care.

Package 4: Care of Healthy Newborn

Priority actions

- Recruitment and rational deployment of ASHAs as per the population norm capacity-building of ASHAs to provide newborn care at the community level
- Ensure uninterrupted supply of ASHA HBNC kits and replenishment thereof, from PHC inventory
- Ensure timely payments of HBNC incentives for ASHAs
- Set up mechanisms for monitoring of HBNC visits, with regards to quality and coverage
- Ensure implementation of standardized training norms and uniform mechanism (formats, checklist) for quality of home visits

- Strengthen and revitalize the role of ANM as supervisor cum mentor to ASHA
- Institutionalize a framework for supportive supervision and mentoring of ASHAs (ARC, DRC, DCM, BCM, Supervisor/Facilitator)
- Build responsive referral system—easy access and availability of referral transport and medical care at the health facilities for all sick/high-risk newborns referred by ASHAs
- Strengthen counselling for breastfeeding, postnatal care, entitlements, and home care practices using counsellors and audiovisuals
- Ensure availability of vaccines and logistic support for immunization at all delivery points.

Package 5: Care of Small and Sick Newborn

Priority actions

- Ensure dissemination of guidelines at all levels of facilities with priority to high caseload facilities and High Priority Districts (HPDs)
- Establish fully functional NBSUs, SNCUs with the requisite HR in blocks/districts with priority to High Priority Districts (HPDs) and scale up KMC unit/wards on the existing FBNC system
- Saturate all districts in the state with fully functional SNCUs followed by all facilities with >3000 deliveries/year
- Upgrade NICUs at the medical colleges/tertiary care facilities to provide referral services for advanced newborn care support (ventilation, surgery) at regional level, and to strengthen linkages with SNCUs and NBSUs
- Operationalize SNCU monitoring software across all SNCUs/NICUs
- Institutionalize network of Regional/State FBNC collaborating centres and Medical Colleges to:
  - Accelerate capacity building of MOs/Staff Nurses/ ANMs posted in NBSUs, SNCUs and KMC units, and of ANMs for IMNCI
  - Develop an integrated framework for supportive supervision
- Ensure mechanisms for timely procurement and supply chain management of equipment, drugs, and laboratory reagents as per the defined norms and technical specifications
- Regularly monitor quality of trainings
- Develop Quality Assurance mechanisms/cells to ensure compliance with norms for quality of care for small and sick newborns, including tools for adherence to admission and discharge criteria, SOPs for clinical management, infection prevention and control

- Conduct regular quality audits of facilities including death audits
- Scale up new operational guidelines, allowing ANMs to administer injectable antibiotics for neonatal sepsis.

Package 6: Care beyond Newborn Survival

Priority actions

- Train all levels of service providers engaged in screening of birth defects and developmental delays
- Deploy trained mobile health teams for screening
- Establish fully functional District Early Intervention Centres (DEICs)
- Institutionalize a robust referral mechanisms between screening points and District Early Intervention Centres (DEICs)
- Establish centres of excellence at tertiary care hospitals for management of conditions, especially the birth defects requiring surgical correction
- Screen birth defects by the service providers at the facility and in community by ASHAs during home visits
- Facility-based follow-up of small and sick babies for developmental delay and appropriate management
- Follow-up of all sick/high-risk newborns discharged from the SNCU for a period of one year by ASHAs
- Develop resource network, including private practitioners, to provide specialized care for identified cases.

INAP—National Targets (Table 4)

Table 4: INAP—National targets

Targets	Current	2017	2020	2025	2030
Impact targets					
NMR (per 1000 live births)	29	24	21	15	<10
SBR (per 1000 live births)	22	19	17	13	<10
Coverage targets					
Safe delivery (institutional + home delivery by SBA (%)	76	90	95	95	95
Initiation of breastfeeding within one hour of birth (%)	–	75	90	90	90

Targets	Current	2017	2020	2025	2030
Women with preterm labour receiving at least one dose of antenatal corticosteroids (%)	–	75	90	95	95
Babies born in health facilities with birth asphyxia received resuscitation (%)	–	75	90	95	95
Babies received complete schedule of home visits under HBNC by ASHA (%)	–	50	75	95	95
Newborn with sepsis in the community received Gentamicin by ANM (%)	–	50	75	75	75
Newborn discharged from SNCU followed until age one (%)	–	35	50	75	75
Newborn with low birth weight/ Prematurity managed with KMC at facility (%)	–	35	50	75	90

Rashtriya Bal Swasthya Karyakram (Table 5)

Under National Rural Health Mission, significant progress has been made in reducing mortality in children over the last seven years (2005-12). Whereas there is an advance in reducing child mortality there is a dire need to improving survival outcome. This would be reached by early detection and management of conditions that were not addressed comprehensively in the past. According to March of Dimes (2006), out of every 100 babies born in this country annually, 6 to 7 have a birth defect. This would translate to around 17 lakhs birth defects annually in the country and accounts for 9.6% of all the newborn deaths. Various nutritional deficiencies affecting the preschool children range from 4 per cent to 70 per cent. Developmental delays are common in early childhood affecting at least 10% of the children. These delays if not intervened timely may lead to permanent disabilities including cognitive, hearing or vision impairment. Also, there are group of diseases common in children viz. dental caries, rheumatic heart disease, reactive airways diseases, etc. Early detection and management diseases including deficiencies bring added value in preventing these conditions to progress to its more severe and debilitating form and thereby reducing hospitalization and improving implementation of right to education. Rashtriya Bal Swasthya Karyakram (RBSK) is an important initiative aiming at early identification and early

Table 5: Target group under child health screening and intervention service categories

Categories	Age group	Estimated coverage		
Babies born at public health facilities and home	Birth to 6 weeks	2 crores		
Preschool children in rural areas and urban slum[1]	6 weeks to 6 years	8 crores		
School children enrolled in class 1st to 12th in government and government aided schools	6 yrs to 18 yrs	17 crores		
Package 5	Care of small and sick newborn			
Package 6	Care beyond newborn survival			

intervention for children from birth to 18 years to cover 4 'D's viz. Defects at birth, Deficiencies, Diseases, Development delays including disability. It is important to note that the 0-6 years age group will be specifically managed at District Early Intervention Center (DEIC) level while for 6–18 years age group, management of conditions will be done through existing public health facilities. DEIC will act as referral linkages for both the age groups. First level of screening is done at all delivery points through existing medical officers, staff nurses and ANMs. After 48 hours till 6 weeks the screening of newborns will be done by ASHA at home as a part of Home Based New-born Care (HBNC) package. Outreach screening will be done by dedicated Mobile Health teams for 6 weeks to 6 years at anganwadis centres and 6–18 years children at school. Once the child is screened and referred from any of these points of identification, it would be ensured that the necessary treatment/intervention is delivered at zero cost to the family.

Health Conditions to be Screened

Child health screening and early intervention services under RBSK envisages to cover 30 selected health conditions for Screening, early detection and free management (Table 6). States and UTs may also include diseases namely hypothyroidism, sickle cell anaemia and beta thalassemia based on epidemiological situation and availability of testing and specialized support facilities within State and UTs.

Table 6: Selected health conditions for child health screening and early intervention services

Defects at birth	Deficiencies
○ Neural tube defect ○ Down's syndrome ○ Cleft lip and plate/cleft palate alone ○ Talipes (club foot) ○ Developmental dysplasia of the hip ○ Congential cataract ○ Congenital deafness ○ Retinopathy of prematurity	○ Anaemia especially severe anaemia ○ Vitamin A deficiency (Bitot spot) ○ Vitamin D deficiency, (Rickets) ○ Severe acute malnutrition ○ Goiter

Disease of childhood	Developmental delays and disabilities
○ Skin conditions (scabies, fungal infection and eczema) ○ Otitits media ○ Rheumatic heart disease ○ Reactive airway disease ○ Dental conditions ○ Convulsive disorders	○ Vision impairment ○ Hearing impairment ○ Neuromotor impairment ○ Motor delay ○ Cognitive delay ○ Language delay ○ Behavior disorder (Autism) ○ Learning disorder ○ Attention deficit hyperactivity disorder

○ **Congenital hypothyroidism, sickle cell anemia, beta thalassemia (optional)**

Kilkari App

Chief Minister of Haryana (**Mahohar Lal Khattar**) launched a mobile app as named "Kilkari" to aware Pregnant Women and Newborn Baby.

Highlights of the Kilkari Mobile App

○ Under this scheme govt. would provide important information to maternity.

○ Kilkari App will awareness pregnant women and Newborn baby.

○ User can register their numbers in this app to get advantage of this scheme.

○ This app will be helpful to care new born baby and pregnant women.

○ Everyone will get messages on mobile through this app.

○ 72 audio massage will be send, from the second trimester of pregnancy until one year of child birth.

○ Time Appropriate Audio Messages will be sent via the app in the Crucial Stages of Pregnancy, Child Birth and Child Care.

Mission Indradhanush

Mission Indradhanush was launched by Ministry of Health and Family Welfare (MOHFW) Government of India on 25th December, 2014.

Objective

To ensure that all children under the age of two years as well as pregnant women are fully immunized with seven vaccine preventable diseases.

The Mission Indradhanush, depicting seven colours of the rainbow, targets to immunize all children against seven vaccine preventable diseases, namely:

1. Diphtheria
2. Pertussis (Whooping Cough)
3. Tetanus
4. Tuberculosis
5. Polio
6. Hepatitis B
7. Measles.

In addition to this, vaccines for Japanese Encephalitis (JE) and Haemophilus influenzae type B (HIB) are also being provided in selected states.

First Phase of Mission Indradhanush

For the first phase, 201 high focus districts across 28 states in the country that have the peak number of partially immunized and unimmunized children were identified by the Government. There were total four rounds in the first phase of the mission. The first round of the first phase was started from 7th April, 2015 and continued for more than a week. Further, second, third and fourth rounds were held for more than a week in the month of May, June and July starting from 7th of each month. The first phase of this mission was very successful.

The main highlights of the first phase of Mission Indradhanush are as given below:

- Total 9.4 lakh sessions were organized during these four rounds of Mission Indradhanush.
- About 2 crore vaccines were given to the children as well as pregnant women.
- Tetanus toxoid vaccine was given to more than 20 lakh pregnant women, 75.5 lakh children were vaccinated and about 20 lakh children were fully vaccinated.
- More than 57 lakh zinc tablets and 16 lakh ORS packets were freely distributed to all the children to protect them against diarrhoea.

Second Phase of Mission Indradhanush

Union Health Minister launches phase-2 of Mission Indradhanush in 352 districts targeting full immunization. The second phase of Mission Indradhanush has been started from 7th October, 2015.

The second, third and fourth rounds of this phase will start from 7th November, 7th December 2015 and 7th January 2016.

Aim

To achieve full immunization in 352 districts which includes 279 mid priority districts, 33 districts from the North East states and 40 districts from phase one where huge number of missed out children were detected.

Objectives and Strategy

General Objective

The objective of Mission Indradhanush is to ensure high coverage of children and pregnant women with all available vaccines throughout the country, with emphasis on the identified 201 high focus districts.

Specific Objectives

With the launch of Mission Indradhanush, the government aims at:

- Generating high demand for immunization services by addressing communication challenges;
- Enhancing political, administrative and financial commitment through advocacy with key stakeholders; and
- Ensuring that the partially immunized and unimmunized children are fully immunized as per national immunization schedule.

Focus Areas

Mission Indradhanush will be a nationwide drive, with focus on 201 identified high focus districts. Key areas reached through Mission Indradhanush will be:

- **Areas with vacant sub-centers:** No auxiliary nurse midwife (ANM) posted for more than three months.
- **Villages/areas with three or more consecutive missed routine immunization (RI) sessions:** ANMs on long leave or other similar reasons.
- High risk areas (HRAs) identified by the polio eradication programme. These include populations living in areas such as:
  - Urban slums with migration
  - Nomadic sites

- ❑ Brick kilns
- ❑ Construction sites
- ❑ Other migrant settlements (fisherman villages, riverine areas with shifting populations)
- ❑ Underserved and hard to reach populations (forested and tribal populations, hilly areas etc.).
- ○ Areas with low RI coverage, identified through measles outbreaks, cases of diphtheria and neonatal tetanus in last two years.
- ○ Small villages, hamlets, dhanis, purbas, basas (field huts), etc., clubbed with another village for RI sessions and not having independent RI sessions.

Strategy for Mission Indradhanush

Mission Indradhanush will be a nationwide intensified RI drive for ensuring high coverage throughout the country and will be conducted between March and June 2015 in the country, with focus on 201 high focus districts. The two main components of this mission will be:

- ○ Operational planning
- ○ Communication planning.

Implementation of Mission Indradhanush

- ○ All ANMs will plan activities for seven days of each drive. This will include 1–2 days of activities in the ANM's own sub-centre area and remaining days in same/adjoining blocks or urban areas of her district.
- ○ All identified areas that require RI strengthening but have no/infrequent RI sessions must be reached through Mission Indradhanush sessions.
- ○ Mission Indradhanush will be implemented according to a roster prepared during the microplanning meetings at block and district levels for each ANM in the district. Once these rosters have been prepared for each ANM in the district for the duration of the Indradhanush week, the DIO must assess the requirement of any hired vaccinators, which if required, should be identified, hired as per NHM financial norms (Annexure 8) and trained by the DIO.
- ○ **Operational planning:** The following two operational mechanisms will be utilized to reach out to the unreached or poorly reached beneficiaries:

Fixed and Outreach Sessions

Medical officer in charge for the block/urban planning unit will conduct a detailed planning for the additional sessions to be conducted in the planning unit. Provision for vaccination should be made at health posts, primary health centers (PHCs) and district hospital.

Sites for Vaccination

In urban areas, urban health posts, post-partum (PP) centers, family welfare centers or local leader's premises in urban slums can also be used as immunization sites. For other areas, primary schools, *anganwadi* centers, private dispensaries, nongovernmental organization (NGO) sites or any other locations that are easily accessible and acceptable to community can be used as immunization sites. Efforts have to be made to provide regular immunization services from these sites even after the Indradhanush weeks are over.

Availability of Human Resources

In addition to health staff available from the same or neighboring community health centre (CHC)/Block PHC, NGOs (LIONS, Rotary etc.), it is necessary to utilize retired health workers, and staff available from other government agencies such as Employee's State Insurance Corporation, Central Government Health Scheme, armed forces, railways, District Urban Development Agency (DUDA)/State Urban Development Agency (SUDA) and community based organizations to reach large number of children.

Timing

The activity will be conducted from 9 am to 4 pm. However, sessions should be planned based on availability of the targeted population to maximize the benefits achieved.

Team

A team will comprise one vaccinator and up to two mobilizers (at least one should be from local mohallas/locality). An additional vaccinator will be included in the team if the estimated injection load is more than 60–70.

Mobile Sessions

Mobile sessions should be planned at places where routine immunization coverage is weak and the small number of beneficiaries does not warrant an independent session. These areas include periurban areas, scattered slums, brick kilns and construction sites. For these sessions, alternate means such as mobile vans should be planned in the attached format.

It is important to ensure that the vials of BCG, measles and JE vaccines that are reconstituted at one site should not be used at the next site. The integrated child development services (ICDS) department may support these mobile clinics through supplementary nutrition services that may be provided to beneficiaries in these difficult-toreach areas.

Planning Considerations

Based on evidence and best practices from the polio eradication programme, following activities will be critical for the successful implementation of Mission Indradhanush:

○ **Meticulous planning of immunization sessions at all levels:** Plan sessions for identified areas with inadequate reach of immunization programme. Ensure availability of sufficient vaccinators and all vaccines during routine immunization sessions.

○ **Effective communication and social mobilization efforts:** Generate awareness and demand for immunization services through need-based communication and social mobilization activities (mass media, mid media, interpersonal communication, school and youth networks and corporates).

○ **Intensive training of health officials and frontline workers:** Build capacity of health officials and workers for routine immunization activities to ensure the highest quality of immunization services delivery to beneficiaries.

○ **Establish accountability framework through task forces:** Enhance involvement and accountability/ownership of state and district administrative and health officials through state and district task forces for immunization. It is important to use concurrent session monitoring data to plug gaps in implementation.

Communication Planning

Need-based communication and social mobilization activities should be planned to achieve the following objectives:

○ Demand generation through increased visibility;

○ Advocacy through media, professional bodies and political leadership;

○ Capacity building of immunization workforce on communication;

○ Social mobilization through interpersonal communication, school and youth networks and corporates; and

○ Monitoring of communication interventions.

Steps for Rollout of Mission Indradhanush

The rollout of Mission Indradhanush requires meticulous planning at all levels. The special sessions under Mission Indradhanush should be conducted in areas that are unreached or poorly reached for routine immunization services to ensure maximum improvement in full immunization coverage of states. Prior to conducting these sessions, headcount must be done in such areas for enlisting beneficiaries and preparing due lists.

Integrated Management of Neonatal and Childhood Illness

Introduction

Government of India recognizes the need to strengthen child health activities in the country. In order to do so and introduce IMCI in the country, a Core Group was constituted which included representatives from Indian Academy of Pediatrics (IAP), National Neonatology Forum of India (NNF), National Anti Malaria Program (NAMP), Department of Women and Child Development (DWCD), Child-in-Need Institute (CINI), WHO, UNICEF, eminent Pediatricians and Neonatologists, and the representatives from Ministry of Health and Family Welfare Government of India. The Adaptation Group developed Indian version of IMCI guidelines and renamed it as Integrated Management of Neonatal and Childhood Illness (IMNCI). The major components of this strategy are:

○ Strengthening the skills of the health care workers
○ Strengthening the health care infrastructure
○ Involvement of the community.

Although the major reason for developing the IMCI strategy stemmed from the needs of curative care, the strategy also addresses aspects of nutrition, immunization, and other important elements of disease prevention and health promotion. The objectives of the strategy are to reduce death and the frequency and severity of illness and disability, and to contribute to improved growth and development. This strategy has been adapted for India as Integrated Management of Neonatal and Childhood Illness (IMNCI). The IMNCI clinical guidelines target children less than 5 years old—the age group that bears the highest burden of deaths from common childhood diseases. The guidelines take an evidence-based, syndromic approach to case management that supports the rational, effective and affordable use of drugs and diagnostic tools. Evidence-based medicine stresses the importance of evaluation of evidence from clinical research and cautions against the use of intuition, unsystematic clinical experience, and untested pathophysiologic reasoning for medical decision-making. In situations where laboratory support and clinical resources are limited, the syndromic approach is a more realistic and cost-effective way to manage patients. Careful and systematic assessment of common symptoms and well-selected clinical signs provides sufficient information to guide rational and effective actions. An evidence-based syndromic approach can be used to determine the:

○ Health problem(s) the child may have;

○ Severity of the child's condition;

○ Actions that can be taken to care for the child (e.g. refer the child immediately, manage with available resources, or manage at home). In addition, IMNCI promotes:

- Adjustment of interventions to the capacity and functions of the health system; and
- Active involvement of family members and the community in the health care process.

The major highlights of Indian adaptation are:

- Incorporation of neonatal care as it now constitutes two-thirds of infant mortality
- Inclusion of 0–7 days
- Incorporating National guidelines on malaria, anemia, vitamin A supplementation and immunization schedule
- Training schedule reduced from 11 days to 8 days
- Training begins with sick young infant up to 2 months
- Proportion of training time devoted to sick young infant and sick child is almost equal. The Government has initiated implementation of the IMNCI strategy in four districts each in nine selected states of Orissa, Rajasthan, Madhya Pradesh, Haryana, Delhi, Gujarat, Uttaranchal, Tamil Nadu and Rajasthan.

Components of the Integrated Approach

The IMNCI strategy includes both preventive and curative interventions that aim to improve practices in health facilities, the health system and at home. At the core of the strategy is integrated case management of the most common childhood problems with a focus on the most common causes of death. The strategy includes three main components:

- Improvements in the case-management skills of health staff through the provision of locally-adapted guidelines on Integrated Management of Neonatal and Childhood illness and activities to promote their use
- Improvements in the overall health system required for effective management of childhood illness
- Improvements in family and community health care practices.

The Principles of Integrated Care

The IMNCI guidelines are based on the following principles:

- All sick young infants age up to 2 months must be examined for signs of "possible serious bacterial infection" and all children 2 months to 5 years must be examined for "general danger signs" which indicate the need for immediate referral or admission to a hospital.
- All sick children must be routinely assessed for major symptoms (for young infants up to 2 months: diarrhoea; and for children age 2 months up to 5 years: Cough or difficult breathing, diarrhoea, fever and ear problem). They must also be routinely assessed for nutritional and immunization status, feeding problems, and other potential problems.

- Only a limited number of carefully selected clinical signs are used, based on evidence of their sensitivity and specificity to detect disease. These signs were selected considering the conditions and realities of first-level health facilities.
- A combination of individual signs leads to a child's classification(s) rather than a diagnosis. Classification(s) indicate the severity of condition(s). They call for specific actions based on whether the young infant or the child
    - Should be urgently referred to another level of care,
    - Requires specific treatments (such as antibiotics or antimalarial treatment), or
    - May be safely managed at home.
- **The classifications are colour coded:** "Pink" suggests hospital referral or admission, "yellow" indicates initiation of treatment, and "green" calls for home treatment.
- The IMNCI guidelines address most, but not all, of the major reasons a sick child is brought to a clinic. A child returning with chronic problems or less common illnesses may require special care. The guidelines do not describe the care at birth and the management of trauma or other acute emergencies due to accidents or injuries.
- IMNCI management procedures use a limited number of essential drugs and encourage active participation of caretakers in the treatment of children.
- An essential component of the IMNCI guidelines is the counselling of caretakers about home care, including counselling about feeding, fluids and when to return to a health facility.

The Case Management Process

The case management process is presented on a series of charts, which show the sequence of steps and provide information for performing them. The charts describe the following steps:

- Assess the young infant or child
- Classify the illness
- Identify treatment
- Treat the infant or child
- Counsel the mother
- Give follow-up care.

EXPANDED PROGRAM ON IMMUNIZATION

Smallpox eradication in India revealed the greatest cost effective work of immunization to the world. WHO launched the "Expanded Program on Immunization" (EPI). This program primarily initiated to provide vaccines against major preventable six killer diseases, i.e. diphtheria, pertussis, tetanus, poliomyelitis, tuberculosis and measles in children. From the start of this program UNICEF had extended its constant support.

World Health Organization defined "expanded" as adding more disease controlling agents to vaccination schedules extending its coverage to the entire country and spreading services to reach less privileged sectors of the society.

Alma-Ata's (1978) primary health care concept highlighted immunization as one of the components of strategies to achieve health for all by 2000 AD.

Mile Stones of the Program

- **1978**—India started "expanded program of immunization (EPI)".
  - This had limited reach and covered mostly urban areas
- **1983**—TT immunization of pregnant women introduced
- **1985**—UNICEF renamed it as "universal immunization program (UIP)."
  - The goal was reduce the mortality and morbidity due to 6 VPD's
  - Under this indigenous vaccine production capacity was enhanced
  - Cold chain process established to monitor the potency of vaccines and assure quality services
  - Through phased implementation—all districts covered by 1989–90
  - Strict monitoring and evaluation system implemented
- **1986**—Technology mission on immunization initiated
  - Monitoring under PMO's 20-point program
  - Coverage in infants (0–12 months) monitored
- **1992**—Child survival and safe motherhood (CSSM)
  - Included both UIP and Safe motherhood program
- **1997**—Reproductive child health (RCH Phase 1)
- **2005**—National rural health mission (NRHM)
- **1995**—Pulse polio immunization program launched. All the children under five years are given additional dose of polio drops in the months of December and January on fixed dates.
- **2010–2011**—Introduction of Hepatitis B vaccine. It is given at 6, 10 and 14 weeks along with primary vaccines DPT and OPV.
- **2006**—Japanese encephalitis vaccine introduced in endemic districts with 2 doses at 9–12 months and 16–24 months
- **2011**—India introduced pentavalent vaccine that consists of DPT, Hepatitis B, and Hib vaccines in two states Kerala and Tamil Nadu. Addition of these vaccines

Hep B and Hib protects against the diseases hepatitis B and haemophelous influenza type B respectively

- **2013**—Multi-dose vial policy for vaccines introduced
- **2013**—To doses of JE introduced in endemic areas
- **2014**—Mission Indradhanush was introduced on 25th December 2014. The goal is to vaccinate all under fives by the year 2020. Under this program 4 special vaccine camps will be conducted in between January and June 2015. This is technically supported by WHO, UNICEF and Rotary international and other donor partners.
- **2015**—IPV introduced in six states in 2015 and being expanded to all states in 2016.
- **2016**—Rotavirus vaccine introduced in four states.

Objectives of EPI

- To reduce the mortality and morbidity occurring from vaccine preventable diseases
- India to become self-sufficient in vaccine production.

Components of Universal Child Immunization

The components of universal child immunization (UCI) had two major components: (1) Immunization of pregnant women against tetanus and (2) Immunization of children in their first year of life against EPI target-diseases.

The UCI aimed to achieve 100% coverage of pregnant women two doses of tetanus toxoid or a booster dose, 85% coverage of children with 3 doses each of DPT, OPV, one dose of BCG and one dose of measles by 1990. Initially (in 1985) UCI was implemented in 30 selected districts and catchment areas of 50 medical colleges. The program has now been extended to all the districts and all medical colleges. The program implemented through MCH services and there is no specific staffing for this.

Program Implementation Plan (PIP) to Strengthen Routine Immunization

- Supporting alternate vaccine delivery from PHC to sub-center and from sub-center to outreach
- Assigning retired manpower in underserved slum areas
- Mobility support to district immunization officer for supervision
- Review meeting at the state level for the districts
- Support to mobilize children to immunization clinic by ASHA, women self-help group, etc.
- Printing of immunization cards, monitoring sheet, etc.
- Support from Central government-Auto disposable syringes, downsizing BCG ampoule from 20 to 10 doses, Cold chain maintenance.

Immunization Schedule 2017 (Tables 7 and 8)

Recommended Immunization Schedule, as per current Universal Immunization Program (**UIP**) by Govt. of India and Indian Academy of Paediatrics revised schedule 2017 (**IAP**), on the guidelines of **WHO**.

*Mandatory vaccines: Vaccines to be administered compulsorily to each child in the country.

Recommended Vaccines: Available Vaccines, recommended by **IAP** for preventing various diseases, administered on the basis of individual's demographics, environmental conditions and medical history.

W – Weeks, **M** – Months, **Y** – Years

Table 6: Recommended Immunization Schedule, as per current Universal Immunization Program (UIP) by Government of India

Vaccine	Birth	6 w	10 w	14 w	6m	7 m	9 m	10 m-12 m	12 m	15 m	16-18 m	18 m	2 y	4 y-6 y	10 y-12 y
*BCG Vaccine	1#														
*Hepatitis B Vaccine	1#	2#			3#										
*OPV	0	1 drop	2 drops	3 drops	1 drop		2 drops							3 drops	
*IPV		1#	2#	3#							4##				
*DTP (DTwP / DTaP) Vaccine		1#	2#	3#							4##			5##	
*Hib Vaccine		1#	2#	3#							4##				
Pneumococcal Vaccine		1#	2#	3#						4##					
*Rotavirus Vaccine		1 drop	2 drops	3 drops											
Influenza Virus Vaccine					1#	2#	1#								
*MMR Vaccine							1#			2#				3#	
Typhoid Conjugate Vaccine								1#					2##		
Hepatitis A Vaccine									1#			2#			
Chickenpox (Varicella) Vaccine										1#				2#	
*Tdap Vaccine															1#
HPV															1# 2#

#	Routine Injectable Dose	##	Booster Injectable Dose

Note: Immune response is best achieved if Immunization is carried out as per schedule without any lapses.

Table 8: Routine dose and catch-up dose for different vaccines

Vaccines	Routine dose (Should be given as per schedule)	Catch-up dose (Can be given if the doses as per schedule are missed)
bCG*	○ At birth or at 6 weeks of age	○ Up to 5 years
Hepatitis B*	○ 1st dose of monovalent Hep B at Birth, followed by 2nd dose at 6 weeks and 3rd dose at 6 months of age (2nd and 3rd dose can be monovalent/pentavalent) ○ Alternatively, 3 primary doses of pentavalent vaccine, including Hep B at 6, 10 and 14 weeks after birth dose	○ If a birth dose is missed, monovalent Hep B before 4 weeks of age ○ Next dose after 1 month, followed by a third dose after 6 months of first dose (0, 1, 6 month schedule)
OPV*	○ OPV 0 is given at birth, followed by OPV1 at 6 months, OPV2 at 9 months and OPV3 at 4-6 years of age ○ OPV can be given for all the primary doses in cases where IPV is not possible	○ Additional doses of OPV on all pulse polio days for children till 5 years of age
IPV*	○ 3 Primary doses at 6, 10 and 14 weeks of age ○ If IPV is not possible for all the primary doses, **give at least one dose of IPV along with OPV primary dose at 14 weeks** ○ Booster dose of IPV at 12-18 months of age if primary doses of IPV are given	○ 2 doses at 2 months gap followed by a booster dose at 6 month gap after the previous dose
DTP (DTwP or DTaP)*	○ 3 primary doses at 6 weeks, 10 weeks and 14 weeks of age ○ First booster at 16-24 months of age, followed by a second booster at 4-6 yrs of age	○ Missed primary doses can be completed till 1 year of age ○ The 1st Booster dose can be given up to 4 years ○ 2nd Booster dose can be given before 7 years of age
Hib*	○ 3 doses of Hib or Hib conjugate vaccine at 6 weeks, 10 weeks and 14 weeks of age ○ Booster dose at age 12 -18 months	○ For age < 12 months; 2 doses at 4 weeks interval, with a booster at age 12-18 months ○ For child 12-15 months; 1 dose only followed by a booster dose after at least 4 weeks ○ Above 15 months; single dose ○ No catch up above 5 years of age
Pneumococcal Conjugate (PCV)	○ 3 primary doses at 6 weeks,10 weeks and 14 weeks of age ○ Booster dose at 15 months of age	○ For infants of age 6-12 months, 2 doses can be given at 4 week gap followed by 1 booster dose. ○ For children of age 12-23 months, 2 doses can be given at 8 week gap. ○ For children of age 2 – 5 years, single dose can be given
Rotavirus*	○ 3 primary doses at 6 weeks, 10 weeks and 14 weeks of age	○ Missed doses can be given before 8 months of age at a minimum gap of 4 weeks ○ No catch-up after 8 months
Influenza	○ 2 doses starting at 6 months of age at 4 week gap for the first time vaccination ○ Single dose every year for age group 1–9 years	○ 2 doses can be given at 4 week gap at any time for children less than 1 year
MMR*	○ 1 dose of MMR vaccine at a minimum age of 9 months (270 completed days) through 12 months of age ○ The 2nd dose at 15 months through 18 months of age or at anytime 4-8 weeks after the 1st dose ○ 3rd dose should be given at 4-6 years of age (According to IAP revised Schedule 2016-17)	○ All school children and adolescents who did not have natural infection or received the vaccine earlier should be immunized with 2 doses of MMR at minimum 4 weeks interval ○ Monovalent measles/measles containing vaccine can be administered to infants aged 6 through 8 months during measles outbreaks. However, this dose should not be counted.

Contd…

Vaccines	Routine dose (Should be given as per schedule)	Catch-up dose (Can be given if the doses as per schedule are missed)
Typhoid Vi PS Conjugate	○ Primary dose at 9-12 months (an interval of minimum 4 weeks should be maintained with the MMR1 dose while following the schedule). ○ Booster dose at 2 years of age with either Typhoid conjugate (Typbar-TCV*) or Typhoid polysaccharide ○ Booster doses every 3 years if Typhoid polysaccharide vaccine is used ○ No further boosters are required if Typhoid Vi PS Conjugate is used	○ Doses can be given till 18 years of age
Hepatitis A	○ Only one dose of Hep A live attenuated vaccine staring at 12 months through 23 months of age ○ First dose of Hep A killed vaccine starting at 12 months through 23 months of age ○ 2nd dose of Hep A killed vaccines at 18 months of age or at minimum interval of 6 months from 1st dose. Gap is flexible anytime between 6-18 months	○ 2 doses for killed vaccine can be administered at minimum 6 months gap to unvaccinated persons ○ Only single dose of live attenuated H2-strain need to be given to unvaccinated persons ○ Hepatitis A vaccine can be given till 18 years of age
Chickenpox	○ First dose at 12 – 15 months ○ Second dose at 4 – 6 years	○ For children aged 7-12 years, 2 doses can be given at a minimum gap of 3 months ○ For persons aged 13 years and older, 2 doses can be given at a minimum gap of 4 weeks
Tdap*	○ 1 single dose at age of 11 years-12 years	○ Can be given up to 18 years ○ Tdap can be given to 7-10 year old kids who are not fully immunized against pertussis
HPV	○ Only 2 doses of either of the two HPV vaccines (HPV2/HPV4) for girls aged 9-14 years. The minimum interval between the two doses should be atleast 6 months ○ 3 doses are recommended for girls aged 15 years and older. 2nd dose is given 1 to 2 months after the 1st dose and the 3rd dose 6 months after the 1st dose (at least 24 weeks after the first dose). Either HPV4 (0, 2, 6 months) or HPV2 (0, 1, 6 months) is recommended in 3-dose schedule	○ Vaccination can be done till 26 years of age, maintaining the minimum intervals between the doses

ADOLESCENT HEALTH PROGRAMS

RASHTRIYA KISHOR SWASTHYA KARYAKRAM

Introduction

The Ministry of Health and Family Welfare has launched a health programme for adolescents, in the age group of 10–19 years, which would target their nutrition, reproductive health and substance abuse, among other issues.

The Rashtriya Kishor Swasthya Karyakram (RKSK) was launched on 7th January, 2014. The key principles of this programme is adolescent participation and leadership, equity and inclusion, gender equity and strategic partnerships with other sectors and stakeholders.

The programme envisions enabling all adolescents in India to realize their full potential by making informed and responsible decisions related to their health and well being and by accessing the services and support they need to do so.

Purpose: Guidance on preparation of the adolescent health (AH) related components of state and district NHM PIPs including budgets and reporting on progress/indicators.

To guide the implementation of this programme, MOHFW in collaboration with UNFPA has developed a National Adolescent Health Strategy. It realigns the existing clinic-based curative approach to focus on a more holistic model based on a continuum of care for adolescent health and developmental needs.

The RKSK (National Adolescent Health Programme), will comprehensively address the health needs of the 243 million adolescents. It introduces community-based interventions through peer educators, and is underpinned by collaborations with other ministries and state governments.

Objectives

Improve Nutrition

○ Reduce the prevalence of malnutrition among adolescent girls and boys

○ Reduce the prevalence of iron-deficiency anaemia (IDA) among adolescent girls and boys.

Improve Sexual and Reproductive Health

○ Improve knowledge, attitudes and behaviour, in relation to SRH

○ Reduce teenage pregnancies

○ Improve birth preparedness, complication readiness and provide early parenting support for adolescent parents.

Enhance Mental Health

Address mental health concerns of adolescents.

Prevent Injuries and Violence

Promote favourable attitudes for preventing injuries and violence (including GBV) among adolescents.

Prevent Substance Misuse

Increase adolescents' awareness of the adverse effects and consequences of substance misuse.

Address Non-communicable Diseases

Promote behaviour change in adolescents to prevent NCDs such as hypertension, stroke, cardio-vascular diseases and diabetes.

Target Groups

The new adolescent health (AH) strategy focuses on age groups 10–14 years and 15–19 years with universal coverage, i.e. males and females; urban and rural; in school and out of school; married and unmarried; and vulnerable and under-served.

Strategies

Strategies/interventions to achieve objectives can be broadly grouped as:

○ Community-based interventions

○ Peer Education (PE)

○ Quarterly Adolescent Health Day (AHD)

○ Weekly Iron and Folic Acid Supplementation Programme (WIFS)

○ Menstrual Hygiene Scheme (MHS).

Facility-based Interventions

Strengthening of Adolescent Friendly Health Clinics (AFHC).

Convergence

○ **Within health and family welfare:** FP, MH (including VHND), RBSK, NACP, National Tobacco Control Programme, National Mental Health Programme, NCDs and IEC.

○ **With other departments/schemes:** WCD (ICDS, KSY, BSY, SABLA), HRD (AEP, MDM), Youth Affairs and Sports (Adolescent Empowerment Scheme, National Service Scheme, NYKS, NPYAD).

SCHOOL HEALTH PROGRAMME

Introduction

National Rural Health Mission (NRHM), has taken cognizance of the potential impact of the school health programme on the health of the students, their families and the generations to come and brought this initiative to forefront within the context of the Reproductive and Child Health (RCH) Programme.

Providing easy access to health, nutrition and hygiene education and services to children in schools is a simple and a cost effective tool which can go a long way in the prevention and control of communicable and non-communicable diseases. It also enables revitalization of local health traditions and the mainstreaming of AYUSH and promotion of healthy life styles in the health curriculum programme in schools.

As NRHM promotes flexibility in the states, under the school health programme, the states have been given an option to implement the programme comprehensively. According to the needs of the children, institutional capacity and available service delivery options 26 States have provisioned for the School Health Programme in their programme implementation plans. It is expected that all the states that have taken up this challenge and introduced a school health programme from the year 2008 will continue with this initiative, expanding it as per the need so that ultimately it has a universal coverage. It is also expected that the other states will start providing school health services in the near future. It is envisaged that all schools, both rural and urban, will be covered under various aspects of the school health programme in all parts of the country.

Objectives

The main objectives of this service is the prevention of illness as well as the promotion of health and well-being of the students through:

○ Early detection and care of students with health problems

- Development of healthy attitudes and healthy behaviors by students
- Ensure a healthy environment for children at school
- Prevention of communicable diseases at school.

Essential Elements

Essential elements of school health are:

- **Health-related school policies** that include children of all communities, encourage healthy lifestyles, address priority public health problems and promote collaboration among teachers. It also enables students and their parents on one side and departments like health, education, women and child development on the other side to bring about convergence.
- **Provision of safe (physically and psycho-socially) and supportive environment** to ensure healthy development of students and provide a healthy learning environment. Provision of nutrition relieves the hunger of the child coming from deprived circumstances and provision of safe water and adequate sanitation reinforces hygienic behaviour. It is especially important to provide privacy (functional women toilets and support for menstrual management) and safety to promote participation of adolescent girls in education. Keeping the school free of violence and various forms of discrimination is also an important dimension.
- **Health, hygiene and nutrition education** that focuses upon the development of age appropriate knowledge, attitudes, values and life skills needed to establish lifelong healthy practices. Additionally, the school environment must provide opportunities to practice the acquired healthy behaviour on order to reduce the vulnerability of youth and teachers to common health risks. For example, mid-day school meal programmes cooked and served hygienically, sanitary toilets/latrines with running water supplies soap and water for hand washing adequate supply of potable water provision of sanitary napkins for girls and kitchen garden to demonstrate feasibility of growing healthy food.
- **School-based health and nutrition services** that are equitable, simple, sustainable, safe and familiar and address problems that are prevalent and recognized as important within the community, e.g. Mid-day meal scheme, mid-day school meals.

Operational Framework

School age population is extremely vulnerable to health risks and illness. Illnesses and behaviour formed during this period can have a detrimental effect on health during the adult years of an individual's life.

Services

Health Screening and Referral Linkage with Health Services for Remedial and Preventive Measures

Screening helps in early detection and the timely institution of treatment for the most-common causes of morbidity.

Opthalmic and dental conditions, skin lesions and nutritional problems in particular are conditions where early identification can affect cure and prevent further progress and complications. By attending to some health determinants like anaemia and malnutrition, it could play a preventive role in addressing these critical problems.

It also helps identify children with refractive errors and hearing deficits, which are a major source of learning difficulties and by arranging to correct them, can dramatically improve school performance. Identification and support to children with disabilities is another major role that screening can play.

It is, therefore, recommended to carry out health checkups of all students at least once in a year, but preferably twice a year. Much of the success of school health screening programmes lies in constructing effective post screening referral arrangements. This is needed to ensure that the roughly 1–1% of children who are identified during the screening process as having serious but correctable ailments receive the higher level of clinical care that they need.

Health Education

This ensures the provision of age appropriate information on health, hygiene and nutrition, and to put it simply, education about the physical and mental aspects of growing up. It has great potential on promotion of healthy development and preventing risk behaviour. There are four broad activity groups that constitute school health education. One is the form of incorporation of a better.

Promote Health and Hygiene Practices within Schools

Understanding of health issues in the formal curriculum. The second is the construct of a series of informal sessions for students on specific necessary health issues which are not part of the formal learning system. This form of communication inculcates interest and enhances retention. It is effective for issues which require interpersonal dialogue, like life skills education and menstrual hygiene or for issues which require demonstrations, for instance, first aid education.

The third is the use of the school for behaviour change communication to disseminate health information and mould health related behaviours through extra curricular activities like poster making, plays, competitions, quiz contests. Finally, it is also the health and hygiene related practices that the school consciously inculcates in its students; for example, the use of toilets, hand washing before meals, the disposal of waste and the cleanliness of class-rooms and school campus.

Addressing Nutritional Issues, Particularly Anaemia and Malnutrition

Health department can assist in providing specific in interventions in the school setting for the priority areas or micro- and macronutrients deficiency. This includes identification and correction of anaemia, periodic treatment for worm infestation, the promotion of use of iodised salt, organizing talks on relevant nutrition issues and a linkage with the school mid-day meal programme to ensure that this acts as the critical supplement to correct macro-nutritional deficiency, rather than being a substitute for food intake at home. School health programme offers a unique opportunity to reach students end through them, their families at home. The nutrition counselling given herein has the potential to last through to the next generation as these students are the parents of tomorrow.

Providing Safe and Supportive Environment in Schools

It is a given pre-requisite that schools need to provide the basic amenities like potable drinking water, separate sanitary toilets for boys and girls and clean classrooms.

It is also necessary that schools strive to ensure safety of their students and staff from physical injuries, stress, corporal punishment and abuse. The school environment needs to be supportive of its teachers and students and also to be sensitive and alert to the manifest signs and symptoms of these conditions and provide the opportunity to seek appropriate help in effective and confidential management.

Service Provision

Services for minor ailments like headache, fever, cuts can be provided by the trained teachers while all other services can be offered through health care providers. **Following activities need to be ensured to provide these services.**

Capacity Building

This is needed to ensure that both school teachers as well as the health staff and their supervisors comprehend the school health programme and are equipped with the knowledge, skills and systems support needed to implement this programme optimally.

As teachers are required to participate actively, nodal teachers need to be identified by principals headmistress and

their training planned and organised. Each school has to have at least one designated nodal teacher for the school health programme and in large schools there has to be one nodal teacher per 250 students, with a school level coordinator. Based on these norms, the number of teachers from each school who act as nodal officers are identified. Ongoing refresher training of those trained before is essential as also is the continuous enrolment and training of new teachers to ensure adequate replacement of those staff members who are transferred or retire in their service tenure.

Monitoring and Evaluation

It is essential that the school health programme put in place is implemented with the requisite quality and scale needed to reach all students and make a significant impact. This system would not only measure the functioning of the programme but is an essential tool for further fine tuning and improvement. For monitoring and evaluation to become operational, a system needs to be developed and incorporated in the routine health monitoring system.

Core Management Group

A core management group responsible for overseeing the implementation of school health programme needs to be constituted at state, district, block and village levels with representatives from various departments and stakeholders like:

o   Department of health, including the AIDS control division

o   Department of education

o   Department of women and child development (WCD)

o   Principal and teachers

o   Parents' representative

o   Students' representative

At the state and district levels overall oversight may be provided by the NRHM Mission Director/District Magistrate/local body and at the village level by Village Health and Sanitation Committee.

Components of the School Health Programme

Health Screening and Remedial Measurers

The students would be screened at least annually by medical and paramedical personnel assisted by school teachers trained for this purpose. Ideally screening should be done twice a year. Since the number of students to be screened is massive the critical limitation is the availability of skilled human resource for this task.

Health Conditions to be Screened

Under this programme all students would be screened for a minimum set of pre-defined conditions, which would include:

General Health and Personal Hygiene

Weight and height recording would be done with computation of BMI and identification of underweight or overweight children. Such children need to be managed by counselling along with their caregivers. In the underweight child, support is needed to ensure that adequate food is being accessed and medical examination rules out secondary causes of malnutrition.

Clinical/Laboratory Assessment of Anaemia

Over 70% of children could be anaemic. Incase of children with anaemia of mild and moderate severity, we also need to note response to treatment and those who fail to respond should be referred since they need to be explored for non-dietary causes of anaemia. Most cases, however, are due to dietary gaps and worms infestation and could be treated in the school setting itself. Case of severe anaemia must be urgently referred to hospital.

Eye Examination

- Eyes should be checked for refractory errors, night blindness, trachoma, conjunctivitis.
- Refractory errors are a major treatable cause of learning problems.

Ear Discharge and Hearing Problems

Repeated ear discharge can lead to deafness. Many times deafness remains unnoticed but contributes to poor scholastic performance. Screening proformas designed under the national programme would be used for those students who have any such suspicion during health screening.

Common Dental Conditions

Dental caries and periodontal disease are common ailments and detected early, further progression can be prevented.

Common Skin Diseases and Infestations

Scabies, pyoderma and lice are some of the most common diseases. These are contagious and simultaneous treatment of all those affected is the easiest and the surest way to cut down the spread.

Heart Defects—Rheumatic and Congenital

There have been successful incidences where these have been detected and managed appropriately through school health programmes in our country.

Disabilities

Visual, hearing, locomotor, others: Children with disabilities have special needs to be able to keep up with the class. Equipment, as well as support and guidance could help them. It is crucial for school health programmes to detect these as well as to create awareness about the special needs of people with disabilities.

Learning Disorders/Problem Behaviours/Stress/Anxiety

Teachers need to be sensitized to identify children with such problems at an early stage and send them to appropriate referral centres. These conditions may not be detected during health screening, but a trained teacher would notice it during the regular course of school.

Planning the Screening and the Referral

A school-wise schedule of visits of the health personnel needs to be drawn up and communicated to the school authorities, students, parents and local government well in advance so that all preparations can be made. The students would be examined, screened and treated/referred/counseled as necessary on the prescribed dates.

A resource manual would be prepared and distributed to all the providers (health staff and teachers) so that they are aware of the interventions, methodology and responsibilities. After screening, the students found to be suffering from any disease/abnormality would be referred to the designated health facilities for each type of illness. A list of such referral facilities would be drawn up. The list will include adolescents health clinics that may have been established in nearby health facilities under RCH-II ARSH strategy. The minimum that states would need to do is to provide referral slips to the students with information to them and their parents as to which centre to go to and when.

Planning for Remedial Action at the School Itself

There is also considerable remedial action that would be taken at the school level itself. Appropriate first-line treatment for small cuts and injuries and certain common illnesses like skin aliments, which would otherwise become septic. For this a first aid kit should be put in place. This is useful irrespective of screening.

Immunization with DT at 6 years and with tetanus toxoid at 10 and 16 years is also another action but this would need the nurse and could be combined with the health screening.

Documentation and Health Records

Teachers would maintain the health record of each student in the school on a child health card and a school health register that ensurers that each child who has been screened gets the follow-up required.

It is also valuable for every school after the screening to provide information of common illnesses detected. The very presentation of this record indicates the seriousness with which the screening was carried out. It also tells us what was screened for and what was not. Tamil Nadu is one State that regularly compiles such statistics and it is an example that is worth emulating.

Equipment and Supplies for Health Screening

Health department would provide the equipment and supplies required for health screening. This would include a functional weighing scale and height measurement equipment (Stadiometer or a wall mounted one). Health department would also provide a Snellen's Chart for testing visual acuity. For smaller schools health team would carry these equipments during the screening visits to schools. For bigger schools the health department could supply these equipments to schools who would ensure safe keeping of the equipments.

Health department would supply first-aid kits containing common medicines like paracetamol for mild pain, headache, fever and dysemorrhea, ORS packets for diarrhea; dressing material and antiseptic solution and antibiotic cream for managing minor wounds.

School health register is a record kept by the school on the results of the screening and helps in organizing the follow-up.

Transport for Screening and Referrals

Adequate provision for funds would be ensured to provide appropriate transport (including provision for hiring vehicle, if necessary) to health staff to visit the schools and more important, to take children for referrals.

SCHEME FOR PROMOTION OF MENSTRUAL HYGIENE

Introduction

The Ministry of Health and Family Welfare has introduced a scheme for promotion of menstrual hygiene among adolescent girls in the age group of 10–19 years in rural areas.

Scheme for promotion of menstrual hygiene: The scheme aims at ensuring that adolescent girls in the target group have adequate knowledge and information about menstrual hygiene and the use of sanitary napkins, that high quality, safe products are made available to them, and that environmentally safe disposal mechanisms are readily accessible. The scheme has been launched as part of the adolescent reproductive and sexual health (ARSH) component under RCH II.

Objectives

The major objectives of the scheme are:

○ To increase awareness among adolescent girls on menstrual hygiene
○ To increase access to and use of high quality sanitary napkins to adolescent girls in rural areas.
○ To ensure safe disposal of sanitary napkins in an environmentally friendly manner.

Under the scheme a pack of 6 sanitary napkins is provided under the NRHMs brand 'Freedays'.

These napkins are sold to the adolescents girls at ₹ 6 for a pack of 6 napkins in the village by the accredited social health activist (ASHA). On sale of each pack, the ASHA gets an incentive of ₹1 per pack besides a free pack of sanitary napkins per month.

In the first phase, the scheme is expected to cover approximately 25% of the country's adolescent girl population (aged 10–19 years), i.e. 1.5 crore girls in 152 districts across 20 States. Out of these, supply of sanitary napkins in 107 districts was envisaged initially in a central supply mode, wherein sanitary napkins were to be supplied by the Government of India. The supply of sanitary napkins in the remaining 45 districts was envisaged in a self help group (SHG) mode, wherein SHGs were to manufacture the sanitary napkins that are to be sold to adolescent girls. Procurement of sanitary napkins, whether through central supply by the Government of India, or through SHGs, has to be done at a fixed price of ₹ 7.50/- per pack of six sanitary napkins. The sanitary napkins are provided under NHM's brand, 'Freedays'. These napkins are being sold to adolescents girls at the rate of ₹ 6 per pack of six napkins by accredited social health activists (ASHAs). From out of the sale proceeds, the ASHA gets an incentive amount of Re. 1 per pack, besides getting a free pack of sanitary napkins per month and the balance ₹ 5 is to be deposited in the state/district treasury. The scheme has taken off in 107 districts in the 17 States that are being supplied sanitary napkins through central procurement.

Target Group

This programme will be targeted at adolescent girls in the age group of 10–19 years, residing in rural areas, to ensure that they have adequate knowledge and information about the use of sanitary napkins, that high quality safe products are made available to them, and that environmentally safe disposal mechanisms are readily accessible. Based on data from Census 2001, there are an estimated 225 million adolescents comprising nearly one-fifth (22%) of India's total population. The projected rural population of girls (10–19 years) is 8.55 crore, of which 2.42 crore belong to the below poverty line (BPL) category and 6.13 crore to the above poverty line (APL) category.

In the first phase, 150 districts are to be covered, i.e. there will be 25% geographic coverage. Therefore, of the total adolescent girl population of 8.55 crore girls, the coverage (at 25%) for the first year amounts to 2.14 crore girls in the target group. Assuming that approximately 70% of population of 2.14 crore of adolescent girls is to be reached, and given varying ages of onset of menarche between 10–12 years, the calculation in this programme is based upon a target population of 1.5 crore girls in the age group of 10–19 years. Out of these 1.5 crore girls, the approximate proportion of APL girls is about 70% (105 lakh) and that of BPL girls is 30% (45 lakh).

Overall Strategy

The scheme adopts two key strategies: Demand generation through ASHA and other community mechanisms such as Women's Groups/Kishori Mandals. An additional mechanism for in-school youth would be that of the AEP through the life skills courses for Classes IX and XI. Supply side intervention through ensuring a supply of a product (sanitary napkin) which is reasonably priced and of high quality.

Selection of Districts

The initiative will be rolled out in phases, with 25% of the country being covered in the first phase, i.e. 150 districts in selected states. The following criteria are suggested to the states for selection of districts where this intervention may be taken up:

- Existing adolescent health programme
- Strong AEP intervention
- Active Self-Help Group (SHG) federations
- Effective ASHA training and support systems.

In the selected districts, the states would cover approximately 70% of the adolescent girl population because of the varying ages of onset of menarche between 10 years and 12 years.

Components of the Programme (Tables 9 and 10)

- Community-based health education and outreach in the target population to promote menstrual health
  - Outreach through ASHA/other community mechanisms
  - Outreach through schools
- Ensuring regular availability of sanitary napkins to the adolescents

- In the community
- In the school
- Sourcing and procurement of sanitary napkins
  - Training of ASHA in menstrual hygiene
  - Behaviour change communication
  - Safe disposal of sanitary napkins.

Table 9: Service delivery framework: Roles and responsibilities at various service delivery levels

Level of care	Service provider	Service package
Village	ASHA/ CBOs/ SHGs	• Mobilise adolescent girls. Conduct monthly meetings. Provide health education to adolescent girls • Conduct women's group meetings • Distribute sanitary napkins to adolescent girls • Ensure regular refill and supply of sanitary napkins to the village from the sub-centre. Sell sanitary napkins and maintain accounts • Track supplies and estimate requirement for the following month • Submit progress report on key indicators
Sub-centre	ANMs	• Training of the ASHA on menstrual hygiene booklet, and conduct periodic refreshers • Monitor the monthly meetings periodically • Transport the sanitary napkin stock from block PHC to sub-centre • Ensure safe storage of the sanitary napkin stock • Supply requisite number of sanitary napkin packs to ASHA in her sub-centre area • Provide imprest funds and transportation costs to ASHA • Conduct spot checks during regular field visits and village health and nutrition day (VHND) • Review and validate ASHA tracking system and accounts register • Maintain inventory, tracking and accounts register
PHC	Medical officer/ Block account officer	• Ensures that ASHA training on menstrual hygiene takes place. • Ensure safe storage of sanitary napkins. • Conduct spot checks during regular field visits. • Maintain inventory, tracking and accounts register.

Contd…

Level of care	Service provider	Service package
District	CMHO/ CS/DPM	○ Serve as the nodal point for the programme. ○ Engage the services of a bookkeeper on a contractual basis to train MO/ Block accounts officer and ANM in all blocks on maintaining inventory and accounts for the scheme. ○ Ensure remittance of funds obtained to district health society through the block. ○ Ensure safe storage of sanitary napkins. ○ Monitor the programme on a regular basis. ○ Monthly programme and financial review of the scheme along with other health programmes. ○ Manage convergence of various departments
State	Mission director, NRHM	○ Organise sourcing of sanitary napkins from SHGs/bidding process ○ Set up quality cell to ensure conformity with prescribed standards ○ Ensure sound logistics systems for smooth supply to district and below

Table 10: Operationalisation of the programme at the district and sub-district levels

Step 1	Sanitary napkins are supplied to the block warehouse. Storage will need to be organised by states at the block level. Such storage needs to be clean, dry, rodent-free and secure
Step 2	The ANM will collect the sanitary napkins from the block during her monthly meeting visit and transport it to the sub-centre. Even when packaged for delivery at the level of the PHC, the commodity is lightweight but bulky, needing adequate space which is free of moisture and pests/rodents. It will be stored at the sub-centre or at a place rented for this particular purpose, if the space in the sub-centre is insufficient. Such storage will need to be organised by states
Step 3	The ANM will provide the ASHA with a one-time imprest fund of ₹ 300 (or more if decided by the State Steering Committee) which she will take from the untied funds pool of the sub-centre
Step 4	The ASHA will use the imprest funds to purchase sanitary napkins from the ANM. ASHA will also get a pack of sanitary napkins free every month for her own use to be able to become an effective change agent
Step 5	The ASHA will sell sanitary napkins to the adolescent girls at a price decided by the Government

Contd…

Step 6	In case ASHA is selling the sanitary napkin packs, she will retain an incentive for every pack sold, the incentive amount being decided by the state steering committee
Step 7	The ASHA will retain the amount recovered from the sale to replenish the imprest amount which the ASHA will use for subsequent purchase
Step 8	The ANM will deposit the funds obtained from the sale of napkins to the ASHA in the united funds of the sub-centre
Step 9	These funds will be used for meeting the costs of transportation from Block to sub-centre and then to the village and rental to store the sanitary napkins at the Sub-Centre level if required
Step 10	The balance fund, if any after, meeting the above costs will be returned to the district health society through the block. The district health society should use these funds for programmes for adolescents

NUTRITION RELATED PROGRAMS

NATIONAL NUTRITIONAL PROGRAMS

Malnutrition is one of the huge burdens faced by India. India introduced many nutritional programs through various ministries to combat malnutrition.

Undernutrition is a condition that occurs as a result of inadequate intake of food or more essential nutrient(s) that may end up in deterioration growth and health. Good nutritional status enhances the health of the individual. In 1993 India introduced national nutrition policy. The policy has direct and indirect intervention strategies.

Direct Intervention (Short-Term)

○ Nutrition intervention for specially vulnerable groups-
  ❏ *Expanding the safety net*: The universal immunization program, oral rehydration therapy and the integrated child development services (ICDS) have had a considerable impact on child survival and extreme forms of malnutrition.
  ❏ *Improving growth monitoring by including mothers of 0–3 years old*
  ❏ Reaching the adolescent girls: Including the adolescent girls within the domain of ICDS should be intensified to enhance their readiness for a safe motherhood
  ❏ *Ensuring better coverage* of expectant women in order to the incidence of low birthweight babies
○ Fortification of essential foods: Essential food items shall be fortified with appropriate nutrients. For example, salt with iodine and/or iron.
○ Popularization of low-cost nutritious food.
○ Control of micro-nutrient deficiencies amongst vulnerable groups.

Indirect Policy Instruments: Long-term Institutional and Structural Changes

- Food security to attain per capita availability of 215 kg/person/year of food grains
- Improvement of dietary pattern through production and demonstration
- Improving the purchasing power through poverty alleviation programs, like the integrated rural development program (IRDP)
- Public distribution system to ensure an equitable food distribution
- Land reform
- Health and family welfare
- Bask health and nutrition knowledge
- Prevention of food adulteration
- Nutrition surveillance
- Monitoring of nutrition programs
- Research
- Equal remuneration
- Communication: Communication through established media for the effective implementation of the nutrition policy
- Minimum wage administration
- Community participation
- Education and literacy
- Improvement of the status of women

Nutritional Programs—Milestones

- During first (1951–1956) and second (1956–1961) five-year plans—Nutrition activities aimed at (1) increased production of food items, (2) supplementary feeding, (3) nutritional surveys and (4) prevention of food adulteration
- During third five-year plan, 1962—applied nutrition program and midday meal program started
- During fourth five-year plan—special nutrition program (1970), integrated child development services (1975) were started
- During 6th and 7th five-year plans—essential measures taken to convert special nutrition program centers to ICDS pattern by linking it with health, sanitation, water supply, hygiene and education.

MIDDAY MEAL PROGRAM (MDMP)

The midday meal program is otherwise known as school lunch program. The school midday meal program is in practice in India since 1961.

Objectives

- To enhance admissions of children in the school
- To enhance students' attendance and retention
- To improve literacy of the children.

Principles of Midday Meal for School Children

- The meal should be a supplement not a substitute to the home diet
- The meal should supply at least one-third of the total energy requirement and half of the protein need
- The cost of the meal should be reasonably low
- The meal should be of that which can be easily prepared
- Made out of locally available foods to reduce the cost
- Frequent changes in the menu to avoid boredom.

The midday meal program became part of the minimum needs program in the fifth five-year plan.

Midday Meal Scheme

Centrally sponsored scheme, the "National Program of Nutritional Support to Primary Education (NP-NSPE)" was launched on 15th August 1995. It was initially implemented in 2408 blocks in the country. By 1997–98, this program was implemented in all over the country. Initially it served only classes I–V of government, government aided and local body schools. Later, in 2002 children studying in Education guarantee school (EGS) and alternative and innovative education (AIE) centers were also covered.

Central assistance under the scheme consisted of free supply of food grains at 100 grams per child per school day, and subsidy for transportation of food grains.

The scheme was revised in 2004 to provide **cooked midday meal** that would yield 300 calories and 8–12 grams of protein to all children studying in classes I–V.

As per the revision made in October 2007, the scheme was extended to cover children in upper primary (classes VI to VIII) of educationally backwards blocks (EBBs).

Purposes

- To enhancing enrollment of children in the school
- To enhance students' attendance retention
- To improve nutritional status of children.

Objectives

- Improving the nutritional status of children of classes I–VIII studying in government, local body and government aided schools, and EGS and AIE centers.

○ Encouraging poor children, belonging to disadvantaged sections, to attend school more regularly and help them concentrate on classroom activities.

○ Providing nutritional support to children of primary stage in drought affected areas during summer vacation.

Benefits of Midday Meal Scheme

○ Admissions in schools will be enhanced

○ Children attend school regularly

○ Facilitate healthy growth of children

○ It is an opportunity to impart various good habits in children (handwashing)

○ Fosters social equality

○ Helps to enhance gender equity

○ Facilitates cognitive, emotional and social development of children

Nutritive values of mid-day meal scheme in school (Table 11)

Applied Nutrition Program (ANP)

Applied nutrition program was first started in Orissa and Andra Pradesh in the year 1963. By 1973 it was extended to whole India. Though it was considered as one of the best nutritional program it could not yield the expected results because of failure in management of the program. It was started centrally sponsored program, but now handed over to states.

It is considered as a low priority program comparing to other nutritional programs. This program aimed at creating self-reliance among community.

Aim

The principal objective is to improve the nutritional status of people by encouraging them to involve production of foods and consumption of the self-produced foods.

Objectives

○ To make people conscious of their nutritional needs

○ To increase production of nutritious foods and its consumption

○ To provide supplementary nutrition to vulnerable groups using local production of foods.

Table 11: Nutritive values-mid-day meal scheme provided in school

Components	Primary child	Upper primary child
Calories	450	700
Protein	12 g	20 g
Micronutrients	Adequate quantities of micronutrients like iron, folic acid and vitamin A	

Beneficiaries

○ Children between 3 and 6 years

○ Pregnant and lactating mothers

Organization

Block development officer supervises the program. Balsevikas play a key role in implementing the program at the community.

Activities

○ Poultry farming

○ Horticulture

○ Beehive keeping

○ Kitchen gardening

○ Supplementary nutrition

○ Nutrition education.

Vitamin A Prophylaxis Program

○ Launched in the year 1970 as a centrally sponsored scheme by Ministry of Health and Family Welfare, Government of India.

○ Component of National program for control of blindness (1976)—under this program a single dose of oily preparation of "vitamin A"—mega dose (200,000 IU), administered orally to all preschool children in the community once in every 6 months.

○ During 1980, the Department of Food introduced a scheme of fortification of milk with vitamin A to prevent nutritional blindness.

○ At present the country is implementing this scheme through dairies.

INTEGRATED CHILD DEVELOPMENT SERVICES SCHEME

Integrated child development services (ICDS) scheme was initiated on 2 October, 1975 during 5th five-year plan period under "Ministry of social welfare" in pursuance of nutritional policy for children. Initially ICDS was started in 33 community development blocks as experimental projects during 1975–76 and expanded to 2,765 projects by the year 1992. This experimental project was implemented in 4 urban, 19 rural and 10 tribal areas in 22 states and the Union Territory of New Delhi.

ICDS Center

ICDS center is called "Anganwadi center (AWC)."

Population norms for AWC in Rural/Urban areas:

○ For 400–800 population—1 AWC

○ For 800–1,600 population—1 AWC

- For 1,600–2,400 population—1 AWC
- Thereafter 1 AWC for multiples of 800 population
- For 150–400 Population—1 Mini AWC
- Population norms for AWC in Tribal/Desert/Hilly and other difficult areas:
- For 300–800—1 AWC
- For 150–300—1 Mini center.

Objectives

- Improve nutritional and health status of children of 0–6 years age group
- To lay the foundations for proper psychological, physical and social development of child
- Reduce incidence of mortality, morbidity, malnutrition and school dropout
- Enhance the capability of mother and nutritional needs of the child through proper nutrition and health education
- Achieve effective coordination among various departments which are working toward the promotion of child development.

Under ICDS various services included to provide as an integrated package to children below the age of 6 years, pregnant and nursing mothers (Fig. 3).

Beneficiaries and Services in ICDS

- *Children <3 years:* Supplementary nutrition, immunization, health checkup and referral services
- *Children in the age group of 3–6 years:* In addition to above services nonformal education is provided
- *Adolescent girls (in selected Blocks):* Supplementary nutrition and health education
- *Pregnant women:* Health check, immunization against tetanus, supplementary nutrition and health education

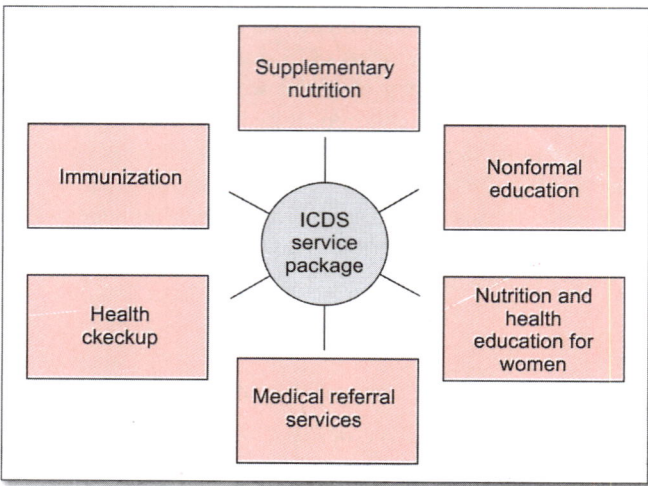

Figure 3: ICDS service package

Table 12: Provision of energy and protein in ICDS

Beneficiaries/age	Calories/day	Protein/day	Expenditure/day
6-72 months	500/child	12–15 g/child	₹4/child
Severely malnourished-6–72 months	800/child	20–25 g/child	₹6/child
Pregnant and nursing women	600/pregnant/nursing mother	18–20 g	₹5/child

- *Lactating women:* Health check, supplementary nutrition and health education
- *Women in reproductive age group (15–44 years):* Nutrition and health education.

Delivery of Services under ICDS

Supplementary Nutrition

The type of foods served is depending upon availability in the area, type of beneficiary and the project type, etc. Provision of energy and protein under ICDS given in (Table 12).

- The revised nutritional and feeding norm provides more than one meal to a child who attends AWCs. This may include a morning snack (milk/banana/egg/seasonal fruit/micronutrient fortified food) followed by a hot cooked meal
- Children below 3 years, pregnant and lactating women are provided with "take home ration"
- ICDS scheme is universal and all are eligible irrespective of the economic status
- Supplementary nutrition is provided for 300 days/year
- Weighing of children monthly.

Guidelines

- Child with first degree malnutrition—Nutritional education and health education to mothers
- 2nd and third degree malnutrition—Supplementary nutrition
- 4th degree malnutrition—Hospitalization.

Nutritional and Health Education

- Nutrition and health education given to all women of age 15–45 years
- Main focus on pregnant and nursing mothers
- Special classes conducted by *anganwadi* workers during home visits.

Immunization

- Children: Vaccines against six vaccine preventable diseases
- Pregnant women—tetanus toxoid.

Health Checkup

- Antenatal care, postnatal care and care of children under 6 years of age
- Immunization, iron and folic acid along with protein supplements to expectant mothers
- Three antenatal visits and physical examination
- Referral to high-risk mothers
- Care to children below 6 years of age:
  - Measuring weight
  - Immunization
  - Periodical general checkup to screen for disease
  - Treatment to prevailing infections like diarrhea, ARI etc.
  - Deworming
  - Prophylaxis against deficiency of vitamin A and anemia
  - Referral services to hospital
  - Health card to mother and child.

Nonformal Education

- Preschool education to children of 3–6 years in AWC in every village with 1,000 population
- The primary idea is to develop good attitude, values, and behavior in children
- Locally manufactured low-cost toys are used for play.

Schemes for Adolescents

There are two special schemes run for adolescent girls using the infrastructure of ICDS. The schemes are:

- Kishori shakti yojana
- Nutrition program for adolescent girls.

Kishori Shakti Yojana

This program addresses the nutrition, health and developmental needs, literacy and numerical skills of girls aging between 11 and 18 years.

Nutrition Program for Adolescent Girls

This program was initiated in 2009–2010 as pilot project. It is being implemented in 51 districts of major states.

Aims

- To improve the nutritional and health status of adolescent girls.
- To provide nutrition and health education to the adolescents.
- Empower adolescent girls to care their personal health and nutrition needs.

Beneficiaries

Under nourished adolescent girls of age 11–15 years with weight <30 kg

Under nourished adolescent girls of age 15–19 years with weight <35 kg.

Services

- 6 kg free food grain per month/adolescent
- Weight measuring four times in a year.

Role of Anganwadi Worker (AWW)

The trained local woman who is the center point for delivery of services under ICDS is knows as "Anganwadi worker (AWW)."

Functions of AWW

- She is the multipurpose agent works close with the community
- Direct link to child and mother
- Assists in the survey of community and beneficiaries
- Organizes non-formal education sessions
- Provides health and nutrition education to mothers
- Assists PHC staff in provision of health services
- Maintains records like immunization, feeding and attendance
- Liaises with members from various disciplines—block administrator, village health nurse, ASHA, with local schools, etc.

NATIONAL NUTRITIONAL ANEMIA PROPHYLAXIS PROGRAM (NNAPP)

Nutritional anemia is the most prevalent problem among women, adolescents, under-five and old people. The NNAPP is a centrally sponsored scheme started in the year 1970. The prevalence of anemia was 70% in children aged 6–59 months, 55% in females aged 15–49 years, and 24% in males aged 15–49 years (NFHS-3). It functions with the general goal of reduction in prevalence and incidence of anemia in women of reproductive age group specifically pregnant and lactating mothers and preschool children.

Objectives

- To assess the baseline prevalence of nutritional anemia in mothers and young children through estimation of hemoglobin (Hb) levels.
- To place anemic mothers and children with low Hb levels (<10 g and <8 g respectively) on antianemia treatment.
- To start prophylaxis program for mothers with Hb level >10 g/dL and children with Hb >8 g/dL and assess their Hb levels periodically.
- Health educate and encourage the mothers to consume the tablets.

Beneficiaries

- Children in the age group of 1–5 years
- Pregnant and nursing mothers
- Female acceptor of terminal methods of family planning and IUDS.

Target to Cover Beneficiaries

- 50% of total pregnant and nursing mothers
- 25% of total women acceptors of terminal methods and IUDs
- 50% of total population in the age group of 1–5 years.

Services

- Promoting the regular inclusion and consumption of foods rich in iron.
- Iron and folate supplementation to the target group.
- Identifying and treating of severely anemic cases.

The recommended daily dosages of iron and folic acid (IFA) tablets:

Adult women : 60 mg elemental iron + 0.5 mg folic acid

Children (1–5 years) : 20 mg elemental iron + 0.1 mg folic acid.

This program activities are carried out in subcenter and PHCs by utilizing multipurpose health workers—females and males.

VARIOUS COMMUNICABLE AND NON-COMMUNICABLE DISEASES HEALTH PROGRAMS

ACUTE RESPIRATORY INFECTION CONTROL PROGRAM

Acute respiratory infections (ARTs) is the most prevalent among children. It is a huge burden on the family and country causing high rates of under-five mortality specifically with pneumonia.

Acute respiratory infection control program was initiated as a pilot project in 14 districts in the year 1990. The main objective was to bring down the child mortality that accused as a result of ARI. The program was incorporated in child survival and safe motherhood (CSSM) program in the year 1992 later on with reproductive and child health (RCH) phase-I in the year 1997. Now ARI control is one of the components of RCH phase-II.

The major strategies implemented to reduce child mortality are:

- Training of medical and health care personnel to provide standard case management for pneumonia in under-five children using set guidelines.
- Training health care personnel to manage pneumonia
- Enhancing maternal knowledge on home management of cough and cold
- Creating awareness among mothers on identifying signs and symptoms of pneumonia
- Exclusive breastfeeding for first 4–6 months
- Awareness on weaning the child
- Administration of vitamin A solution to prevent vitamin A deficiency leading to blindness

Note: Since 1997 the components of the ARI control program is implemented under RCH phase-II

REVISED NATIONAL TUBERCULOSIS CONTROL PROGRAM (RNTCP)

Around 38% morbidity and 39% mortality of the world tuberculosis burden is found in South-East Asia Region (SEAR) of world health organization. The National tuberculosis program of 1962 did not achieve fruitful results in reducing the TB burden. There were many defaulters and rise in multidrug resistance cases on TB. After 30 years of work the Government of India tried reviewing the TB scenario along with and Swedish-international development cooperation agency (SIDA) in the year 1992. The review revealed certain important reasons. They were: (1) Inadequate funding, (2) overreliance on X-rays for diagnosis, (3) interrupted supplies of drugs, and (4) low treatment completion rates.

In 1993, the program was named as "Revised NTCP" with new strategies to control the burden of tuberculosis. RNTCP is building upon the basic infrastructure available from initial NTP. This RNTCP had incorporated the elements of internationally recommended directly observed treatment short course (DOTS). This was started in phased manner and the whole country was covered by the year 2006.

Organization Set-up

At state level there is a state tuberculosis office headed by state TB officer.

State TB training and demonstration center-Director

At district level—medical officer for TB control activities. Under him, one senior treatment supervisor and a senior TB laboratory supervisor are functioning. In addition, there are microscopy centers, treatment centers and DOT providers.

Objectives

- To achieve the cure rate of not less than 85% through short course chemotherapy
- To detect 70% of the estimated cases through sputum smears
- To involve nongovernmental organizations (NGOs)
- Use DOTS as community based treatment.

Strategies

- Increased organizational support at the central and state level for meaningful coordination
- Increase in budgetary outlay
- Use of sputum microscopy as a primary method of diagnosis among self-reporting patients
- Standardized tuberculosis treatment regimens
- Enhancement of peripheral level supervision through the creation of a sub-district supervisory unit
- Ensuring a regular uninterrupted supply of drugs up to the most peripheral level
- Emphasis on training, IEC, operational research and NGO involvement in the program.

Prevention and Control

The control measures: Case finding and TB treatments as curative measure and BCG vaccination as preventive measure.

Case Finding

Under RNTCP active case finding not pursued.

Early detection of all cases means finding people whose sputum is positive for TB bacilli. Finding the suspects means whose sputum is negative but X-ray shows suggestive shadows of TB.

Note: Under RNTCP active case findings are not pleasured

The patients seeking medical advice voluntarily with chest symptoms like persistent cough and fever are the most appropriate target group for case finding.

Sputum Examination

Sputum examination is the cheapest and most suited tool for finding the cases. Sputum smears collected from suspected persons should be collected early in the morning on three successive days. The presence of at least 10,000 organisms per mL of sputum is considered "TB positive."

As per RNTCP, priority for sputum smear examination should be given to patients who come on their own to hospital or health center with the following symptoms:

- Persistent cough of 3–4 weeks duration
- Continuous fever
- Chest pain
- Hemoptysis

Sputum Culture

- It is a long process and needs to perform in trained people
- It is delivered only as centralized service in district hospitals
- Advised for the patients whose sputum smear is negative but has chest symptoms.

Mass Miniature Radiography

This is abandoned as a case finding measure because of its poor yields with high cost.

Chest X-ray

Chest X-ray is recommended as additional method to diagnose pulmonary tuberculosis when only one smear is positive.

Tuberculin Test

This test does not have much value as a case-finding tool.

Chemotherapy

Effective treatment is available to treat tuberculosis. The main aim is to eliminate fast and slowly multiplying bacilli from a case and provide cure. Chemotherapy is readily available, free of cost to every detected case. Patient or the case is the core component of the success of the treatment because it requires strict compliance from the patient. Most often tuberculosis patients default since they start to feel good and active only by completing with 2 weeks of medicine at start.

Anti-TB drugs: Categorized into first-line drugs and Second-line drugs. First-line drugs are further grouped into:

Bactericidal drugs: INH, Rifampicin, pyrizinamide and streptomycin

Bacteriostatic drugs: Ethambutol and thioacetazone

A combination of these are used to treat TB patients.

Domiciliary Treatment

It is the method of self-consumption of prescribed anti-TB drugs by the patients without getting admitted to the hospital. Domiciliary treatment includes only oral drugs.

Short Course Chemotherapy (SCC)

Wallace Fox and his colleagues from British medical research council added (1972) Rifampicin and Pyrazinamide to anti TB regimen and reduced the duration of treatment from 18 months to 6–8 months.

In short course chemotherapy the drugs are given in two phases.

Intensive Phase

This is the initial phase lasts for 2 months; a combination of 3 or 4 drugs are given. During this phase a combination of three or more drugs are used to kill off as many bacilli as possible.

Continuation Phase

This is the maintenance phase lasts for 4–6 months under short course chemotherapy in which a combination of 2 or 3 drugs are given.

Treatment is given daily or biweekly (Intermittent).

Drug Administration in Directly Observed Treatment Short Course Chemotherapy (DOTS)

○ In intensive phase of treatment a health worker or trained person closely watches the patient swallowing the drug in his presence

○ During continuation phase the patient is issued 1 week medicine in a multiblister combipack. The first dose is swallowed by the patient in front of health worker

○ The drug consumption in the continuation phase is counter-checked by return of empty multiblister combipack while collecting the drugs for next week

○ The drugs are provided in patient-wise boxes with sufficient shelf life.

○ Tuberculosis cases are divided into three categories for the sake of putting them under different regimens based on specific criteria.

Interpretation of the Numbers and Letters Placed in the Regimens

○ Prefix number indicates the number of months for that regimen.

○ Suffix number indicates the frequency of administration in a week.

  □ No suffix means given daily

  □ R-Rifampicin

  □ H-Isoniazid

  □ S-Streptomycin

  □ Z-Pyrazinamide.

Chemoprophylaxis

This preventive treatment is administered to contacts: INH for 1 year or INH and Ethambutol are given for 9 months.

Surveillance

○ This focuses on the continuous monitoring and measurement.

○ It closely monitors and measures the rates of incidence, prevalence and other rates like TB death rates. It helps the epidemiologist to have current knowledge about what is happening and what he has to do to control the diseases.

WHO's Stop TB Strategy

World health organization recommends all countries, public and private sectors functioning at national, local levels to implement the following to bring down the burden of TB:

○ Practice high-quality of "DOTS" expansion and enhancement.

○ Secure political commitment with enough and continued financing

○ Ensure early detection of cases and diagnosis and maintain quality

○ Provide standardized treatment with suitable supervision and patient support

○ Assure effective drug supply and management

○ Continuous monitoring and evaluation.

New Initiatives

○ **Nikshay:** *TB surveillance using case-based web-based IT system*

○ *Web-based resource center: This is a case based, web based software application launched in May 2012. The functional components of it include: Master management, user details, TB patient registration details, DOT provider, HIV status, follow-up, contact tracing and outcomes.*

- *This also includes mobile application for notification and SMS to patient and TB program officers.*
- *Automatic periodic reports on case finding, sputum conversion and treatment outcome.*
- Communication facilitators provided to support IEC at district level
- Capacity building of program managers to plan and implement need-based IEC activities
- Well-defined IEC strategies.

Role of Community Health Nurse in RNTCP

- Immunize with BCG at birth
- Under RNTCP active case-finding is not pursued. However, people found to be with symptoms of tuberculosis in the clinic and during the home visits can be encouraged for further investigations
- Convey the message that tuberculosis is curable and free treatment facilities available
- Help to remove fears and taboos about the disease
- Advising on balanced diet to protect from infections
- Motivating the people with symptoms to clinic
- Collecting thorough history
- Show high-level of interest in contact screening
- Teaching on how to take out sputum by coughing when test for AFB suggested
- Administer tuberculin test, if ordered
- Stress on importance of continuation of regular treatment as prescribed. Stress on the point "not default" which is bad for his family as well to community
- Teach good practices like closing the mouth and speaking, maintaining considerable physical distance to avoid sprinkling of saliva on others
- Teach how to dispose sputum safely
- Close follow-up on treatment compliance.

COMMUNICABLE AND NONCOMMUNICABLE DISEASES

NATIONAL LEPROSY ERADICATION PROGRAM (NLEP)

It is a disease of public health concern because of its potential nature of causing disability and the social stigma and discrimination attached to it. In India, 86,000 cases were on record as on April 1, 2014. The prevalence rate of leprosy was 0.68 per 10,000 population in 2014. In 1955, India launched the National Leprosy Control Program (NLCP) with the features of case detection, treatment with Dapsone and community education. This was changed to the National Leprosy Eradication Program (NLEP) in 1983, with the introduction of multidrug therapy (MDT).

Historical Mile Stones in NLEP

- 1848–Leper Act, British India abolished later
- 1948–Hind Kusht Nivaran Sangh
- 1955–National Leprosy Control Program
- 1980–Dapsone
- 1982–MDT
- 1983–National Leprosy Eradication Program (MDT started)
- 1991–World Health Assembly resolution to eradicate leprosy by 2000 AD.
- 1998-2004 -Modified Leprosy Elimination Program.
- 2005 December—Prevalence rate 0.95/10,000 and government declared achievement of elimination target
- 2005—NRHM covers NLEP
- 2012—Introduction of special action plan for 209 high endemic districts of 16 States/UTs
- National Leprosy Eradication Program under NRHM-Organogram.

12th Five-Year: Implementation Plan (Flowchart 2)

Objectives on NLEP in 12th Five-Year Plan (2012-2017)

- Elimination of leprosy, i.e. prevalence of less than 1 case per 10,000 population in all districts of the country
- Strengthen disability prevention and medical Rehabilitation of persons affected by leprosy
- Reduction in the level of stigma associated with leprosy.

Program Strategies as Per 12th Five-Year Plan

To achieve the objectives of the plan, the main strategies to be followed are:

- Integrated leprosy services through general health care system
- Early detection and complete treatment of new leprosy cases
- Carrying out household contact survey for early detection of cases
- Involvement of accredited social health activist (ASHA) in the detection and completion of treatment of leprosy cases on time
- Strengthening of disability prevention and medical rehabilitation (DPMR) services

Flowchart 2: National leprosy eradication program

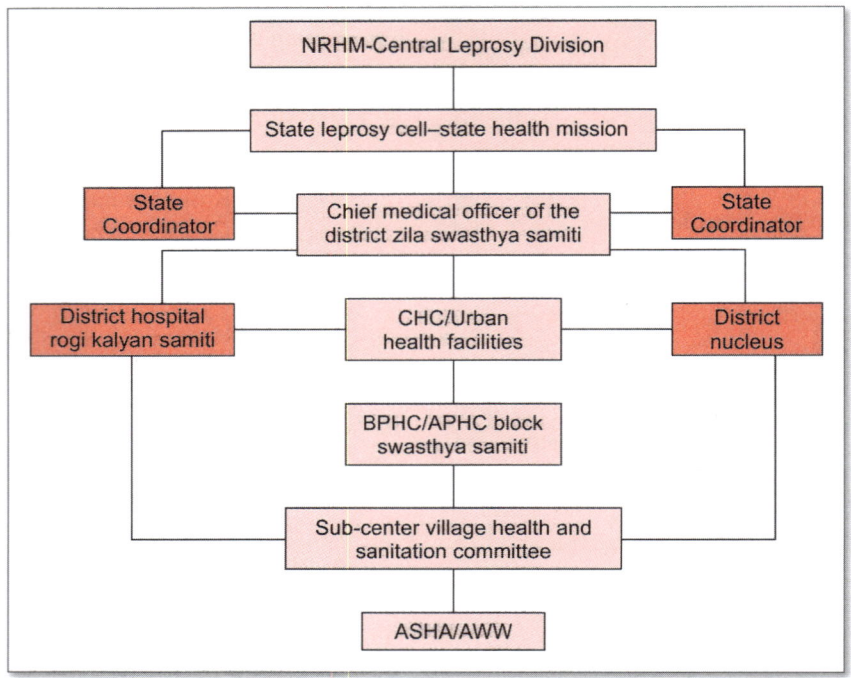

- Information, education and communication (IEC) activities in the community to improve self-reporting to primary health center (PHC) and reduction of stigma
- Intensive monitoring and supervision at block primary health center/community health center.

Case Detection and Management

Social stigma on leprosy is a phenomenon that stops people coming forward to get themselves diagnosed. Detection of the new cases at the early stage is the only solution to cut down the transmission. Early detection would help preventing disabilities in affected individuals. It is therefore suggested that the States will draw up innovative plans:

- To improve access to services
- To involve women including leprosy affected persons in case detection
- To organize skin camps for detecting leprosy patients while providing services for other skin conditions.
- To undertake contact survey to identify the source in the neighborhood of each child or multibacillary case
- To increase awareness through the ANM, AWW, ASHA and other Health Workers visiting the villages and people affected by leprosy to suspect and motivate leprosy affected persons for early reporting to the medical officer.

Services in Urban Area

It is evident from urban statistics that more cases are detected in urban area than the rural. It may be attributed to the quality health facilities and migrating population into urban areas. However, the treatment completion rates is lesser than the rural areas. All the component-wise activities can be carried out as it is in rural areas. Examples are: Training, IEC, procurement and supply of MDT and other required medicines, MCR footwear, aids and appliances, payments of incentive for RCS, etc. However, it is essential to carry out the following additional activities.

Guidelines Provided for Additional Activities in Urban Areas

- Identify human resources available with Government Civil societies, NGOs and private medical practitioners for leprosy services like suspect and referral. Population groups may be allocated to each human resource, and for follow-up of the cases.
- Build capacity of the identified human resources at the time of induction and periodically examination of all household contacts of all new cases at least once before the completion of treatment of index case.
- Identify one referral center in each urban location for diagnosis and to manage leprosy with or without complications.
- Supervision and monitoring of the program is the responsibility of the district leprosy officer, and medical officer of the referral center.
- Mobile health clinics of general health services include leprosy services on their visit to slums, periurban villages and migrant agglomerations.

- Develop a system of record keeping and reporting by each participating center.
- Develop a system of regular MDT supply to each health center.
- Procure additional requirement of drugs, dressing material, aids and appliances for inhabitants of leprosy colony requiring regular care for their disabilities.
- Organize sensitization meetings for IEC and advocacy, participate in exhibitions, quiz competition for awareness to reduce stigma.

ASHA Involvement

- Accredited social health activists (ASHA) will be involved during 12th plan to bring out suspected cases from their villages for diagnosis at PHC and after confirmation of diagnosis, will follow-up the patients for completion of treatment.
- The ASHA will be entitled to receive incentive as below:
- At confirmation of diagnosis ₹250
    - On completion of full course of treatment in time –
    - Pauci Bacillary (PB)—additional ₹400/-
    - Multi Bacillary (MB)—additional ₹600/-

Activities to be performed by ASHAs

- Search for suspected cases of leprosy, i.e. before any sign of disability appears. Such early detection will help in prevention of disability and also cut down transmission potential.
- Follow-up all cases for completion of treatment in scheduled time. During follow-up visit, also look for symptoms of any reaction due to leprosy and refer them to the Health Workers/PHC for treatment. This will again reduce chances of disability occurring in cases under treatment.
- Advise and motivate self-care practices by disabled cases for proper care of their hands and feet during the follow-up period. This will improve quality of life of the affected persons and prevent deterioration of disabilities.
- Spreading awareness.
- The involvement of ASHAs will be monitored by the concerned PHC medical officers.
- Records of cases referred by ASHAs will be maintained properly and incentive will be paid on time and regular monthly report will be submitted to the district leprosy officer.

SET Scheme

- The NGOs under the SET scheme are working for:
- Disability prevention and ulcer care

- IEC activities
- Referral of suspected cases, and reconstruction surgeries (RCS)
- Research and rehabilitation.
- The NGO support is mainly required to follow-up of the under treatment cases particularly in urban locations and in difficult to access areas.

Disability Prevention and Medical Rehabilitation (DPMR)

Patients are provided with services like self-care services, MCR footwear, aids and appliances at medical college and hospital/central leprosy institutes.

Role of Community Health Nurse in NLEP

- Educate community about cause, spread, prevention and management of the disease
- Try to assist in changing their misperceptions and stigma about the disease
- Stress on importance of early detection of the disease that helps in prevention of deformity
- Teach on how deformities are prevented and corrected
- Regular examination of skin surfaces and report if anything new or abnormal. Particularly contacts must be alerted on this
- Advise the cases to take MDT regularly as advised
- Cases should be careful while working in the kitchen because lack of sensation may cause fire accidents and burns
- Rats and rodents should be kept away. Since they may not have sensation in the toes rats may bite. Advise the cases to apply neem- oil over the toes and fingers before going to bed
- Individual/group/Mass education should be conducted.
- Follow-up through home visits—Identify and advise on regular treatment. If needed drugs can be supplied at home
- Patients with any complications should be referred to PHC
- Refer for disability prevention and medical rehabilitation (DPMR).

NATIONAL AIDS CONTROL PROGRAM (NACP)

Human immunity deficiency program (HIV) is a life-threatening infection, claimed 34 million lives so far. In the year 2014 alone 1.2 million people died due to HIV and its related causes, globally. Acquired immunodeficiency Syndrome (AIDS) is the most advanced stage of HIV infection.

Table 13: Historical milestones of the program

Years	Event
1986	First case of HIV detected National AIDS committee established under Ministry of Health
1990	Medium term plan launched for four states and the four metros
1992	NACP-1 launched to slow down the spread of HIV infection National AIDS control board constituted NACO set-up
1999	NACP-II Initiated-Focusing on behavior change State AIDS control societies established
2002	National AIDS control policy adopted National blood policy adopted
2004	Anti-retroviral treatment adopted
2007	NACP-III Launched for 5 years (2007–2012)
2014	NACP-IV launched for 5 years (2012–2017)

India launched National Aids Control Program in the year 1987. The total number of people living with HIV (PLHIV) in India is estimated at 21.17 lakhs in 2015 compared with 22.26 lakhs in 2007. National Aids Control Organization was set by the Ministry of Health and Family Welfare as a separate wing to closely monitor all the components of NACP.

Table 13 shows the important historical milestones of the AIDS and the program

Objectives

- To prevent further transmission of HIV
- To bring down the morbidity and mortality of the infection
- To minimize the socioeconomic impact of the disease

Preventive Services under NACP-IV

Following package of services are provided under NACP-IV.

Prevention Services

- Targeted Interventions for High Risk Groups and Bridge Population [Female sex workers (FSW), Men who have sex with men (MSM), Transgenders/Hijras, Injecting drug users (IDU), truckers and migrants]
- Needle syringe exchange program (NSEP) and opioid substitution therapy (OST) for IDUs
- Prevention interventions for migrant population at source, transit and destination
- Link worker scheme (LWS) for HRGs and vulnerable population in rural areas

- Prevention and control of sexually transmitted infections/reproductive tract infections (STI/RTI)
- Blood safety
- HIV counseling and testing services
- Prevention of parent to child transmission
- Condom promotion
- Information, education and communication (IEC) and Behavior change communication (BCC).
- Social mobilization, youth interventions and adolescent education program
- Mainstreaming HIV/AIDS response
- Work place interventions.

Care, Support and Treatment Services

- Laboratory services for CD4 testing and other investigations
- Free first line and second line anti-retroviral treatment (ART) through ART centers and Link ART centers (LACs), centers of excellence (COE) and ART plus centers.
- Pediatric ART for children
- Early infant diagnosis for HIV exposed infants and children below 18 months
- HIV-TB coordination (Cross-referral, detection and treatment of co-infections)
- Treatment of opportunistic infections
- Drop-in centers for PLHIV networks.

Types of Facilities for HIV Testing and Counseling

The ICTCs are located inside the hospital or health center. Services delivered in two ways: (a) Facility-based services and (b) Community-based services

Facility-based services (screening or confirmation) are offered to individuals accessing healthcare facilities functioning as per the OPD timings of the institution where the center is located.

Community-based screening is conducted by the ANMs in Health Subcenters.

Counseling and Testing Centers (ICTC)

It is of two types. Client oriented on his own will and provider initiated which the doctor advises.

Functions of the center includes early detection of the disease, providing information on modes of transmission and prevention, treatment and care process.

Stand-Alone (SA-ICTC)

The SA-ICTC facility should be located at an easily accessible place with direction signs to guide people to the location. Usually located in medical colleges, district hospitals etc. The SA-ICTC facility should consist of at least two rooms, one for counseling and the other for testing.

Full time counselor and laboratory technician provides counseling and testing respectively.

Mobile ICTC

The activities provided as mobile services in a van. It is mainly to serve hard to reach places. A paramedical team consisting of a counselor, health educator, ANM and a laboratory technician function to provide mobile services.

PPTCT Program

The Prevention of Parent to Child Transmission of HIV/AIDS (PPTCT) program was started in the country in the year 2002. Currently, there are 15,000 integrated counseling and testing centers (ICTCs) in the country, most of these in government hospitals, which offer PPTCT services to pregnant women. These are functioning with aim of universal coverage of all pregnant women to prevent transmission of HIV from mother to child. PPTCT provides HIV diagnostic, prevention, care and treatment to all pregnant women.

Package of PPTCT Services in India

- HIV testing and counseling
- Family centric approach by involving the spouse and family members in care
- Provision of lifelong ART pregnant and HIV infected—lactating women regardless of CD4 count.
- Promotion of institutional deliveries for HIV infected mothers
- Provision of care of associated conditions like STI/RTI, TB and other opportunistic infections
- Provision of nutrition, counseling and psychological support to HIV infected pregnant women
- Provision of counseling to initiate breastfeeding within 30 minutes of birth and continue for 6 months
- Provision of ARV prophylaxis for infants until 6 months
- Follow-up of HIV exposed infants into routine health care services
- Cotrimoxazole prophylactic therapy for infants
- Strengthening community network to support HIV positive pregnant women and their families.

WHO Criteria to Recommend HIV Treatment

HIV treatment recommended when the CD4 test shows less than 500 cells/mm^3 2013.   —(WHO)

Combination Therapy

Treating with two or more antiretroviral drugs at a time is called combination therapy. Taking a combination of three or more anti-HIV drugs is referred to as highly active anti-retroviral therapy (HAART).

Recommendations—Antiretroviral Treatment (WHO, 2013)

For adults and adolescents, they recommend starting on a first line therapy of two nucleoside reverse transcriptase inhibitors (NRTIs) plus a non-nucleoside reverse-transcriptase inhibitor (NNRTI). The favored recommendation is a fixed dose combination (just one pill) of:

TDF—Tenofovir
3TC—Lamivudine or FTC—Emtricitabine
EFV—Efavirenz

First- and Second-line Therapy

- At the commencement of treatment, the combination of drugs that a person is given is called first-line therapy. In case of resistance or any serious drug effects person will be changed to second-line therapy
- Second-line therapy recommendations by WHO suggest two NRTIs and a ritonavir-boosted protease inhibitor (PI).

SEXUALLY TRANSMITTED DISEASE (STD) CONTROL PROGRAM

Sexually transmitted disease control is now, linked with AIDS control program activities. As per WHO estimates around 10% of all adults are infected with curable STI (sexually transmitted infection) each year. Department of NACO coordinates RTI and STD at all levels of the health care: Free standardized STI/RTI services provided through 1160 clinics situated at government health care facilities, at district hospital level, and above. These clinics named as "Suraksha Clinics" provide sexual and reproductive health services.

Facilities in Surakhsha Clinics

- Standardized training to the medical and paramedical personnel based on syndromic case management approach
- Counseling services from trained counselors in Suraksha clinics.
- Color coded syndromic drug kits and rapid plasma reagin (RPR) test kits are being centrally procured and supplied to these clinics (Table 14).

Table 14: Syndromic management using pre-packed suraksha kit

Kit Number	Syndrome	Color	Content
1	UD, ARD, Cervicitis	Grey	Tab Azithromycin (1 g) 1 stat Tab Cefexime 400 mg 1 stat
2	Vaginitis	Green	Tab Secnidazole 2 g (1) stat Cap. Fluconazole 150 mg (1) Stat
3	Genito ulcerative disease (GUD) -non herpetic	White	Benzathine Penicillin (2.4 MU)-1 Vial Tab Azithromycin (1 g) single dose
4	Genito ulcerative Disease (GUD) -non herpetic-For patients allergic to penicillin	Blue	Doxcycline 100 mg BD × 15 days Azithromycin 1 g (single dose)
5	Genito ulcerative disease (GUD) -non herpetic	Red	Tab Acyclovir 400 m TDS for 7 days
6	Lower abdominal pain (LAP)	Yellow	Tab Cefexime 400 m OD stat Tab Metronidazole BD for 14 days, Doxcycline 100 m BD for 14 days
7	Inguinal Bubo	Black	Tab Azithromycin 1 g OD Stat Tab Doxcycline 100 mg BD for 21 days

Requirements to Manage Sexually Transmitted Infections (STIs)

- Accurate diagnosis
- Treatment at first encounter
- Rapid cure with effective drugs
- Condom promotion
- Partner notification
- Education/counseling

Essential Steps in STI Management

- Contact tracing
- Compliance
- Confidentiality
- Condom use
- Counseling

Information, Education and Communication Activities (IEC)-NACP-IV

- Create awareness among general population specifically to youth and women on safe sexual behavior
- Enhance behavioral change in the population
- To generate awareness to opt for care and support services
- Create awareness to wipe away stigma and discrimination among the public.

Adolescence Education Program

This program is mainly conducted with the objectives of building life skills in adolescents to prepare them cope with physical and psychological changes that accompanies while growing up.

- Conducted in secondary and senior secondary schools
- Sixteen hours session planned for 9th and 11th standard students.
- This program is offered in 23 states of India.

Red Ribbon Club Activities

- To encourage peer to peer message on HIV prevention
- To provide safe space for young people to clarify their doubts on HIV/AIDS
- Promotion of blood donation among youth
- Conduction of blood donation.

NATIONAL PROGRAM FOR CONTROL OF BLINDNESS (NPCB)

India is the first country to initiate a program for controlling blindness. India started "Trachoma control program" in 30th March 1963. Later this program was subsumed in to NPCB. National program for visual impairment and blindness was started with 100% assistance from the central government. Later it was named as National program for control of blindness (NPCB). The organizational structure of NPCB is shown in Flowchart 3.

Objectives for NPCB Under 12th Five-Year Plan

- To reduce the backlog of avoidable blindness through identification and treatment of curable blind.
- "Eye Health for All" through comprehensive universal eye care services.
- Strengthening and upgradation of Regional Institutes of Ophthalmology (RIOs) and also the other partners like medical colleges, district hospitals, etc.

Flowchart 3: Organizational structure of NPBC

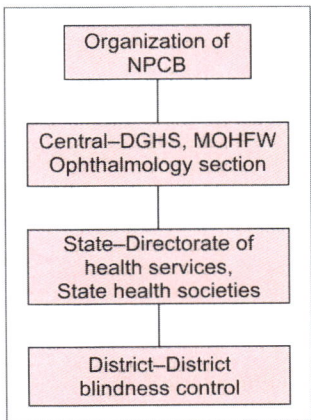

Abbreviations: DGHS, director general of health services; MoHFW, ministry of health and family welfare; NPCB national programs for control of blindness

- Strengthening of existing infrastructure and developing additional human resources.
- To enhance community awareness on eye care and lay stress on preventive measures.
- Increase and expand research for prevention of blindness and visual impairment.
- To secure participation of voluntary organizations/ private practitioners in delivering eye-care.

Strategies

- Continued emphasis on free cataract surgeries through health care delivery systems and NGOs.
- Emphasis on comprehensive eye care by showing attention on diabetic retinopathy, glaucoma, corneal transplantation, vitreoretinal surgeries, childhood blindness, etc. eliminate avoidable blindness.
- To reduce backlog of blind persons through active screening of population above 50 years of age through camps.
- Screening of school children for identification and treatment of refractory errors and provision of free glasses.
- Coverage of underserved areas for eye care through public-private partnership.
- Capacity building of health personnel
- IEC activities for creating awareness in the community.
- Strengthening regional institute of ophthalmology (RIOs) and medical colleges of states and district hospitals through provision of latest equipment and training of the staff.
- Continuing emphasis on primary eye care by establishing vision centers in PHCs.
- Multipurpose district mobile ophthalmic units for better coverage.
- Participation of community and panchayatraj institutions in organizing services in rural areas.

- Involvement of public-private partnership.
- Central ophthalmology section DGHS, MOHFW.
- State—state ophthalmic cell, Directorate of health services, State health societies
- District—district blindness control societies.

Referral System and Service Delivery

Referral System

Tertiary Level

- Apex, regional institutes
- Medical colleges.

Secondary Level

- District hospital and NGO eye
- Hospital

Primary Level

- Sub-district level hospitals/CHC
- Mobile ophthalmic units
- Upgraded PHCs
- Link workers
- Panchayat

Services

School Eye Screening Program

- Around 6–7% of school-children have problem with their eye sight
- Teachers screen the children for eye problems and suspected children with refractive errors are referred to ophthalmic assistants.
- Following corrective spectacles prescribed or provided free of cost to children below poverty line.

Collection and Utilization of Donated Eyes

- Hospitals motivate the relatives of the patients like terminally ill, accident victims and one with grave diseases.
- Eye donation fortnight is organized between 25th August to 8th Sep every year to promote eye donation/eye banking.
- Encouraging the involvement of voluntary organizations like Rotary clubs to conduct eye camps as per the guidelines.
- Community health education on eye donation.

Vision 2020: The Right to Sight

- This is global initiative to avoid preventable blindness by the year 2020. India has committed itself with the following plan of action.

o The targetted diseases are: Cataract, refractive errors, childhood blindness, corneal blindness, glaucoma and diabetic retinopathy.

o Proposed four tier structure to achieve the target includes (1) centers of excellence-20, (2) Training centers-200, (3) service centers-2000 and (4) Vision centers 20000.

Universal Health—Global Action Plan (2014–2019)

o To reduce the prevalence of avoidable visual impairment by 25% by the year 2019 taking baseline from 2010

o The number of eye care personnel to number of cataract surgeries.

IODINE-DEFICIENCY DISORDER PROGRAM (IDD)

Iodine-deficiency disorder is a major public health problem. A large segment of population in all continents of our planet are affected by this disorder. As per the sources reviewed, globally, there are more than 1.5 billion people are at risk of IDD. The surveys conducted by ICMR and medical institutes have clearly demonstrated that not even a single state/union territory is free of IDD in India.

Considering the magnitude of the IDD, India launched a 100% centrally assisted National Goiter Control Program (NGCP) in 1962. In August 1992, National Goiter Control Program (NGCP) was renamed as the National Iodine Deficiency Disorder Control Program (NIDDCP) with a view to cover a wide spectrum of iodine deficiency disorders like mental and physical retardation, deaf-mutism, cretinism, stillbirths, abortion etc.

The objectives of the program are:

o Survey to assess the magnitude of the iodine deficiency disorder

o Supply of iodized salt in place of common salt

o Resurvey after every 5 year to assess the extent of iodine deficiency disorder and the impact of iodized salt

o Laboratory monitoring of isolated salt and urinary iodine excretion.

o Health education and publicity.

At the central level adviser, Directorate general of health services, manages IDD control program. Independent nutrition and IDD cell functions under the deputy assistant director general (IDD) supported by a research officer (IDD) and a team. States have their own IDD cell.

Activities

o Formulated policy statements established the consumption of iodized salt is the best and simplest way to prevent and control IDD.

o In 1984, as per the recommendations from central council of health, India took a policy decision to iodize the edible salt in the country by 1992 in a phased manner. The program initiated in 1986.

o It was notified that the sale of noniodized salt was banned for direct human consumption in India with effect from 17th May, 2006 under the Prevention of Food Adulteration Act 1954.

IDDCP in 12th Five-Year Plan (2012–2017) — Goals

Universal use of iodine fortified salt.

o To bring down prevalence of IDD below 5% in the entire country by 2017 AD.

o To ensure 100% consumption of adequately iodized salt (15 PPM) at the household level.

Strategies

o IDD survey

o Establishment of IDD control cells

o Establishment of IDD monitoring labs.

o Training program

o Production and distribution of iodized salt

o Health education and publicity

o Community level iodized salt testing

o Incentive to ASHA for community level awareness of iodized salt

o Strengthening of central IDD control cell.

NATIONAL WATER SUPPLY AND SANITATION PROGRAM

o This program was launched in the year 1954. The basic aim was to provide safe drinking water supply and drainage facilities to entire rural and urban population of India. Accelerated rural water supply program initiated in 1972 as a supplement to national water supply and sanitation program. During 5th five-year plan period, the accelerated rural water supply program included in to the minimum needs program of the State Plan. Following the central government extended its assistance to states identifying the "Problem-villages."

o Criteria for selecting "problem village" where no source of safe water available in a distance of 1.6 km, or at the depth of 15 m or has the source of extreme salinity, iron, fluorides and other toxic elements or where water is exposed to the risk of cholera.

Swajaldhara

Swajaldhara was launched on 25th December 2002. It was community led participatory program with certain guidelines to be adhered by the states.

Fundamental reform principles, to State Governments:

- Empowerment of villagers with full participation in the project of drinking water scheme
- Full ownership of drinking water assets with appropriate levels of panchayats
- Involve panchayats/communities to have the powers to plan, implement, operate, maintain and manage all water supply and sanitation schemes
- It is an integrated service delivery mechanism
- Conservation measures through rainwater harvesting and groundwater recharge systems for sustained drinking water supply
- Changing the role of government from direct service delivery to that of planning, policy formulation, monitoring and evaluation, and partial financial support
- Swajaldhara was revised in 2009 and renamed as National Rural Drinking Water Program.

Bharat Nirman

- India launched this program in 2005 to build rural infrastructure. This program was mainly concentrated on water quality.
- It had was implemented in two phases
  - **2005–06** to **2008–09**: Bharat Nirman-Phase-I
  - **2009–10** to **2011–12**: Bharat Nirman-Phase-II

New Initiatives in 12th Five-year Plan

- The rural domestic water supply should cover all rural households with safe piped drinking water supply at 70 lpcd.
- At least 50% of the rural population should have the access to water within their household premises or within 100 m radius.
- At least 30% having individual household connections against 13% of today.
- For villages with lower household coverage of toilets a public hand pump should be provided within 100 m of every household.
- Construction of toilets should be completed within 3–6 months.

Rural Sanitation Program

Swachh Bharat Mission (SBM): Prime Minister Narendra Modi launched "Cleanliness drive" in the country on 2nd October 2014. This program envisages to cover the entire community for saturated outcomes with a view to create Nirmal Gram Panchayats.

Nirmal Bharat Abhiyan

Main Objectives

"Nirmal Bharat Abhiyan" (NBA): The objective is to accelerate the sanitation coverage in the rural areas so as to comprehensively cover the rural community through renewed strategies and saturation approach.

- Bring about an improvement in the general quality of life in the rural areas.
- Accelerate sanitation coverage in rural areas to achieve the vision of Nirmal Bharat by 2022.
- Sustainable sanitation facilities through awareness creation and health education.
- To promote hygiene in anganwadi centers and schools not covered under sarva shiksha abhiyan (SSA) in the rural areas with proper sanitation facilities.
- Develop community managed environmental sanitation systems focusing on solid and liquid waste management for overall cleanliness in the rural areas.

Principles

Provision of individual household latrine (IHHL) of both below poverty line (BPL) and identified above poverty line (APL) households within a gram panchayat.

MINIMUM NEED PROGRAM

Minimum need program was introduced in 1st year of 5th Five year plan period (1974–78). This program focuses on social and economic development of the community especially the underprivileged and underserved population.

Objective

To raise the standards of living by providing minimum needs.

Components of "Minimum need program" to raise the standard of living:

- Rural health
- Rural water supply
- Rural electrification
- Elementary education
- Adult education
- Nutrition
- Environmental improvement of urban slums
- Houses of landless laborers.

Principles Observed in Providing Services

○ Priority is given to underserved to improve the existing disparities.

○ Facilities are provided as a package through intersectoral coordination.

○ *To improve rural health:* Objectives to be achieved during the 8th five year plan period were: 1 PHC for every 30,000 population in plain areas and 1 PHC for 20,000 population in hilly and tribal areas; 1 subcenter for 5,000 population in plain areas and 1 subcenter for 3000 population in hilly and tribal areas. One community health center in each block covering 1 lakh population. These all were to be achieved by 2000 AD. The State sector of minimum needs program was responsible for the construction of buildings for all these targets.

○ *To improve nutrition:*

  ❑ To extend nutrition support to 11 million eligible persons

  ❑ To expand special nutrition program to all the ICDS centers

  ❑ To consolidate the mid-day meal program and link it to health, potable water and sanitation

20-POINT PROGRAM

After becoming independent nation, India developed five year plans, annual plans and many health-related programs to improve the health status and economic growth of the country. In addition, in 1975, India initiated a special activity called 20-point program. This program was described as an agenda for national action to promote social justice and economic growth. In 1986 the program was restructured.

Objectives

India listed the objectives as "eradication of poverty, raising productivity, reducing inequalities, removing social and economic disparity and improving the quality of life."

This program was restructured on 20 August 1986. Out of 20 points there are close to 8 points directly or indirectly related to health. They are:

○ Point 1 : Attack of rural poverty

○ Point 7 : Clean drinking water

○ Point 8 : Health for all

○ Point 9 : Two children norm

○ Point 10 : Expansion of education

○ Point 14 : Housing for the people

○ Point 15 : Improvement of slum

○ Point 17: Protection of the environment

This restructured program makes the charter for socioeconomic development of the country. This provides the real plan for the poor.

POLIO ERADICATION: PULSE POLIO PROGRAM

Polio has been eradicated from most of the world using several key strategies.

Important Events in Pulse Polio Immunization

○ 1978—Vaccination against polio was initiated under expanded program on immunization (EPI)

○ 1984—Around 40% of all infants received 3 doses of oral polio vaccine (OPV)

○ 1985—Universal immunization program (UIP) was launched under UNICEF

○ 1995—The number of reported cases of polio declined from 28,757 during 1987 to 3,265 in 1995. 1995–1996 Pulse polio immunization (PPI) program was launched to cover all children below the age of 3 years

○ 1996–97—To speedup the pace of polio eradication, the target age group was increased to all children under the age of 5 years

○ 1997—India in collaboration with World Health Organization initiated National Polio Surveillance Project.

Strategies for Polio Eradication in India

○ Monitor the OPV coverage at district level and below

○ Enhanced surveillance to identify all cases of acute flaccid palsy (AFP) that occurs due to polio and nonpolio etiology

○ Speeding the process of investigation that include collection of stool samples for virus isolation

○ Follow all cases of AFP at 60 days to check for residual analysis

○ Control of epidemic through various measures.

In 1988 world health assembly set a goal for eradication of polio and recommended to the member nations. This eradication goal referred to (1): No cases of clinical poliomyelitis associated with wild poliovirus, and no wild poliovirus found worldwide despite intensive efforts to do so.

Attaining high routine immunization: By immunizing every child aged <1 year with at least 3 doses of OPV.

Pulse Polio Immunization Days

○ Plan and implement pulse polio immunization (PPI) days every year as per the national guidelines until poliomyelitis is eradicated.

○ Pulse polio immunization (PPI) program by providing additional OPV doses to every child aged <5 years at intervals of 4–6 weeks.

○ PPI program is intensified through performing extra immunization rounds, house-to-house "search and vaccinate" in addition to immunization at a fixed clinic or camp.

Line Listing of Cases

To avoid duplication in reporting this line listing of cases started in the year 1989. All cases of AFP must be reported immediately to the medical officer with the particulars like name, age, address, sex, vaccination status, date of onset of paralysis and date of reporting, clinical diagnosis and name of the doctor and his address.

Mopping Up

This is being implemented in India. It is the last stage in eradication steps. It involves door-to-door immunization in high-risk districts.

PPI Implementation in India

On 9th December 1995 and 20th January 1996 Government of India performed its first round of PPI that included two immunization days at 6 weeks internal. This first round concentrated on all children below the age of 3 years irrespective of their immunization status. As per the WHO's guidelines, India decided to cover all children below 5 years in subsequent pulse polio rounds.

The term, "Pulse" is used to describe the sudden, simultaneous, mass administration of OPV on a single day to all children below 5 years of age regardless of previous immunization.

The PPI in India planned as two rounds about 4–6 weeks apart during low transmission season of polio (November to February).

Guidelines

○ PPI are only extra doses, which supplement but do not replace the regular doses in the immunization schedule.

○ There is no minimum interval between PPI and scheduled OPV doses.

An important improvement in PPI during 1998 has been the use of vaccine vial monitor.

Start point: Inner square is lighter than outer ring. USE the vaccine, if expiry date not reached.

Inner square is darkening, but still lighter than outer ring. Use the vaccine, if expiry date not reached.

Discard point: Inner square matches the color of outer ring. Do not use the vaccine.

Beyond the discard point: Inner square is darker than outer ring. DO NOT use the vaccine.

On 27th March 2014 India was declared as non-endemic country for polio

Steps Taken by Indian Government to Achieve Polio Eradication

○ Formulation of rapid response team (RRT) to respond to any polio outbreak

○ Development of emergency preparedness and response plan (EPRP) by all states

○ In UP and Bihar every newborn is identified and tracked for all 8 rounds.

○ All the possible measures utilized to reach every child. Like children are immunized in railway station, bus stand, market places, temples, major road crossings, etc.

○ High level vigilance through surveillance.

○ Higher care (Safe water, sanitation, etc.) to 107 high-risk blocks for polio

○ Enhanced community participation in PPI.

Surveillance

Acute Flaccid Paralysis Surveillance

○ Nationwide AFP surveillance is considered the gold standard for detection of cases of poliomyelitis. This involves four steps of surveillance:

○ Identifying and reporting children with acute flaccid paralysis (AFP)

○ Sending stool samples for analysis

○ Isolating and finding out the poliovirus in the laboratory

○ Mapping the virus to find out the place of origin of the virus strain.

AFP Reporting Procedure

○ *Immediate reporting of AFP cases below 15 years of age and paralytic illness in suspected age for polio attack and should be investigated within 48 hours*

○ *Collect two stool specimens 24–48 hours apart and within 14 days of the onset of paralysis.*

Environmental Surveillance

○ Testing sewage and other environmental samples for the presence of poliovirus are the vital measures of environmental surveillance. Generally, environmental surveillance most often helps in identifying poliovirus infections in the absence of cases of paralysis.

- Systematic environmental sampling (e.g. in Egypt and Mumbai, India) provides important supplementary surveillance data.

- Ad-hoc environmental surveillance (especially in polio free regions) provides insights into the international spread of poliovirus.

NATIONAL PROGRAM FOR PREVENTION AND CONTROL OF CANCER, DIABETES, CARDIOVASCULAR DISEASE AND STROKE (NPCDCS)

It is evident from literature that by 2020, cardiovascular disease will be the largest cause for disability and death in comparing to all deaths in India. Around 70% of the world's cancer deaths occur in Africa, Asia and Central and South America. The five major behavioral and dietary risks include increased levels of body mass index, low intake of fruit and vegetables, lack of physical activity, tobacco use and alcohol use. During the year 2005, noncommunicable diseases (NCD) accounted for 53% of all the deaths in the age group 30–59 years in India. Of these, 29% were due to cardiovascular diseases. There are an estimated 25 lakh cancer cases in India. The number of people with diabetes in India is currently around 40.9 million and is expected to rise to 69.9 million by 2025, unless urgent preventive steps are taken. (Diabetes Atlas 2006, International Diabetes Federation). The noncommunicable diseases are taking giant tide in rise. Based on these facts India started National Program on prevention and control of diabetes, cardiovascular diseases and stroke. Later on it was integrated with cancer control program and renamed as "National Program for Prevention and Control of Cancer, Diabetes, Cardiovascular Disease and Stroke (NPCDCS)."

Diabetes, Cardiovascular Disease and Stroke (DCS) Prevention and Control Components Under NPCDCS

The NPCDCS focuses promotion of health and prevention of diseases, strengthening the infrastructure, early diagnosis and management. This will be connected with the primary health care system through NCD cells at various levels to gear up the functioning abilities.

Objectives

- Prevent and control common NCDs through behavior and lifestyle changes

- Provide early diagnosis and management of common NCDs

- Build capacity at various levels of health care for prevention, diagnosis and treatment of common NCDs

- Train human resource within the public health setup viz. doctors, paramedics and nursing staff to cope with the increasing burden of NCDs and

- Establish and develop capacity for palliative and rehabilitative care.

Strategies

The following strategies used to achieve the above objectives:

- Prevention through behavioral modifications by adopting healthy lifestyle—Advise on physical activity, obesity reduction, consuming healthy food items, avoidance of tobacco, alcohol, etc.

- Early diagnosis and treatment

- Strengthening and training of human resource

- Surveillance, monitoring and evaluation

  The above strategies will be implemented in 20,000 sub-centers and 700 community health centers (CHCs) in 100 Districts across 21 States/UTs.

Activities at Subcenter

- Plan health promotional activities—Organizing camps on these disease and performing individual, group and mass education using various audiovisual aids

- Perform opportunistic screening among people above the age of 30 years by assessing the blood pressure measurements and blood glucose levels by strip method

- Referring suspected cases to higher level health care facilities (Community health centers).

Activities at CHC

- Performing investigations like blood sugar, lipid profile, ultrasound, X-ray and ECG

- Management and prevention of complications in CVD, diabetes and stroke

- Referring complicated cases to district hospitals

- Home visit to bedridden patients by one of the staff nurses to assess the care provided by health workers.

Activities at District Hospital

- Screening people above the age of 30 years who are at risk of developing the diseases like diabetes, hypertension, cardiovascular diseases at clinics

- Detailed investigations for those who at risk

- Regular management of patients suffering from cancer, diabetes, hypertension and cardiovascular diseases

○ Home-based palliative care for chronic patients

○ Health education and health promotion activities.

Urban Health Scheme for Diabetes and Hypertension

○ Screening the slum population for diabetes and hypertension

○ To create statistical data base for slum areas

○ Promote healthy lifestyle

○ Blood pressure and blood sugar will be assessed for all the people above 30 years

     The NCD cell at the center will be actively involved in monitoring the control activities.

Cancer Prevention and Control Components under NPCDCS

Cancer is a huge problem all over the world and India is not an exception. It is estimated that there are 2–8 million cases of cancer cases at any given point of time. The cancer control program was started for the prevention and early diagnosis and treatment. Cancer control program was started in the year 1975–76. This program was revised twice (1984–85 and 2004). In 2010, this program was integrated with "National Program for Prevention and Control of Cancer, Diabetes, Cardiovascular Disease and Stroke (NPCDCS)."

Regional centers: The existing centers are strengthened to function as effective referral centers

     Oncology wing development scheme: These are established to make the facilities accessible to people ₹3 crores of central assistance is provided.

The objectives of cancer control are:

○ Primary prevention of cancer by health education

○ Secondary prevention—Early detection and diagnosis of common cancers like cancer of the breast, cervix, mouth by self-examination/screening

○ Tertiary prevention—This is by strengthening the institutions to provide comprehensive therapy and palliative care.

Decentralized NGO Scheme

This is primarily established for IEC activities on cancer. Nodal agencies provide assistance to NGOs for health educating the community.

IEC Activities at Central Level

The IEC activities at central level focuses on wider publicity about the anti-tobacco legislation, e.g. cigarette smoking is injurious to health.

Research and Training

The NCCP had developed manuals for capacity building at district level—Manual for health professionals, manual for cytology, manual for palliative care and manual for tobacco cessation.

Cancer Control Services Under NPCDCS

○ Facilities for diagnosis, surgeries, chemotherapy and palliative care made available in 100 district hospitals

   ❑ Each district is provided with financial support of ₹1,66 crore/year for following activities:

      • Chemotherapy drugs for 100 patients/each district hospital

      • Day care chemotherapy in 100 district hospitals

      • Facilities for investigations (e.g. mammography) provided in 100 district hospitals

○ Home-based palliative care for progressive cancer patients at 100 districts

○ *Contractual manpower support-*

   Medical oncologist-1

   Cytopathologist-1

   Cytopathology technician-1

   Nurses for day care-2

○ To strengthen 45 tertiary care centers for providing comprehensive services at a cost of ₹6 crores in 2011–12

Tobacco Control Legislation

The cigarettes and other tobacco products Act (2003), passed in April 2003. Some of the highlights of it are as follows

○ Prohibition of cigarette smoking in public places

○ Prohibition of direct and indirect advertisement of cigarettes and other products

○ Prohibition of sale of cigarette and other products to person below 18 years of age—"Sale of tobacco products to a person under the age of is years is a punishable offence" in Indian language(s) as applicable.

○ Prohibition of sale of such products near the educational institutions; distance of one hundred yards shall be measured radically starting from the outer limit of boundary wall, fence or as the case may be, of the educational institution.

○ Mandatory depiction of statutory warnings (including pictorial warnings) an tobacco packs.

○ Mandatory depiction of tar and nicotine contents along with maximum permissible limits on tobacco pack.

○ Smoking areas may be created in hotels having 30 rooms, restaurants having seating capacity of 30 persons and in airports.

The legislation on prohibition of smoking in public places came into force since 2nd October 2008. It became mandatory to display smoke free signages at all public places. Labeling and packaging rules mandating the depiction of specified health warnings on all tobacco product packs came into force from 31st March May 2009.

National Tobacco control program: The national tobacco program launched in 2007–08 under 11th five- year plan. India being the member of the WHO framework convention on tobacco control (FCTC) committed to implementing all provisions included in the international treaty.

Followings are the objectives of the program

- Public awareness through mass media campaigns for behavior change
- Establishment of tobacco product testing laboratories, to build regulatory capacity, as required under COPTA, 2003
- Mainstreaming the program component as part of health delivery mechanism under the national rural health mission framework
- Mainstreaming the research and training on alternate crops and livelihood in collaboration with other nodal ministries
- Monitoring and evaluation including surveillance, e.g. Global adult tobacco survey (GATS), India.
- Tobacco control cells to implement and monitor anti-tobacco initiatives
- School health program
- Provision of tobacco cessation facilities.

NATIONAL MENTAL HEALTH PROGRAM

National Mental Health Program (NMHP) is in operation in India since 1982. This was initiated primarily to tackle the problem of huge burden of mental disorders in India.

Important Mile Stones of the Program

1996—The district mental health program was added to the program.

2003—The Program was re-strategized and two new schemes were included: (1) modernization of state mental hospitals and (2) Upgradation of psychiatric wings of medical colleges/ general hospitals.

2009—The manpower development scheme (Scheme—A and B) was included as the part of the program.

Objectives

- To ensure the availability and accessibility of minimum mental health care for all in the foreseeable future

- To encourage the application of mental health knowledge in general health care and in social development
- To promote community participation in the mental health service development and enhance human resource in mental health sub-specialties.

Components

District mental health program (DMHP): This program provides basic mental health care services at the community level. Currently, DMHP is functioning in 241 districts and is proposed to expand it to all districts in a phased manner. Mental health services (in and outpatient) are provided in hospitals with 10 inpatient capacity. Each DMHP is given the financial support of ₹83.2 lakhs.

Staffing: DMHP is staffed with staff on contractual basis. It includes psychiatrist, clinical psychologist, psychiatric nurse, psychiatric social worker, community nurse, monitoring and evaluation officer, case registry assistant and ward assistant/ orderly.

Out-Reach Services

- Four satellite clinics conducted at CHCs/PHCs
- The target interventions are life skills education and counseling in schools and colleges, stress management at sites and services on suicide prevention
- Training of health personnel at the district and sub-district levels
- Conduct awareness camps by including faith healers, teachers, village leaders and influential persons
- Encouraging community participation by linking with self-help groups, family and caregiver and NGOs of mental health
- Sensitization of enforcement officials regarding legal provisions
- As of now, 241 districts have been covered under the scheme and it is proposed to expand DMHP to all districts in a phased manner.

PPP Model Activities (financial support @ ₹5 lakhs per NGO): Under this component, the state governments execute mental health-related activities in partnership with nongovernment organizations as per the guidelines of the NRHM.

Day Care Center

The established day care center is provided with the financial support of ₹50,000 per center per month and that equals the yearly support of ₹6 lakhs. This is basically to provide rehabilitation and recovery services to persons with mental illness.

Residential/Long-term Continuing Care Center

❍ Residential/long-term continuing care center is provided with the financial support of ₹75,000 per center per month that equals ₹9 Lakhs/year.

❍ Chronically mentally ill individuals, whose symptoms are stable but unable to return to their families and are currently the residents of the mental hospitals, will be placed in these centers.

Mental Health Care at Community Health Centers

❍ Outpatient and inpatient services to all emergency psychiatry patients.

❍ Counseling services to all.

Staffing

The CHC staffed with one medical officer and clinical psychologist or psychiatric social worker.

At Primary Health Centers

❍ Outpatient services available

❍ Counseling services in accessing social care benefits

❍ Pro-active case findings and mental health promotion activities.

Staffing

Staffed with two community health workers.

Mental Health Services at Medical Colleges/ Teaching Hospitals

❍ These services are provided under the overall supervision of the head of psychiatry department

❍ Each of such facility receives the financial support of ₹15.00 lakhs per year.

Thrust Areas of Mental Health Services Delivery

❍ Strengthening and modernization of mental health hospitals

❍ Upgrading the psychiatric wing of the medical colleges and improving the psychiatric curriculum in medical education

❍ Enhancing the research and training in the field of community mental health.

YAWS ERADICATION PROGRAM

WHO Expert Committee on venereal infections and treponematoses set the criteria for the eradication of yaws in 1960. Yaws is a disfiguring and disabling non venereal skin infection caused by Treponema pallidum—subspecies pertenue.

Yaws Eradication Program (YEP) was a centrally sponsored scheme first started in 1996–97 in Koraput district of Orissa. During the 9th plan period it was expanded to cover the 10 endemic states—Andhra Pradesh, Orissa, Maharashtra, Madhya Pradesh, Chhattisgarh, Tamil Nadu, Uttar Pradesh, Jharkhand, Assam and Gujarat.

Program Strategies

❍ Manpower development

❍ Detection of cases by active search

❍ Treatment of cases and contacts concurrently

❍ Health education using multisectoral approach

❍ Injection of benzathine penicillin given in single dose.

The number of reported cases in 10 endemic states came down to 46 during 2003 from 3,500 cases in 1996.

No new case of Yaws has been reported after November 2003. On 19th September 2006, India formally declared the elimination of yaws from the country.

> *World health organization targeted to eradicate "Yaws" by 2020.*
>
> Five groups from International Verification Team (IVT) of World Health Organization (WHO) visited India's five yaws endemic states during 4–17 October, 2015. Following this visit, the IVT recommended WHO issuing a "Certificate of Eradication of Yaws" for India.

HEALTH SCHEMES

Employee state insurance scheme and central government health scheme cover two large groups of wage earners in the country.

Employees State Insurance Scheme (ESI Act, 1948)

❍ The Employees State Insurance Scheme Act was passed in the year 1948 and amended in 1975, 1984, 1989 and 2010.

❍ It is a significant social security and health insurance for employees of India.

❍ It provides certain cash and medical benefits to industrial employees in case of sickness, maternity and employment injury.

Scope of ESI Act

The ESI Act of 1948 covers the whole India. The ESI 1948 covered all power using factories other than seasonal factories where more than 10 persons were employed.

The 1975 amendment of ESI Act extended to cover the following too:

- Small factories employing more than 10 persons, irrespective of power usage
- Shops
- Hotels and restaurants
- Cinemas and theaters
- Road-Motor transport establishments
- Newspaper establishments
- Private medical and educational institutions employing 20 or more in some states.

The ESI Act amended (01.05.2010) to cover all employees like manual, clerical, supervisory and technical whose monthly income is up to ₹15,000.

Administration of ESI Corporation (Flowchart 4)

Administration structure of ESI is shown in Flowchart 4 ESI functions under the Chair of Union Minister for Labor. The Secretary to Government of India is the Vice Chairman of ESI. The ESI corporation is represented by members from central, state, employers' and employees' organizations, medical profession and parliament. The standing committee with its members acts as the executive body. The chief executive officer is the Director General who is assisted by various commissioners. There is a medical benefit council functioning under the CEO, assisted by medical commissioner.

Flowchart 4: Organizational structure of ESI

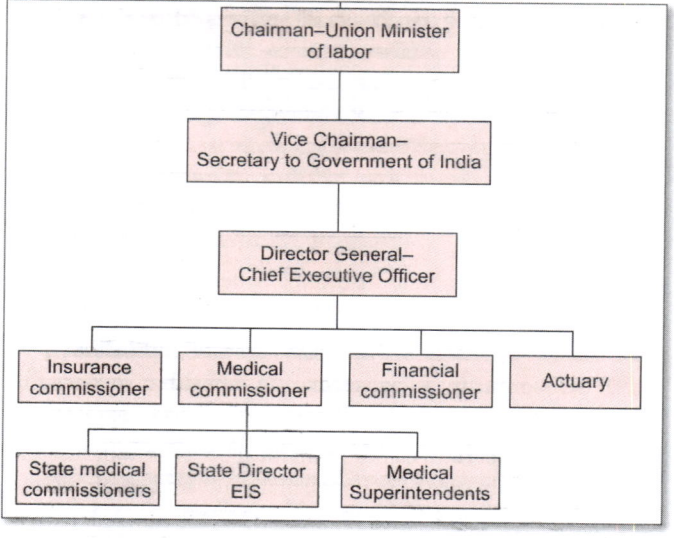

Beneficiaries under ESI Scheme

Corporation has setup a wide spread network of service outlets.

Covers 185 lakh family units of 165 lakh employees.

Medical facilities through:

- 1,427 ESI dispensaries
- 2,100 panel clinics
- 307 diagnostic centers
- 151 ESI hospitals
- 43 hospital annexes
- 27,000 beds.

Finance

ESI scheme is run with the contributions from employers, employees and grants from central and state governments.

Contributions from Sources

- The employer contributes 4.75% of total wage bill
- The employee contributes 1.75% of wages
- *Note:* Employees with daily wages of <₹70/- exempted from payment of contribution
- State government's share on medical expenditure is 1/8th of total cost of medical care
- ESI corporation share on medical expenditure is 7/8th of total cost of medical care.

Benefits to Employees

The insured employees have various benefits under ESI as per the regulations (Fig. 4).

Medical Benefits

Full medical care including hospitalization, free of cost, to the insured persons in case of sickness, employment injury and maternity.

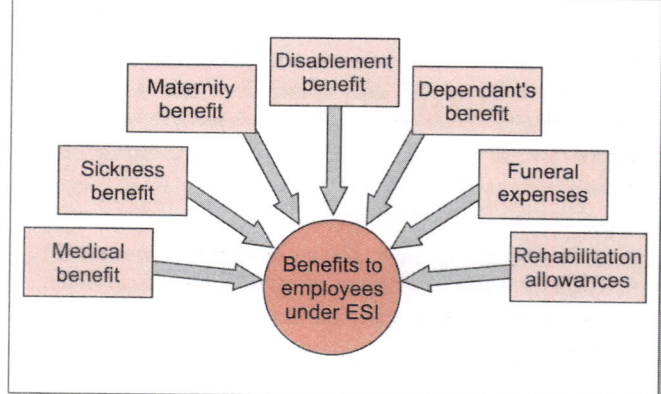

Figure 4: Benefits to employees under ESI

Table 15: Patterns of delivery of medical services

Direct pattern	Indirect Pattern
In areas having 1,000 or above service dispensaries established with medical and paramedical personnel On an average a doctor attends 80 outpatients/day and makes one home visit	A panel of medical practitioners recognized to provide services
In areas with less than 750 employees part time dispensaries are established If employees scattered in a long distance mobile dispensaries established	Registered medical practitioners under this system designated as, "Insurance Medical practitioners" This system is known as "Panel system"

- Outpatient care
- Supply of drugs or dressings
- Specialist services in all branches of medicine
- Pathological and radiological investigations
- Domiciliary services
- Antenatal, natal and postnatal services
- Immunization services
- Family planning services
- Emergency services
- Ambulance services
- Health education
- Inpatient treatment.

Pattern of Delivery of Medical Services

Medical services provided in two ways (Table 15):

1. Direct delivery through ESI facilities—ESI hospitals, ESI dispensaries
2. Indirect delivery through a panel of medical practitioners appointed as "Insurance Medical Practitioners."

Other Medical Facilities

- Dentures, spectacles and hearing aids provided to patients in whom that occurred because of employment injury
- Artificial limbs to those who lost their limb because of employment injury
- Provision of special appliances when prescribed like hernia belts, walking calipers, surgical boots, spinal braces and jackets.

Sickness Benefits

- Periodical cash payment is made to an insured person during his sickness, if his sickness is duly certified by an **Insurance Medical Officer** or **Insurance Medical Practitioner**.
- Payable up to a maximum period of **91 days in any continuous period of 365 days**.

Extended Sickness Benefit

- In addition to above (91 days sickness benefit) insured person suffering with long-term illnesses is eligible to receive extended sickness benefit for a maximum period of **2 years**.
- There are **34 diseases listed** that are eligible for extended sickness benefit (TB, leprosy, AIDS, coronary heart disease, Parkinson's disease, etc.)
- The insured person is protected from dismissal or discharge from service by the employer during the period of sickness.

Maternity Benefits

Payable by cash to an insured women for confinement, miscarriage and sickness arising out of confinement.

Duration of Benefit

- For confinement: 12 weeks
- For miscarriage: 6 weeks
- For sickness arising out of confinement: 30 days
- The benefit is allowed at full wages
- The rate of expenses given per confinement: ₹5000/-

Disablement Benefit

- Cash payment and free medical treatment, in the event of temporary or permanent disablement as a result of employment injury as well occupational diseases.
- 90% of wages paid as long as the temporary disablement lasts.
- In case of total permanent disablement life pension is given on the basis of loss of earning capacity determined by the medical board.
- In case partial permanent disablement a portion of it is given as life pension.

Dependent's Benefit

- The dependents of an insured person are eligible for periodic payments if the insured person die as a result of employment injury.
- Pension at the rate of 90% of wages is payable, dependents share this in a fixed ratio, on a monthly basis.
- An eligible son or daughter is entitled to dependent's benefit up to the age of 18 year; the benefit is withdrawn if the daughter marries earlier.

Funeral Expenses

Cash payment payable on the death of an insured person toward the expenses on his funeral, the amount not exceeding ₹5000 (This is w.e.f. 01-4-2011)

Rehabilitation

On monthly payment ₹10/-, the insured person and his family members continue to get medical treatment after permanent disablement or retirement.

Benefits to Employers

○ Exemption from the applicability of Workmen's Compensation Act, 1923

○ Exemption from Maternity Benefit Act, 1961

○ Exemption from payment of medical allowance to employees and their dependents or arranging for their medical care.

○ Rebate under the Income Tax Act on contribution deposited in the ESI account.

○ Healthy work-force.

Rajiv Gandhi Shramik Kalyan Yojna

○ This scheme was launched on 1st April, 2005 for employees under ESI.

○ This scheme provides **unemployment allowance** for the employees who are unemployed involuntarily due to retrenchment/closure of factory, etc. after fulfilling certain eligibility conditions.

○ The employee should have been contributed a minimum of 5 years of service under the establishment to utilize this facility. In that case, he or she is eligible to claim unemployment allowance for the period of 6 months/ entire service.

○ Under this scheme, he is also eligible for medical care for himself and his dependents.

Central Government Health Scheme in India

This scheme was formerly known as contributory health service scheme. This scheme was first introduced at New Delhi in the year 1954 for providing services to central government employees. This provides comprehensive health services to the CGHS beneficiaries. At start this scheme has had 16 allopathic dispensaries covering 2.3 lakh beneficiaries. Now it covers 42.76 lakhs beneficiaries and provides care through various systems of medicine in 320 dispensaries/hospitals.

Beneficiaries of Central Government Health Scheme

○ All Central Government servants paid from Civil Estimates (other than those employed in railway services and those employed under delhi administration except members of delhi police force).

○ Pensioners drawing pension from civil estimates and their family members

○ Members and ex members of Parliament

○ Judges of Supreme Court of India

○ Ex-Governors and Ex-Vice Presidents

○ Former Prime Ministers, Former Judges Supreme Court and High Courts and freedom fighters

○ It provides services through following allopathic, homeopathic, Indian system of medicines (Ayurveda, Unani, Yoga, and Sidha System)

○ Employees and pensioners of autonomous bodies covered under CGHS.

Services Under the Scheme

○ Outpatient services

○ Domiciliary care

○ Family welfare and MCH services

○ Supply of necessary drugs

○ Specialist consultation facilities at dispensary, polyclinic and hospital

○ Diagnostic facilities like X-ray, ECG and laboratory examinations.

○ Hospitalization at recognized government and private hospitals

○ Emergency treatment

○ Supply of optical dental aids at reasonable cost

○ Health education.

Other Insurance Schemes
Rashtriya Swasthya Bima Yojana (RSBY)

○ Rashtriya Swasthya Bima Yojana was launched on 1st April 2008 by Ministry of Labor, Government of India.

○ The primary aim was to provide health insurance coverage to people **Below Poverty Line (BPL).**

Objective

To meet the financial difficulties that may come from hospitalization.

Beneficiaries

○ This insurance covers five members of the family. This includes head of the family, spouse and up to three dependents.

○ This is unique and beneficial to poor families that migrate.

○ Beneficiary has to pay only ₹30 toward registration.

Salient Features of RSBY

- The beneficiary can choose government or private hospitals according to his choice
- The insurer is paid premium of each household enrolled in RSBY
- Participating hospitals have incentives
- Beneficiary can use his smart card in any of the empanelled hospitals
- RSBY uses a cashless and paperless transaction
- Each beneficiary is issued biometric enabled smart card
- All the health facilities under RSBY are IT enabled so the transactions are very easy
- Government charges a maximum of ₹750 per family to provide care/year

Aam Aadmi Bima Yojana (AABY)

This scheme is a social security scheme for rural landless. It was launched on 2nd October 2007.

Beneficiaries

- The head of the family or one earning member in the family aging between 18 and 59 years covered under this scheme
- The premium of ₹200/person/year is shared equally by state and central governments.

Benefits

- Scholarship to children
- On natural death of the person ₹30,000/- is given
- On death due to accident/permanent disability due to accident ₹75,000/- is given
- On partial permanent disability due to accident ₹37500/- is given.

National Programme for Health Care of the Elderly
Introduction

The National Programme for Health Care of the Elderly (NPHCE) is an articulation of the International and National commitments of the Government as envisaged under the UN Convention on the Rights of Persons with Disabilities (UNCRPD), National Policy on Older Persons (NPOP) adopted by the Government of India in 1999 and Section 20 of "The Maintenance and Welfare of Parents and Senior Citizens Act, 2007" dealing with provisions for medical care of senior citizen.

The programme has envisaged to provide promotional, preventive, curative and rehabilitative services in an integrated manner for the elderly in various Government health facilities. The range of services will include health promotion, preventive services, diagnosis and management of geriatric medical problems (out-and in-patient), day care services, rehabilitative services and home based care as needed. Districts will be linked to regional geriatric centres for providing tertiary level care.

Objectives

- Main objective of the programme is to provide preventive, curative and rehabilitative services to the elderly persons at various level of health care delivery system of the country.
- Other objectives are, to strengthen referral system, to develop specialized man power and to promote research in the field of diseases related to old age.

Vision

The vision of the NPHCE are:

- To provide accessible, affordable, and high-quality long-term, comprehensive and dedicated care services to an ageing population
- Creating a new "architecture" for ageing
- To build a framework to create an enabling environment for "a society for all ages"
- To promote the concept of active and healthy ageing.

Specific Objectives

- To provide an easy access to promotional, preventive, curative and rehabilitative services through community based primary health care (PHC) approach.
- To identify health problems in the elderly and provide appropriate health interventions in the community with a strong referral backup support.
- To build capacity of the medical and paramedical professionals as well as the care-takers within the family for providing health-care to the senior citizen.
- To provide referral services to the elderly patients through district hospital regional medical institutions.
- Convergence with National Rural Health Mission (NRHM), AYUSH and other line departments like Ministry of Social Justice and Empowerment.

Core Strategies

- Community based PHC approach including domiciliary visits by trained health-care workers.
- Dedicated services at PHC/Community Health Centre (CHC) level including provision of machinery,

equipment, training, additional human resources, information, education and communication (IEC), etc.

○ Dedicated facilities at the district hospital with 10 bedded wards, additional human resources, machinery and equipment, consumables and drugs, training and IEC.

○ Strengthening of 8 Regional Medical Institutes to provide dedicated tertiary level medical facilities for the elderly, introducing PG courses in geriatric medicine, and in-service training of health personnel at all levels.

○ IEC using mass media, folk media and other communication channels to reach out to the target community.

○ Continuous monitoring and independent evaluation of the programme and research in geriatrics and implementation of NPHCE.

Supplementary Strategies

○ Promotion of public private partnerships in geriatric health care.
○ Mainstreaming AYUSH—revitalizing local health traditions and convergence with programs of Ministry of Social Justice and Empowerment in the field of geriatrics.
○ Reorienting medical education to support geriatric issues.

Expected Outcomes

○ Regional geriatric centres (RGC) in eight Regional Medical Institutions by setting up RGCs with a dedicated geriatric out-patient department (OPD) and 30-bedded geriatric ward for management of specific diseases of the elderly, training of health personnel in geriatric health care and conducting research.
○ Postgraduates in geriatric medicine (16) from the 8 regional medical institutions
○ Video conferencing units in the 8 regional medical institutions to be utilized for capacity building and mentoring.
○ District geriatric units with dedicated geriatric OPD and 10-bedded geriatric ward in 80–100 district hospitals.
○ Geriatric clinics/rehabilitation units set up for domiciliary visits in community/primary health centres in the selected districts.
○ Sub-centres provided with equipment for community outreach services.
○ Training of Human Resources in the Public Health-Care System in geriatric care.

Package of Services Under NPHCE (Table 16)

In the program, it is envisaged providing promotional, preventive, curative and rehabilitative services in an integrated manner for the elderly in various Government health facilities. The package of services would depend on the level of health

facility and may vary from facility to facility. The range of services will include health promotion, preventive services, diagnosis and management of geriatric medical problems (out- and in-patient), day care services, rehabilitative services and home based care as needed. Districts will be linked to RGCs for providing tertiary level care. The services under the program would be integrated below district level and will be an integral part of existing PHC delivery system and vertical at district and above as more specialized health care are needed for the elderly.

Table 16: Packages of services to be made available at different levels under NPHCE

Health Facility	Packages of Services
Sub-centre	○ Health education related to healthy ageing ○ Domiciliary visits for attention and care to home bound/bedridden elderly persons and provide training to the family care providers in looking after the disabled elderly persons ○ Arrange for suitable callipers and supportive devices from the PHC to the elderly disabled persons to make them ambulatory ○ Linkage with other support groups and day care centres, etc. operational in the area Institutional framework for the implementation of NPHCE
Primary health centre	○ Weekly geriatric clinic run by a trained Medical Officer ○ Maintain record of the elderly using standard format during their first visit ○ Conducting a routine health assessment of the elderly persons based on simple clinical examination relating to eye, BP, blood sugar, etc. ○ Provision of medicines and proper advice on chronic ailments ○ Public awareness on promotional, preventive and rehabilitative aspects of geriatrics during health and village sanitation day/camps ○ Referral for diseases needing further investigation and treatment, to community health centre or the district hospital as per need
Community health centre	○ First referral unit (FRU) for the elderly from PHCs and below ○ Geriatric clinic for the elderly persons twice a week ○ Rehabilitation unit for physiotherapy and counselling ○ Domiciliary visits by the rehabilitation worker for bed ridden elderly and counselling of the family members on their home-based care ○ Health promotion and prevention ○ Referral of difficult cases to district hospital/higher health care facility

Contd...

Health Facility	Packages of Services
District hospital	o Geriatric clinic for regular dedicated OPD services to the elderly. o Facilities for laboratory investigations for diagnosis and provision of medicines for geriatric medical and health problems o 10 bedded geriatric ward for in-patient care of the elderly o Existing specialities like general medicine; orthopaedics, ophthalmology; ENT services etc. will provide services needed by elderly patients o Provide services for the elderly patients referred by the CHCs/PHCs etc. o Conducting camps for geriatric services in PHCs/CHCs and other sites o Referral services for severe cases to tertiary level hospitals
Regional geriatric centre	o Geriatric clinic (specialized OPD for the elderly) o 30-bedded geriatric ward for in-patient care and dedicated beds for the elderly patients in the various specialties viz. surgery, orthopedics, psychiatry, urology, ophthalmology, neurology, etc. o Laboratory investigation required for elderly with a special sample collection centre in the OPD block o Tertiary health care to the cases referred from medical colleges, district hospitals and below

SUSTAINABLE DEVELOPMENTAL GOALS

The **Sustainable Development Goals** (SDGs), officially known as **Transforming our world: the 2030 Agenda for Sustainable Development**, is a set of 17 "Global Goals" with 169 targets among them. At the Sustainable Development Summit on 25 September 2015, UN Member States adopted the 2030 Agenda for Sustainable Development, which includes a set of 17 Sustainable Development Goals (SDGs) to end poverty, fight inequality and injustice, and tackle climate change by 2030.

The SDGs are built upon the Millennium Development Goals (MDGs). The MDGs, adopted in 2000, aimed at an array of issues that included slashing poverty, hunger, disease, gender inequality, and access to water and sanitation. Enormous progress has been made on the MDGs, showing the value of a unifying agenda underpinned by goals and targets.

The new SDGs, and the broader sustainability agenda, go much further than the MDGs, addressing the root causes of poverty and the universal need for development that works for all people.

The 17 SDGs are given in Figure 5.

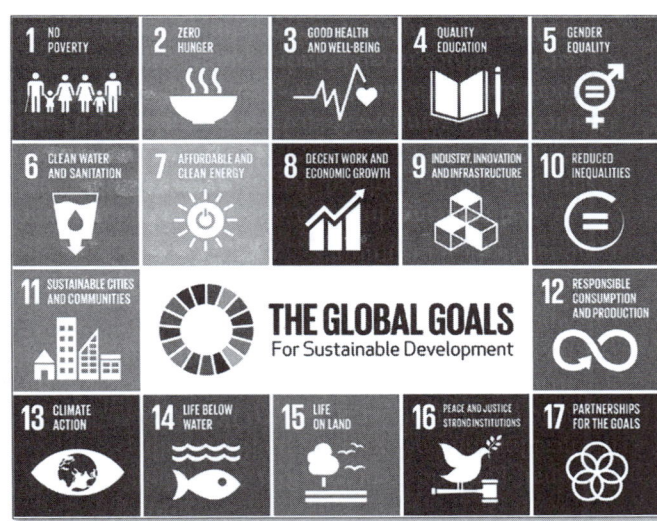

Figure 5: Sustainable development goals

The targets of SDGs pertaining specifically to development of children all over the world are discussed below.

Goal 1: No Poverty

End poverty in all its forms everywhere

o By 2030, eradicate extreme poverty for all people everywhere, currently measured as people living on less than $1.25 a day

o By 2030, reduce at least by half the proportion of men, women and children of all ages living in poverty in all its dimensions according to national definitions

o By 2030, build the resilience of the poor and those in vulnerable situations and reduce their exposure and vulnerability to climate-related extreme events and other economic, social and environmental shocks and disasters

o Create sound policy frameworks at the national, regional and international levels, based on pro-poor and gender-sensitive development strategies, to support accelerated investment in poverty eradication actions

Goal 2 Zero Hunger

End hunger, achieve food security and improved nutrition and promote sustainable agriculture

o By 2030, end hunger and ensure access by all people, in particular the poor and people in vulnerable situations, including infants, to safe, nutritious and sufficient food all year round

o By 2030, end all forms of malnutrition, including achieving, by 2025, the internationally agreed targets on stunting and wasting in children under 5 years of age, and address the nutritional needs of adolescent girls, pregnant and lactating women and older persons

o By 2030, ensure sustainable food production systems and implement resilient agricultural practices that increase productivity and production, that help maintain ecosystems, that strengthen capacity for adaptation to climate change, extreme weather, drought, flooding and other disasters and that progressively improve land and soil quality

o Adopt measures to ensure the proper functioning of food commodity markets and their derivatives and facilitate timely access to market information, including on food reserves, in order to help limit extreme food price volatility

Goal 3 Good Health and Well Being

Ensure healthy lives and promote well-being for all at all ages

o By 2030, reduce the global maternal mortality ratio to less than 70 per 100,000 live births

o By 2030, end preventable deaths of newborns and children under 5 years of age, with all countries aiming to reduce neonatal mortality to at least as low as 12 per 1,000 live births and under-5 mortality to at least as low as 25 per 1,000 live births

o By 2030, end the epidemics of AIDS, tuberculosis, malaria and neglected tropical diseases and combat hepatitis, water-borne diseases and other communicable diseases

o By 2030, reduce by one third premature mortality from non-communicable diseases through prevention and treatment and promote mental health and well-being

o Strengthen the prevention and treatment of substance abuse, including narcotic drug abuse and harmful use of alcohol

o By 2030, ensure universal access to sexual and reproductive health-care services, including for family planning, information and education, and the integration of reproductive health into national strategies and programmes

o Achieve universal health coverage, including financial risk protection, access to quality essential health-care services and access to safe, effective, quality and affordable essential medicines and vaccines for all

o Strengthen the implementation of the World Health Organization Framework Convention on Tobacco Control in all countries, as appropriate

o Support the research and development of vaccines and medicines for the communicable and noncommunicable diseases that primarily affect developing countries, provide access to affordable essential medicines and vaccines, in accordance with the Doha Declaration on the TRIPS Agreement and Public Health, which affirms the right of developing countries to use to the full the provisions in the Agreement on Trade Related Aspects of Intellectual Property Rights regarding flexibilities to protect public health, and, in particular, provide access to medicines for all

o Strengthen the capacity of all countries, in particular developing countries, for early warning, risk reduction and management of national and global health risks

Goal 4 Quality Education

Ensure inclusive and quality education for all and promote lifelong learning

o By 2030, ensure that all girls and boys complete free, equitable and quality primary and secondary education leading to relevant and Goal-4 effective learning outcomes

o By 2030, ensure that all girls and boys have access to quality early childhood development, care and preprimary education so that they are ready for primary education

o By 2030, ensure equal access for all women and men to affordable and quality technical, vocational and tertiary education, including university

o By 2030, substantially increase the number of youth and adults who have relevant skills, including technical and vocational skills, for employment, decent jobs and entrepreneurship

o By 2030, eliminate gender disparities in education and ensure equal access to all levels of education and vocational training for the vulnerable, including persons with disabilities, indigenous peoples and children in vulnerable situations

o By 2030, ensure that all youth and a substantial proportion of adults, both men and women, achieve literacy and numeracy

o By 2030, ensure that all learners acquire the knowledge and skills needed to promote sustainable development, including, among others, through education for sustainable development and sustainable lifestyles, human rights, gender equality, promotion of a culture of peace and non-violence, global citizenship and appreciation of cultural diversity and of culture's contribution to sustainable development

o Build and upgrade education facilities that are child, disability and gender sensitive and provide safe, nonviolent, inclusive and effective learning environments for all

o By 2020, substantially expand globally the number of scholarships available to developing countries, in particular least developed countries, small island developing States and African countries, for enrolment in higher education, including vocational training and information and communications technology, technical, engineering and scientific programmes, in developed countries and other developing countries

○ By 2030, substantially increase the supply of qualified teachers, including through international cooperation for teacher training in developing countries, especially least developed countries and small island developing states

Goal 5 Gender Equality

Achieve gender equality and empower all women and girls

○ End all forms of discrimination against all women and girls everywhere

○ Eliminate all forms of violence against all women and girls in the public and private spheres, including trafficking and sexual and other types of exploitation

○ Eliminate all harmful practices, such as child, early and forced marriage and female genital mutilation

○ Recognize and value unpaid care and domestic work through the provision of public services, infrastructure and social protection policies and the promotion of shared responsibility within the household and the family as nationally appropriate

○ Ensure universal access to sexual and reproductive health and reproductive rights as agreed in accordance with the Program of Action of the International Conference on Population and Development and the Beijing Platform for Action and the outcome documents of their review conferences

○ Adopt and strengthen sound policies and enforceable legislation for the promotion of gender equality and the empowerment of all women and girls at all levels

Goal 8 Decent Work and Economic Growth

Promote inclusive and sustainable economic growth, employment and decent work for all

○ Sustain per capita economic growth in accordance with national circumstances and, in particular, at least 7 per cent gross domestic product growth per annum in the least developed countries

○ Promote development-oriented policies that support productive activities, decent job creation, entrepreneurship, creativity and innovation, and encourage the formalization and growth of micro-, small- and medium-sized enterprises, including through access to financial services

○ By 2030, achieve full and productive employment and decent work for all women and men, including for young people and persons with disabilities, and equal pay for work of equal value

○ By 2020, substantially reduce the proportion of youth not in employment, education or training

○ Take immediate and effective measures to eradicate forced labour, end modern slavery and human trafficking and secure the prohibition and elimination of the worst forms of child labour, including recruitment and use of child soldiers, and by 2025 end child labour in all its forms

○ Protect labour rights and promote safe and secure working environments for all workers, including migrant workers, in particular women migrants, and those in precarious employment

○ By 2020, develop and operationalize a global strategy for youth employment and implement the Global Jobs Pact of the International Labour Organization

Goal 10 Reduced Inequalities

Reduce inequality within and among countries

○ By 2030, progressively achieve and sustain income growth of the bottom 40 per cent of the population at a rate higher than the national average

○ By 2030, empower and promote the social, economic and political inclusion of all, irrespective of age, sex, disability, race, ethnicity, origin, religion or economic or other status

○ Ensure equal opportunity and reduce inequalities of outcome, including by eliminating discriminatory laws, policies and practices and promoting appropriate legislation, policies and action in this regard

○ Adopt policies, especially fiscal, wage and social protection policies, and progressively achieve greater equality

○ Facilitate orderly, safe, regular and responsible migration and mobility of people, including through the implementation of planned and well-managed migration policies

○ Implement the principle of special and differential treatment for developing countries, in particular least developed countries, in accordance with World Trade Organization agreements

○ By 2030, reduce to less than 3 per cent the transaction costs of migrant remittances and eliminate remittance corridors with costs higher than 5 per cent

Goal 16 Peace and Justice Strong Institutions

Promote just, peaceful and inclusive societies

○ Significantly reduce all forms of violence and related death rates everywhere

○ End abuse, exploitation, trafficking and all forms of violence against and torture of children

- Promote the rule of law at the national and international levels and ensure equal access to justice for all
- Ensure responsive, inclusive, participatory and representative decision-making at all levels
- Broaden and strengthen the participation of developing countries in the institutions of global governance
- By 2030, provide legal identity for all, including birth registration

- Ensure public access to information and protect fundamental freedoms, in accordance with national legislation and international agreements
- Strengthen relevant national institutions, including through international cooperation, for building capacity at all levels, in particular in developing countries, to prevent violence and combat terrorism and crime

Summary

National health programs were launched time to time to prevent, control, eliminate or eradicate certain communicable and noncommunicable diseases.

Acute respiratory infection (ARI) control program was initiated as a pilot project in 14 districts in the year 1990.

It was incorporated into CSSM program in the year 1992 later on with RCH phase-I in the year 1997. Now ARI is component of RCH phase-II.

Reproductive and child health program phase-I—This program incorporated family planning, CSSM, prevention and management of reproductive tract infections (RTIs), sexually transmitted diseases (STDs), aquired immuno-deficiency syndrome (AIDS).

Reproductive and child health program phase II—This RCH phase—II was launched on 1 April 2005 with the aim to reduce maternal and child mortality and morbidity while concentrating on rural health care. Revised National Tuberculosis Control Program (RNTCP). Around 38% morbidity and 39% mortality of the world tuberculosis burden is found in South-East Asia Region (SEAR) of world health organization.

National Vector-Borne Disease Control Program (NVBDCP). In India, the Directorate of National Vector-Borne Disease Control Program (NVBDCP) is the central agency for the prevention and control of the six most common VBDs in the country. They are: malaria, dengue, lymphatic filariasis, kala-azar, Japanese encephalitis and chikungunya.

Integrated accelerated action toward reducing mortality of malaria, dengue and JE by half, elimination of Kala-azar by 2010, elimination of lymphatic filariasis by the year 2015.

Malaria: Malaria control program was launched during first five-year plan, in 1953. The increased success rates motivated India to convert the program into eradication program.

Since 1955, National Filarial Control Program in operation (NFCP). In June 1978, NFCP was merged with Urban Malarial scheme. In 2003 it was included in NVBDCP.

National Health Policy 2002 set the goal to eliminate lymphatic filariasis by 2015.

Kala-azar—Prior to introduction of DDT, Kala-azar was highly endemic in India and had disturbed the economic growth of country due to its high morbidity and mortality rates. Kala-azar is a centrally sponsored program, launched in 1990–91.

Last case of guinea worm disease in India was identified in 1996. The International certification team (ICT), presented its report on guinea worm disease status in India to the ICCDE in the meeting held in February 2000 in Geneva. On the basis of ICT report, India was declared as guinea worm disease free country by international commission for certification of dracunculiasis eradication (ICCDE).

National leprosy eradication program (NLEP): In 1955, India launched the **National Leprosy Control Program (NLCP)** with the features of case detection, treatment with Dapsone community education. This was changed to the National Leprosy Eradication Program (NLEP) in 1983, with the introduction of multidrug therapy (MDT).

Accredited Social Health Activists (ASHA) will be involved during 12th plan to bring out suspected cases from their villages for diagnosis at PHC and after confirmation of diagnosis, will follow-up the patients for completion of treatment. The ASHA will be entitled to receive incentive: At confirmation of diagnosis ₹250/- On completion of full course of treatment in time for Pauci Bacillary (PB)- additional ₹400/- Multi Bacillary (MB).

India launched national aids control program in the year 1987. Sexually transmitted disease control is now, linked with AIDS control program activities. Department of NACO coordinates RTI and STD at all levels of the health care: Free standardized STI/RTI services provided through 1160 clinics situated at government health care facilities, at district hospital level, and above. These clinics named as "Suraksha Clinics" provide sexual and reproductive health services.

India started **"Trachoma control program"** in 30th March 1963. Later it was named as National program for control of blindness (NPCB).

Iodine deficiency disorder program (IDD)—Iodine deficiency disorder is a major public health problem. A large segment of population in all continents of our planet are affected by this disorder. Considering the magnitude of the IDD, India launched a 100% centrally assisted national goiter control program (NGCP) in 1962. In August 1992, NGCP was renamed as the national iodine deficiency disorder control program (NIDDCP) with a view to cover a wide spectrum.

World Health Organization (WHO) defined **"expanded"** as adding more disease controlling agents to vaccination schedules extending its coverage to the entire country and spreading services to reach less privileged sectors of the society. In **1978**, India started "expanded program of immunization (EPI)".

The components of universal child immunization (UPI)-UCI had two major components: (1) Immunization of pregnant women against tetanus and (2) Immunization of children in their first year of life against EPI target-diseases.

National water supply and sanitation program: This

program was launched in the year 1954. The basic aim was to provide safe drinking water supply and drainage facilities to entire rural and urban population of India. **Swajaldhara** was launched on 25th December 2002. It was community led participatory program with certain guidelines to be adhered by the states.

Bharat Nirman: India launched this program in 2005 to build rural infrastructure. This program mainly concentrated on water quality.

Rural Sanitation Program

Swachh Bharat Mission (SBM): Prime Minister Narendra Modi launched "Cleanliness drive" in the country on 2nd October 2014. This program envisages to cover the entire community for saturated outcomes with a view to create Nirmal Gram Panchayats.

"Nirmal Bharat Abhiyan" (NBA): The objective is to accelerate the sanitation coverage in the rural areas so as to comprehensively cover the rural community through renewed strategies and saturation approach.

Minimum Need Program

Minimum needs program was introduced in 1st year of 5th five-year plan period (1974–78). This program focuses on social and economic development of the community especially the underprivileged and underserved population.

Polio Eradication: Pulse Polio Program

Polio has been eradicated from most of the world using several key strategies.

1978—Vaccination against polio was initiated under expanded program on immunization (EPI).

1984—Around 40% of all infants received 3 doses of oral polio vaccine (OPV)

1985—Universal immunization program (UIP) was launched under UNICEF.

Pulse polio immunization (PPI) program by providing additional OPV doses to every child aged <5 years at intervals of 4–6 weeks.

India started National Program on prevention and control of diabetes, cardiovascular diseases and stroke. Later on it was integrated with cancer control program and renamed as "National Program for Prevention and Control of Cancer, Diabetes, Cardiovascular Disease and Stroke (NPCDCS)."

The cancer control program was started for the prevention and early diagnosis and treatment cancer control program was started in the year 1975–76. This program was revised twice (1984–85 and 2004). In 2010 this program was integrated with "National Program for Prevention and Control of Cancer, Diabetes, Cardiovascular Disease and Stroke (NPCDCS)."

Tobacco Control Legislation

The cigarettes and other tobacco products Act (2003), passed in April 2003. Some of the highlights of it: Prohibition of cigarette smoking in public places, prohibition of direct and indirect advertisement of cigarettes and other products. The National Tobacco Program launched in 2007–08 under 11th five-year plan.

National mental health program (NMHP): National Mental Health Program (NMHP) is in operation in India since 1982. This was initiated primarily to tackle the problem of huge burden of mental disorders in India.

1996—The district mental health program was added to the program.

Yaws eradication program: WHO expert committee on venereal infections and treponematoses set the criteria for the eradication of yaws in 1960. Yaws is a disfiguring and disabling non-venereal skin infection caused by treponema pallidum—subspecies pertenue.

The number of reported cases in 10 endemic states came down to 46 during 2003 from 3,500 cases in 1996. On 19th September 2006, India formally declared the elimination of yaws from the country.

Vitamin A Prophylaxis Program

Launched in the year 1970 as a centrally sponsored scheme by Ministry of Health and Family Welfare, Government of India.

Component of National program for control of blindness (1976)—under this program a single dose of oily preparation of "vitamin A"—mega dose (200,000 IU), administered orally to all preschool children in the community once in every 6 months.

Integrated child development services (ICDS) scheme was initiated on 2 October, 1975 during 5th five-year plan period under "Ministry of social welfare" in pursuance of nutritional policy for children. ICDS center is called "anganwadi center (AWC)."

○ For 400–800 population—1 AWC
○ For 800–1600 population—1 AWC

Delivery of services under integrated child development services (ICDS) scheme include: Supplementary nutrition, nutritional and health education, immunization, health checkup nonformal education and schemes for adolescents.

Health schemes—Employee state insurance scheme and central government health scheme cover two large groups of wage earners in the country.

The employees state insurance scheme Act was passed in the year 1948 and amended in 1975, 1984, 1989 and 2010.

○ It is a significant social security and health insurance for employees of India.

○ It provides certain cash and medical benefits to industrial employees in case of sickness, maternity and employment injury.

The 1975 amendment of ESI Act extended to cover the following too: Small factories employing more than 10 persons, irrespective of power usage, shops, hotels and restaurants, cinemas and theatres, road-motor transport establishments, newspaper establishments and private medical and educational institutions employing 20 or more in some states.

Central Government Health Scheme in India

This scheme was formerly known as contributory health service scheme. This scheme was first introduced at New Delhi in the year 1954 for providing services to central government employees. This provides comprehensive health services to the CGHS Beneficiaries.

The services under the scheme—Outpatient services, domiciliary care, family welfare and MCH services, supply of necessary drugs, other insurance schemes, Rashtriya Swasthya Bima Yojana (RSBY), Rashtriya Swasthya Bima Yojana was launched by ministry of labor, government of India. The primary aim was to provide health insurance coverage to people below poverty line (BPL).

Aam Aadmi Bima Yojana (AABY)

This scheme is a social security scheme for rural landless launched on 2nd October, 2007.

The Beneficiaries are the head of the family or one earning member in the family aging between 18–59 years covered under this scheme. The premium of ₹ 200/person/year is shared equally by state and central governments.

Assess Yourself

I. Multiple Choice Questions (Choose the Correct Answer)

1. **Currently the acute respiratory infection control (ARI) program is the component of:**
   a. CSSM
   b. RCH-Phase-I
   c. RCH-Phase-II
   d. Maternal and child health

2. **RMNCH+A Strategy was introduced in the year:**
   a. 2011
   b. 2012
   c. 2013
   d. 2014

3. **Family planning program in India, was implemented in the year:**
   a. 1941
   b. 1951
   c. 1961
   d. 1971

4. **Reproductive and child health Program Phase-I was launched in the year:**
   a. 1997
   b. 1987
   c. 1993
   d. 2003

5. **The Employees State Insurance Scheme Act was passed in the year:**
   a. 1938
   b. 1948
   c. 1958
   d. 1968

6. **Rashtriya Swasthya Bima Yojana aims to provide health insurance coverage to:**
   a. Adolescents
   b. Women
   c. Below poverty line
   d. All people

7. **Aam Aadmi Bima Yojana (AABY) was launched in the year:**
   a. 1997
   b. 2007
   c. 1992
   d. 2002

8. **Which of these schemes provides unemployment allowance to involuntarily-unemployed employees?**
   a. Rajiv Gandhi Shramik Kalyan Yojna
   b. Rashtriya Swasthya Bima Yojana
   c. Aam Aadmi Bima Yojana
   d. ESI Scheme

9. **The Central Government Health Scheme was first launched in India in the year:**
   a. 194
   b. 1954
   c. 1964
   d. 1974

10. **Which of these programs referred to adolescents?**
    a. Kishori Shakthi Yojana
    b. Rashtriya Swasthya Bima Yojana
    c. Aam Aadmi Bima Yojana
    d. ESI Scheme

11. **Which of the following is *not* the component of ICDS scheme?**
    a. Nonformal education
    b. Nutrition
    c. Immunization
    d. Poverty eradication

12. **The population norm for AWC in rural area refers to:**
    a. For 100–400 population—1 AWC
    b. For 200–500 population—1 AWC
    c. For 300–700 population—1 AWC
    d. For 400–800 population—1 AWC

13. **The population norm for mini AnganWadi Center (AWC) in *tribal area* refers to:**
    a. For 150–300–1 Mini center
    b. For 200–300–1 Mini center
    c. For 250–300–1 Mini center
    d. For 300–400–1 Mini center

14. **India formally declared the elimination of yaws from the country in the year:**
    a. 1986
    b. 1996
    c. 2006
    d. 2016

15. **Which of the following would you advise for the 9 months infant?**
    a. 1 lakh international units of vitamin A solution
    b. 2 lakh international units of vitamin A solution
    c. 3 lakhs international units of vitamin A solution
    d. 4 lakhs international units of vitamin A solution

16. **Which of the following dose per day would you administer for children of 6 months to 5 years?**
    a. 20 mg of elemental iron and 100 mcg of folic acid
    b. 30 mg of elemental iron and 250 mcg folic acid
    c. Adult dose will be given
    d. None of the above

17. **Anemia prevention under RCH program supplements iron to children for the period of:**
    a. 100 days/year
    b. 150 days/year
    c. 200 days/year
    d. 250 days/year

18. **Which of these belongs to the components of essential obstetric care?**
    a. Institutional delivery
    b. Operationalizing first referral units
    c. Operationalizing Primary Health Centers (PHCS)
    d. All of the above

19. **Which of the following would be correct about your interpretation about the prefix number written on the TB drug regimen?**
    a. Indicates the number of months
    b. Indicates the dosage per day
    c. Indicates the frequency in a week
    d. Indicates the number of weeks

20. **Which of the following would be correct about your interpretation about the suffix number written on the TB drug regimen?**
    a. Indicates the number of months
    b. Indicates the dosage per day
    c. Indicates the frequency in a week
    d. Indicates the number of weeks

Health Agencies

21. The "Revised strategy of eradication of Kala-azar" was launched in the year:
    a. 2004
    b. 2014
    c. 2006
    d. 2016

22. Which of the program uses "Prepacked color coded kits" for treatment?
    a. AIDS control program   b. STD control program
    c. Cancer control program   d. Malaria control program

II. Short Answer Questions

1. List down the health programs which were independent earlier and now incorporated into RCH.
2. List the health programs incorporated into CSSM until 1997.
3. List four major interventions under RCH-I.
4. Write down the frequency and age wise dosages of vitamin A prophylaxis to children.
5. State the anemia management in children with iron and folic acid.
6. List four components of RCH phase-I.
7. List the strategies for essential newborn care under RCH phase-I.
8. List the four criteria for health facility to function as a first referral unit (FRU).
9. List four services under Emergency obstetric care.
10. List the recent initiatives under RCH phase-II.
11. List the objectives of RNTCP.
12. List the facilities in suraksha clinics.
13. List essential steps in sexually transmitted infections (STI) management.
14. Information, education and communication activities (IEC)-NACP-IV.
15. List the functions of anganwadi worker.
16. State four benefits of ESI Act.
17. List four principles of midday meal program.

III. Write Short Notes

1. Historical development to reach upto RCH phase-II
2. Reproductive and Child Health Program—phase-II.
3. Revised National tuberculosis control program (RNTCP).

4. National vector borne disease control program (Malaria, filaria, kala-zar, japanese encephalitis, dengue, chikungunya)
5. National guinea worm eradication program
6. National leprosy eradication program
7. Lymphatic filariasis—elimination strategies
8. National AIDS control program
9. STD control program
10. National program for control of blindness
11. Iodine deficiency disorder program
12. Expanded program on immunization
13. National water supply and sanitation program
14. Minimum needs program
15. 20-point program
16. National program for prevention and control of diabetes, cardiovascular disease and stroke
17. Polio eradication: Pulse polio program
18. Yaws eradication program
19. National mental health program
20. National nutritional programs
21. ICDS program
22. Midday meal scheme
23. Health schemes
24. ESI
25. Central Government Health Scheme (CGHS)
26. Health Insurance
27. Tobacco Control Legislation
28. District mental health program

IV. Write Essays

1. Explain the Reproductive and Child Health Program and describe the role of community health nurse in RCH program.
2. Describe the "Revised National Tuberculosis Control Program (RNTCP)" and the role of community health nurse in RNTCP.
3. Describe the National Vector Borne Disease Control Program (NVBDCP) and the role of community health nurse in NVBDCP.
4. Describe the role of community health nurse in malaria prevention and control.

ANSWERS

I. 1. c   2. c   3. b   4. a   5. b   6. c   7. b   8. a
9. b   10. a   11. d   12. d   13. a   14. c   15. a   16. a
17. a   18. a   19. a   20. c   21. b   22. b

Learning Objectives

At the end of this unit the learners will be able to:

- Explain the significant milestones before the genesis of world health organization
- List the international agencies
- State the meaning of multilateral, lateral and non-governmental agencies
- State the objectives in the preamble of world health organization
- Describe the administrative structure of world health organization
- State the functions of world health organization
- Describe the services of UNICEF
- Describe the functions of FAO
- List the functions of UNDP
- Explain the pattern of work of ILO
- Describe the functions of UNIFPA
- United Nations Fund for Population Activities (UNFPA)
- Explain the Colombo Plan
- List the functions of European Commission
- Explain "United Nations Educational, Scientific and Cultural Organization (UNESCO)"
- Describe the activities of "United States agency for International Development (USAID)"
- List the functions of "Danish International Development Agency (DANIDA)"
- List the assistance of "Swedish International Development Agency (SIDA)" to India
- Explain about Rockefeller foundation
- Explain Ford Foundation
- Explain Cooperative for Assistance and Relief Everywhere (CARE)
- Describe International Red Cross
- Describe the functions of voluntary health agencies
- Explain the activities of Indian Red Cross Society
- Highlight the importance of Hind Kusht Nivaran Sangh
- Explain about Indian Council for Child Welfare (ICCW)
- State the services of "Tuberculosis Association of India (TAI)"
- Explain the activities of Bharat Sevak Samaj (BSS)
- List the functions of Central Social Welfare Board (CSWB)
- State the aim of Kasturba Memorial Fund
- Describe the activities of Family Planning Association of India (FPAI)
- State the activities of All India Women's Conference (AIWC)
- Explain about "All India Blind Relief Society"

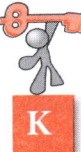

KEY TERMS

- First International sanitary conference, Pan American sanitary Bureau (PASB), Office International D' Hygiene Publique (OIHP), The Health Organization of the League of Nations, The United Nations Relief and Rehabilitation administration (UNRRA)
- World Health Organization (WHO), UNICEF (United Nations Children's Emergency Fund), United Nations Development Program (UNDP),
- Food and Agricultural Organization (FAO)
- The International Labor Organization (ILO)
- World Bank, United Nations Fund for Population Activities (UNFPA), The Colombo Plan, European Commission
- United Nations Educational, Scientific and Cultural Organization (UNESCO), United States agency for International Development (USAID),
- DANIDA, SIDA
- Rockefeller foundation, Ford Foundation
- Cooperative for Assistance and Relief Everywhere (CARE)
- International Red Cross, Indian Red Cross Society
- Hind Kusht Nivaran Sangh
- Indian Council for Child Welfare (ICCW)
- Tuberculosis Association of India (TAI)
- Bharat Sevak Samaj (BSS), Central Social Welfare Board (CSWB), The Kasturba Memorial Fund
- Family Planning Association of India (FPA)
- All India Women's Conference (AIWC)
- All India Blind Relief Society
- Professional bodies
- International agencies

INTRODUCTION

A health problem of one geographical region makes its journey to another region through global trades and communication and as well by other means. Centuries ago, the most important reason for which people travelled from one place to another is trades and business choosing the available modes of communication (road, air, water or nomadic movements). Religion, language and culture definitely had their boundaries but diseases not. Some of the most prominent and popular examples that saddened the world were plague and cholera. People traveled were branded infecting others created a great fear in the world. Severe acute respiratory distress syndrome (SARS) pandemic of recent decades had caused lots of fear in people of the world. During 14th century, Europe had used "Quarantine", for the first time to protect against bringing in of plague from other countries. There was great opposition to quarantine since detention of people for the period of 40 days caused lot many inconveniences to trades and travelers.

There were series of efforts taken by individual rulers, specific countries and countries in collaboration to control communicable diseases and promote international health. Before the genesis of "World Health Organization (WHO)" there were many significant events took place: New conferences organized with great efforts to develop new organizations for the promotion of international health. These significant events are real milestones to reach to the creation of world health organization.

First International Sanitary Conference

This conference was held in 1851 to bring about uniformity in implementing quarantine measures in all the countries. This was mainly attended by the European nations. This conference and the following conferences held from 1851 to 1902 did not yield any consensus among the countries.

Pan American sanitary Bureau (PASB)

Pan American Sanitary Bureau (PASB) was established in America in the year 1902 with the basic intention to coordinate quarantine procedures among American states.

PASB was the world's first international health agency.

"The Pan American Sanitary Code" released in 1924 is still in force in American states. The PASB reorganized and renamed as the, "Pan American Sanitary Organization (PASO) in 1947. In 1949 as agreed upon PASO started to serve as the regional office for World Health Organization. PASO renamed into, "Pan American Health Organization (PAHO)" in 1958.

Office International D' Hygiene Publique (OIHP)

In 1907, office international D' Hygiene Publique (OIHP) generally known as, "Paris Office," established mainly to supervise international quarantine measures. It was purely European and later had extended cooperation to PASB. Sixty countries including British India entered joined OIHP. This existed till 1950 and then on WHO had taken over its responsibilities.

Health Organization of the League of Nations

This was established after the world war (1914–1918) with the primary aim to building a better world. Later it also included, "health organization," to international concerns on prevention and control of diseases. This also paid attention to housing, nutrition, rural hygiene and training of public health workers. In 1939 the league nations was dissolved. However, it continues its work in Geneva with its component of "health organization," publishing weekly epidemiological records and provides other information at requests.

United Nations Relief and Rehabilitation administration (UNRRA)

This was setup in 1943 with the aim to organize recovery from the bad consequences of world war. The world campaign on "malaria eradication" with the joint efforts from UNRRA, the Rockefeller foundation and the Italian Government initiated in Sardinia. In 1946, UNRRA terminated its official existence and its activities were taken over by interim commission on the WHO.

INTERNATIONAL AGENCIES

The scope and intensity of global health challenges are multitude in nature. No single country or agency can tackle or find solutions for this. Multiple international agencies and institutions extend their help and cooperation in shaping the global health polices, funding, implementation and evaluation of the programs that work for international health.

Types of International Health Agencies

Generally, international health agencies are of three groups. They are:

1. **Multilateral agencies or organizations:** These types of agencies receive funds from multiple governments and nongovernmental sources and distribute among many different countries. For example, World Health Organization, World Bank, United Nations Children's Fund, etc.

2. **Bilateral organizations:** A bilateral organization is a government agency or not-for-profit organization based in a single country and provides funding to developing countries. For example, United States Agency for International Development, Centers for Disease Control and Prevention (CDC), etc.

3. **Nongovernmental organizations (NGOS):** Nongovernmental organization (NGO) is any non-profit, task oriented, voluntary citizens' group that is organized at the local, national or international level. For example, CARE International.

MULTILATERAL AGENCIES OR ORGANIZATIONS

World Health Organization

The origin of WHO dates back to April 1945 during the conference held at San Francisco to setup the United Nations. WHO was formally established on 7th April 1947. Hence, every year 7th April is celebrated as "WHO Day" by focusing on specific theme.

The main objective of WHO is "the attainment by all people of the highest level of health" which is setout in the preamble of the constitution. The current objective of WHO is the attainment by all people of the world a level of health that will permit them to lead a socially and economically productive life.

Objectives in the Preamble of WHO

- Health is a complete state of physical, mental and social well-being and not merely the absence of disease or infirmity
- Attainment of highest standard of health is the fundamental right without discrimination
- The health of people is fundamental for attainment of peace and security
- Achievement of any state in promotion and protection of health is of value to all
- Unequal development in different countries in promotion and control of disease is danger to all
- Extension to all people of the benefits of medical, psychological and related knowledge is essential to the fullest attainment of health
- Informed opinion and active cooperation of public is at most importance to improve the health of people
- Governments have a responsibility on people's health that can be achieved by provision of adequate health and social measures.

Major Policies and WHO

The two major policies that have influenced WHO are the Alma-Ata conference in 1978 on "primary health care" and the "global strategy for health for all by 2000 AD" and the millennium development goals. More recent "sustainable development goals" is a comprehensive one, which may also have strong influence on activities of WHO.

Structure of World Health Organization

The WHO includes three principal organs, they are: The World Health Assembly, the Executive Board and the Secretariat.

World Health Assembly

This is the highest governing body and the "health parliament of nations." Holds annual meeting in the month of May, usually at the headquarters Geneva. However, it holds meetings in other countries too. The assembly is composed of delegates representing member states each has one vote.

Functions of World Health Assembly

- Decides on international health policy and programs

- Review the work of the past year
- Approve the budget for the following year
- To elect member states to designate a person to serve for three years on the executive board
- To replace the retiring members
- To appoint Director General on the nomination of executive board
- To conduct technical discussions on specific area of world interest.

Executive Board

- Executive board has 18 members each designated by a member state subsequently it was raised to 30. Currently it has 34 members.
- The executive board meets twice in a year. The board enrolls only qualified people from health field as Board-members.
- One-third of the membership renewed yearly.

Functions of the Executive Board

- To give effect to the decisions of the assembly
- Has power to take decisions in emergencies. For example, disaster.

Secretariat

The Director General who functions as the chief technical and administrative officer of the organization chairs the Secretariat.

Functions of the Secretariat

- To provide technical and managerial support to member states for their national development programs.
- Five Assistant Director Generals deal with different divisions.

Divisions of the Secretariat

There are 14 divisions in Secretariat and each deal with specific function. They are:

- Epidemiological surveillance and health situation and trend assessment
- Communicable diseases
- Vector biology and control
- Environmental health
- Mental health
- Diagnostic and rehabilitation
- Strengthening of health services

- Family health
- Noncommunicable diseases
- Information systems support
- Personnel and general services
- Budget and finance

Functions of World Health Organization

- **Prevention and control of specific diseases:**
  - The global eradication of smallpox is the best example of WHO's work in disease control
  - Now it is actively involved in eliminating/eradicating some of the diseases
  - Collection and dissemination of epidemiological information automatic telex reply service (ATRS) and weekly epidemiological record
  - WHO emergency scheme for epidemics is useful to all countries
  - Apart from concentrating on communicable disease control it also attends noncommunicable diseases like cancer, diabetes, hypertension, cardiac diseases, etc.
  - Quality control drugs
  - Immunization against common diseases of childhood
- **Development of comprehensive services:**
  - Health policy and development of health programs—organizing health system based on primary health care, motivating member states to build infrastructure and develop staffing.
  - Appropriate technology for health (ATH) is launched encourage self-sufficiency in solving health problems.
- **Family health:** Since 1970 WHO is concentrating on human reproduction, maternal and child health, nutrition and health education to improve the quality of life.
- **Biomedical research:**
  - Stimulates and coordinates research work
  - Established worldwide network centers for research collaboration
  - Award of grants to researchers and institutions
- **Health statistics:** Disseminates information on morbidity and mortality statistics—The data is published in various publications of WHO. WHO publishes:
  - Weekly epidemiological record
  - World health statistics quarterly
  - World health statistics annual
  - International classification of disease and is updated every 10th year

- The data from WHO helps to compare between the nations
- It also supports the countries in planning and operating health information systems.
- **Environmental health:**
  - Encourages the countries to provide basic sanitation
  - Stresses on improvement of the environment—quality of air, housing, ventilation, food protection, injury prevention, protection at work and early identification of disease or hazards
  - WHO developed programs like WHO environmental health criteria program and WHO environmental health monitoring program to improve environmental health
- **Cooperation with other organization:**
  - World health organization collaborates with the United Nations and with other specialized agencies
  - Maintains relationship with international governmental organizations.

WHO Regional Centers

To meet the special health needs of different areas WHO established its regional centers in six places:

1. South-East Asia-New Delhi (India)
2. Africa-Brazzaville-Congo
3. The Americas-Washington DC (USA)
4. Europe-Copenhagen (Denmark)
5. Eastern Mediterranean-Alexandria (Egypt)
6. Western Pacific-Manila (Philippines)

The regional organizations play an important role in implementing the policies and programs. The Regional Director heads the Regional Office. Technical and administrative officers and members of the secretariat assist him. A regional committee composed of members of representative-countries functions at each region. The regional committee meets once in a year for reviewing and further planning in the region. Regional plans sent to head quarters and amalgamated after scrutiny by Director General of WHO.

UNICEF

United nations children's emergency fund (UNICEF) was one of the specialized agencies of United Nations formed in 1946 to provide relief to children of devastated countries of world war-II. After 1950 once, the relief functions were over the fund was utilized for helping the children's welfare, in less developed countries. In 1953, the general assembly renamed it as "United Nations Children Fund" and retained the initials

UNICEF. UNICEF awarded with the Nobel Prize for Peace in 1965. UNICEF has its headquarters in New York.

UNICEF works in close collaboration with WHO, FAO, UNDP and UNESCO.

Goals

To provide enduring care to mothers and children in developing countries.

To emphasize community level services to promote health and well-being of children.

Services of UNICEF (Fig. 1)

○ **Child health:** UNICEF provided extensive support in the field of maternal and child health. UNICEF gave higher level priority to child health, nutrition, family and child welfare, breastfeeding and growth monitoring, prevention of vaccine preventable diseases, prevention of diarrhea and oral rehydration.

  ❑ Supported India's BCG vaccination program from the time of its inception

  ❑ Provided assistance in establishing penicillin plant near Pune

  ❑ Donated DDT plant

  ❑ Provided two plants for manufacturing triple vaccine and iodized salt

  ❑ Assistance in water supply in rural areas

  ❑ Assistance in safe drinking water

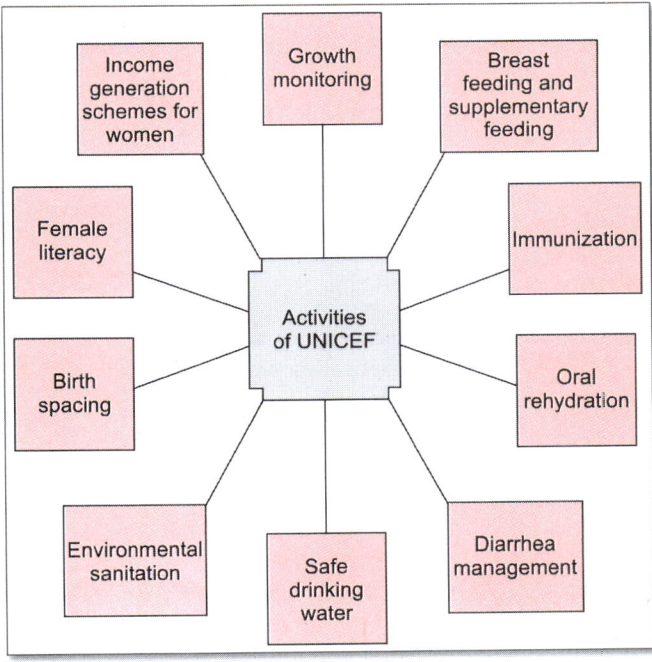

Figure 1: Overall activities of UNICEF

❑ Primary health care to mothers and children

❑ Child care

❑ Immunization

❑ Family planning services

❑ Safe water and adequate sanitation

❑ Motivation on community participation.

○ **Child nutrition:** Supplementing child feeding as measure to improve the nutritional status of children began in 1950 and slowly reached to the level of preparing low-cost protein rich foods.

  ❑ UNICEF in collaboration with FAO started "Applied nutrition program' (Food and Agricultural Organization) as a part of community development

  ❑ Took initiative in supplying equipment for modern dairy plants in various parts of India

  ❑ Provision of large doses of vitamin A in areas where xeropthalmia was prevalent

  ❑ Iodization of salt in goiter endemic areas

  ❑ Provision of iron and folate supplements to combat anemias.

○ **Family and child welfare:**

  ❑ UNICEF aimed at improving the care of children not only at home but also outside their homes.

  ❑ UNICEF had taken efforts to attain the above objective through provision of education to parents, day care centers, child welfare and youth welfare agencies and women's clubs. These projects are merged with other programs on health, nutrition and education.

○ **Education**

  ❑ **Formal and nonformal education:** UNICEF in collaboration with UNESCO helps India in the expansion and improvement of teaching science

  ❑ UNICEF provides support in supplying laboratory equipment, library books, and audio-visual aids to the institutions

  ❑ **Promotion of "GOBI-FFF campaign"** to encourage four basic strategies for a "child health revolution."

  G–*Growth charts* to better monitor child development

  O–*Oral rehydration* to treat all mild and moderate dehydration

  B–*Breastfeeding* is the best possible food which gives great immunity to fight against common infections that occur in the first six month of life

  I–*Immunization* against measles, diphtheria, pertussis, tetanus, poliomyelitis and tuberculosis

  F–*Female education*—educating females is the vital instrument to reduce under-five mortality.

A child born of a mother with no education has twice the chance to die in infancy than a child born of a mother who has four years of schooling. **F–***Family spacing*—Infant and child deaths have been found to be, on average, twice as high when the interval between births is less than two years

F–*Food supplements*—Provision of a handful of extra food each day for at-risk pregnant women has been shown to reduce the risk of low birth–weight. The babies of low–birthweight are at two or three times of greater risk to die in infancy. Since 1976 UNICEF participates in **urban basic services (UBS)**—This also focuses on health, nutrition, water supply, education and basic sanitation.

United Nations Development Program

- United Nations Development Program (UNDP) was established in the year 1966.
- The main goal of UNDP is to help poorer nations develop their human and natural resources more fully.
- The UNDP projects provides support to every economic and social sector like agriculture, industry, education and science, health, social welfare, etc.

Activities of UNDP

- UNDP's network links and coordinates global and national efforts to attain the above said goals.
- UNDP helps countries to build and share solutions to meet the challenges in the fields of:
  - Democratic governance
  - Poverty reduction
  - Crisis prevention and recovery
  - Environment and energy
  - HIV/AIDS

Food and Agricultural Organization

The food and agriculture organization (FAO) was formed in the year 1945 with headquarters in Rome. This United Nations organization specialized look after several areas of world co-operation. FAO is the lead United Nations (UN) agency for agriculture, fisheries, forestry and rural development.

Major Aims of FAO

- To help nations raise living standards
- To improve the nutritional status of people of all countries
- To increase the efficiency of farming, forestry and fisheries
- To improve the condition of rural people through providing opportunity of productive work.

Functions

The core functions of the FAO include:

- Collecting, analyzing and disseminating information
- Developing international instruments, norms and standards
- Providing advice and capacity-building for agricultural policy makers
- Contributing to emergency and post-emergency assistance at member states' request, through its global network of experts
- Ensuring that the food is consumed by people who need it
- Increases the food production to balance with ever growing population
- Collaboration with other agencies in applied nutrition programs
- Training and research on brucellosis and other zoonosis.

International Labor Organization

The international labor organization (ILO) was established in the year 1919 as an affiliate to league of nations to improve the living conditions of the working populations all over the world. The headquarters of ILO is in Geneva, Switzerland.

In 1969, the organization received the Nobel Peace Prize for improving peace among classes, pursuing justice for workers, and providing technical assistance to other developing nations. Currently, 185 of the 193 UN member states are members of the ILO.

Purposes of ILO

- To help in developing lasting peace through promotion of social justice
- To improve through international action, labor conditions and living standards
- To improve economic and social stability.

Services

- The ILO is a United Nations agency that deals about labor issues. ILO specifically looks observes international labor standards and to provide decent work for all
- It also extends assistance to organizations interested in improving living and employment standards
- ILO collaborates with WHO in matters related to health and labor.

World Bank

The World Bank, was established in the year 1944 with the headquarters in Washington, DC.

This is a specialized agency of United Nations. The World Bank functions as a main source of financial and technical assistance to developing countries, globally. World bank's controlling authority is the Board of Governors.

Objectives

○ To fight poverty with passion and professionalism for long-term results.

○ To equip people to help themselves and their environment by providing resources, sharing knowledge, building capacity and forging partnerships in the public and private sectors.

Services

World Bank provides low-interest loans, interest-free credits and grants to developing countries for various purposes. The purposes may include: (1) Investments in education, (2) Health, (3) Public administration, (4) Infrastructure, (5) Financial and (6) Private sector development, (7) Agriculture, (8) Environmental and natural resource management.

Provision of loans for projects that helps in economic development of the country (e.g. India Population project).

World Bank works in close collaboration with WHO. For example, projects for water supply, world food program, population control and control of onchocerciasis program in west Africa.

World bank also works in close collaboration with FAO, UNICEF, etc.

United Nations Fund for Population Activities

The united nations fund for population activities (UNFPA) is an international development agency, created in 1968 to support the execution of projects and programs in the area of population and sexual and reproductive health. UNFPA has been providing assistance to India since 1974.

It provides assistance in:

○ Intensive development of health and family welfare infrastructure

○ Development of national capability in manufacturing contraceptives

○ Development of population education program

○ To improve the output of gross-root level workers

○ Introduction of innovative approaches to family planning and MCH care.

Support to Promote Healthy Families

○ Training health workers to deliver quality family planning services and supply contraceptives in emergency situations

○ Ensuring youth-friendly reproductive health care

○ Providing counseling to women who want to avoid or delay pregnancy

○ Educating men on the benefits of birth spacing.

Support to Promote Maternal Health

○ Training midwives and health workers

○ Supplying clean birthing kits following disasters

○ Strengthening emergency obstetric care

○ Ensuring reliable supplies of essential medicines and equipment

○ Enabling birth spacing.

UNFPA Advocates for the Welfare of Young People

○ Promoting the human rights of adolescents

○ Preventing HIV infection

○ Engaging young people in decisions that affect them

○ Supporting age-appropriate comprehensive sexuality education

○ Creating safe spaces for adolescent girls

○ Encouraging abandonment of harmful practices

○ Encouraging leadership.

Colombo Plan

The Colombo plan was one of the oldest regional intergovernmental organizations dates back to 1950 specifically the idea emerged to enhance economic and social development of the countries of the region. The Colombo Plan for Cooperative Economic and Social Development in Asia and the Pacific intended to work on a partnership concept of self-help and mutual-help in development aimed at socioeconomic progress of its member countries. The Colombo Plan was established on 1 July 1951 by Australia, Canada, India, Pakistan, New Zealand, Sri Lanka and the United Kingdom. Now, this has 26 member countries including non-Common wealth countries and countries belonging to regional groupings such as Association of South-East Asian Nations (ASEAN) and South Asian Association for Regional Cooperation (SAARC).

Objectives

○ To promote interest and support for the economic and social development of Asia and the Pacific

○ To promote technical cooperation and assist in the sharing and transfer of technology among member countries

○ To keep under review of relevant information on technical cooperation between the member governments, multilateral and other agencies in order to accelerating development through cooperative effort

○ To facilitate the transfer and sharing of the developmental experiences among member countries within the region with emphasis on the concept of South-South cooperation.

Organizational Structure of the Colombo Plan

The Consultative Committee (CCM), is the highest review and policy making body of the Colombo Plan. It comprises of all member governments. Its biennial meetings serve as a forum for the exchange of views on current development problems in member countries. It also reviews the work of the Colombo Plan in economic and social development within the region.

The Colombo Plan Council, comprises heads of diplomatic missions of member governments who are resident in Colombo, Sri Lanka. The President of the Council is nominated from among member countries annually on an alphabetical rotational basis. Quarterly meeting by council to identify important issues in member countries and implementation of the committee's decisions.

The Colombo Plan Secretariat is located in Colombo, Sri Lanka, since 1951 and functions as the secretariat for the Consultative Committee and the Council. The Secretary General heads the Secretariat. The Secretariat is responsible program administration of the Colombo Plan, for in partnership with member countries and collaborating agencies.

Funding

The administrative costs of the Council and the Secretariat are borne equally by all member countries. The traditional and emerging donors of member countries fund the training activities of Colombo plan. Developing member countries are encouraged to meet local expenditure of training programs held in their respective countries. The non-member governments and regional/international organizations also funds the Colombo Plan training programs.

Programs

The colombo plan has 4 permanent programs. They are:

○ Drug advisory program (DAP)

○ Program for public administration and environment (PPA and ENV)

○ Program for private sector development (PPSD)

○ Long-term scholarships program (LTSP).

European Commission

The European Commission is the European Union's executive body and represents the interests of Europe as a whole (as opposed to the interests of individual countries). It is responsible for proposing legislation and implementing decisions. The European Commission is located in Brussels in Belgium. In addition, it has offices in Luxembourg. Governments of the Member States nominate the President of the Commission by consulting with the European Parliament. Currently it has 28 Commissioners, one from each Member State. Each commissioner is given the portfolio of his responsible area. Members of the Commission are appointed for a renewable term of 5 years. Present commission will be in office from 2014 to 2019.

Functions

○ It is responsible for initiating legislation and submitting proposals for European laws

○ The Commission functions as a guardian of the European Union (EU) treaties

○ It is responsible for ensuring that all Member States apply EU legislation

○ It can initiate actions against Member States or businesses that fail to comply with EU law

○ It is responsible for formulation of policies and the annual budget

○ It represents the EU on the international stage

○ It negotiates trade and cooperation agreements with non-EU countries.

United Nations Educational, Scientific and Cultural Organization

The United Nations Educational, Scientific and Cultural Organization (UNESCO) is a specialized agency of the United Nations system based in de Fontenoy, Paris. The organization emerged more than a half century ago, with the mission to build the defences of peace in the minds of men. Its Constitution states that: "Since wars begin in the minds of men, it is in the minds of men that the defences of peace must be constructed". This constitution was adopted by the London Conference in November 1945. UNESCO currently has 188 Member States.

The main objective of UNESCO is to contribute **peace and security** in the world by promoting international collaboration through education, science, culture and communication irrespective of race, sex, language or religion.

Principal Functions of UNESCO

○ Provides a platform for promoting and strengthening of democratization, the rule of law and respect for human rights in Africa and the Arab region

- Helps in strengthening the Arab-African relations and promote cooperation
- Involved in strengthening the existing research networks, undertake research and studies, disseminate the findings
- Encourage policy-makers to promote the participation of women and youth in political, legislative, social, economic and cultural processes
- Promotes democracy and respect for human rights
- Encourage and fosters implementation of the Forum's recommendations
- To establish a sound communication program through different media and IT channels.

BILATERAL ORGANIZATIONS

United States Agency for International Development (USAID)

United Nations government extends its help and support to Indian projects through three agencies, they are: (1) USAID; (2) The Public law 480 program; (3) US export-import bank.

The USAID is the United States Government agency, that is responsible for administering civilian foreign aid. In 1961, President John F Kennedy created the USAID. USAID's mission statement highlights two goals. They are: (1) ending extreme poverty, (2) promoting the development of resilient, democratic societies that are able to realize their potential.

The US government assists India in a number of projects:

- Malaria eradication
- Medical education
- Nursing education
- Health education
- Water supply and sanitation
- Control of communicable diseases
- Nutrition
- Family planning

Most recently high-level support is extended on agriculture and family planning by reducing on general health fund

Danish International Development Agency

Danish international development agency (DANIDA), is the brand that the Denmark uses for providing humanitarian aid and development assistance to other countries. It mainly focuses on developing nations. Hence, there is no separate DANIDA organization within the Ministry of Denmark. Denmark has been granting development assistance to different developing countries since the end of the Second World War. It is one of the five countries in the world that meets the United Nation's target of granting 0.7% of gross national income to development assistance. Denmark disbursed roughly US$2.98 billion for development assistance to countries in Africa, Asia, Latin America and Middle east and Denmark's European union neighbors.

Since 1978 India receives DANIDA's assistance for blindness control program.

Aim

The aim of Denmark's development cooperation is to reduce poverty through the promotion of human rights and economic growth. It is focused on some of the poorest countries in the world.

Four Main Priority Areas

- Human rights and democracy
- Green growth
- Social progress
- Stability and protection

Swedish International Development Agency

Swedish International Development Agency (SIDA) is a government agency works on behalf of the Swedish parliament and government with head office at Valhallavägen in Stockholm, SIDA works with the mission "to reduce poverty in the world." SIDA has eight departments, Internal Audit and the Director-General's Office. Five departments work toward implementing the development assistance and the rest three with support, steering and control.

Assistance to India

- SIDA is assisting India's National Tuberculosis control program since 1979.
- SIDA's assistance is utilized for purchasing supplies to X-ray unit, microscope and antituberculosis drugs
- SIDA also helped in pilot project of Short Course Chemotherapy drug regimens (1983–84) and pilot phase-I of revised strategy of national TB control program in 5 sites (since 1993).

NONGOVERNMENTAL AND OTHER AGENCIES

Rockefeller Foundation

- Rockefeller foundation is a philanthropic organization started in 1913 by Mr John D Rockefeller. It was started with the basic aim of promoting the well-being of mankind all over the world. At its start, primary focus was on public health and medical education. Later, this foundation attended to other areas like the life sciences, social sciences, the humanities and the agricultural sciences.

- Rockefeller foundation initiated its work in India in 1920 in control of hookworm infestation.
- From then, it had close association in extending support to many programs in India.

Activities

- The establishment of All India Institute of hygiene and public health at Kolkatta
- Setting up of field demonstration area to department preventive and social medicine and All India Institute of Medical Sciences
- Provision of training to competent teachers and research workers
- Training of Indian candidates abroad through fellowships and travel grants
- Sponsoring of large number of medical students from USA to visit India
- Provision of grant in aids to selected institutions
- Development of medical college libraries
- Assistance to research projects
- Currently this foundation provides support in the activities related to agriculture, family planning, medical education and rural training.

Ford Foundation

The Ford Foundation is a private, non-profit, philanthropic organization founded in 1936. Since then, this operated in the state of Michigan, USA, as a local philanthropy. In 1950 the foundation became popular and expanded to become a national and international foundation. The Foundation, works to promote international peace and welfare of people all over the world. It takes efforts in identifying the problems of national and international importance and helps to find solution for the same. The Foundation aims at providing support innovative works in the field of applied research, training, experimentation, advocacy and developmental efforts. It also prefers to choose projects that ensure significant advances.

The Foundation established its office at New Delhi, India in 1952 following the receipt of an invitation from Prime Minster Jawaharlal Nehru. This is Foundation's first program outside the United States and the largest among overseas operations. The office in New Delhi, also serves in Nepal and Sri Lanka.

Goals of the Foundation

- Strengthen democratic value
- Reduce poverty and injustice

- Promote international cooperation; and
- Advance human achievement.

Functions of Ford Foundation

- Environment development
- Community-based natural resource management
- Promotion and utilization of local knowledge and appropriate technology for better management of resources
- Making micro-finance more accessible to people
- Promoting peace and social justice
- Encouraging appropriate strategies for poverty reduction.

Assistance by Ford Foundation in Various Projects in India

- Establishment of orientation training centers at various places (Singur, Poonamallee, Najafgarh) to train medical and paramedical personnel all over India, in the field public health
- Establishment of research cum action centers to solve basic problems in environmental sanitation. For example, hand flushed latrines in rural areas
- Pilot projects in rural health services—Establishment of coordinated health service model for 1 lakh population at Gandhigram, Tamil Nadu
- Establishment of National Institute of Health Administration and Education (NIHAE) at Delhi to provide training for senior health administrators
- Preparation of master plan for water supply, sewerage and drainage for the city Kolkata
- Enhancement of research in reproductive biology and family planning through fellowship programs.

Cooperative for Assistance and Relief Everywhere

Cooperative for assistance and relief everywhere (CARE), was formerly known as "Cooperative for American Remittances to Europe." CARE is the world's largest independent, nonsectarian, nongovernmental organization founded in 1945. CARE is a major international humanitarian agency that extends emergency relief and assistance to long-term international development projects. CARE is currently working in 79 poor and developing countries. The main aim is to help poorest people.

Mission of Care

"To save lives, defeat poverty and achieve social justice"

CARE places women and girls as the core of their service because they believe that to overcome poverty all people should have equal rights and opportunities.

Services in India

CARE was in operation since 1950 in India. Until 1980, the primary focus of "CARE" in India was providing food to children of 6–11 years. From 1980, it started to support ICDS project and showed interest in developing health programs and income supplementation schemes. CARE-India works in partnership with government of India, state governments and NGOs.

Currently CARE supports in the following projects in India:

- Integrated nutrition and health project
- Better health and nutrition project
- Anemia control project
- Improving women's health project
- Improved health care for adolescent girls project
- Child survival project
- Improving women's reproductive health and family spacing project.

International Red Cross

Jean Henry Dunant was a young Swiss businessman. He happened to see the wounded soldiers in the battle field of Solferino, Italy in 1859 during the Franco–Austrian war. He was shocked to see the conditions of the soldiers and tried arranging for relief services by getting the help of the local community. His experience compelled him to write the book "Memory of Solferino." In the book he suggested for establishing a neutral organization to aid the wounded soldiers in times of war. Just a year after the release of the book, an international conference held in Geneva. In this conference, suggestions of Henry Dunant considered and this made the pavement for the birth of Red Cross Movement. Geneva Convention of 1864 established international "Red Cross Movement". The international committee of red cross (ICRC) the independent neutral institution developed. The name and the emblem of the movement are derived from the reversal of the Swiss national flag, to honor the country in which Red Cross was found. In 1919 the League of the Red Cross Society was created functions at Geneva to coordinate the work of national societies. Its mission is to alleviate human suffering, protect life and health, and uphold human dignity, especially during armed conflicts and other emergencies.

Services

Initially, confined to humanitarian services focused on serving the victims of war. Later the services extended to meet various challenges:

- Services to armed forces
- Service to war veterans
- Disaster service
- First aid and nursing
- Health education
- Maternity and child welfare services.

VOLUNTARY HEALTH AGENCIES

Voluntary health agencies hold very important place in supporting and uplifting the health and economic status of a country through established associations/council with specific or multiple objectives. "A voluntary health agency may be defined as an organization that is administered by an autonomous board which hold meeting, collects funds for its support chiefly from private sources and expands money, whether with or without paid workers, in conducting a program directed primarily to furthering the public health by providing health services or health education, or by advancing research or legislation for health, or by a combination of these activities."

United States is the place where many voluntary agencies emerged and flourished. In 1945 itself United States had more than 20,000 voluntary health agencies.

Areas of Functions of Voluntary Health Agencies

Voluntary health agencies have been involved in providing various services. The services can be grouped under the following headings:

Supplementing the Work of Government Agencies

It is not possible for the government sectors to fulfill all the needs of the community since they work with financial and statutory constraints. Hence, voluntary agencies help in strengthening the work of government by providing personnel, contribution of funds for procuring equipment, and supplies.

Pioneering-ways and Means of doing New Things

- Voluntary health agencies are interested in novelty and innovation that would help the countries in finding a solution for a problem.
- Pioneering with new projects is one of its passions. For example, the family planning program in India was pioneered by voluntary health agencies. Once it started to yield good results India came forward to take over the project.

Education

India needs much in the field of health education. This humongous work cannot be carried out in solo. Voluntary agencies extends its support in this area.

Demonstration

○ The new track selected by voluntary health agencies to achieve public health was through demonstrations in community.

○ It came out with a solution through demonstration of bore hole latrines to prevent hookworm problems.

Guarding the Work of Government Agencies

Being as a pioneer and a role model it is possible to criticize and guide governmental projects.

Advancing Health Legislation

Helps in mobilizing public opinion and promotes legislation for the sake of people.

INDIAN RED CROSS SOCIETY

Young, Swiss-executive, Jean Henry Dunant to alleviate human suffering, established Indian Red Cross Society in 1920. Since its inception it has been serving for promoting health, preventing disease and mitigation of suffering. During the world war-I (1914), there was no organization for providing relief services to the affected soldiers in India. Now Red Cross has a network of more than 400 branches throughout India.

Activities

Relief Work

During disasters (earth-quake, floods, drought, epidemics etc.) as an immediate response the Red Cross mobilizes its sources to extend help in rescuing people in disaster affected areas.

Milk and Medical Supplies

Red Cross provides assistance to hospitals, dispensaries, maternity and child welfare centers, schools and orphanages every year, in the form of milk powder, vitamins, medicines and other supplies.

Armed Forces

Its primary function is to care sick and wounded people from military services.

Red Cross Society runs its own hospital (Red Cross Home) in Bengaluru for permanently disabled Ex-servicemen.

Maternal and Child Welfare Societies

Currently there are many maternal and child welfare centers run by Red Cross all over India.

The Bureau of Maternity and Child welfare provide technical advice and finance aids for starting modern maternity and child welfare centers.

Family Planning

Several states have family planning clinics under Red Cross.

Blood Bank and First Aid— St John Ambulance Association

○ Some state branches have blood banks

○ Red Cross has trained several lakh men and women in first aid, home nursing and allied sciences.

Hind Kusht Nivaran Sangh

The Hind Kusht Nivaran Sangh was founded in 1950. Indian Council of the British Empire Leprosy Relief Association (BELRA) renamed as LEPRA in 1950 was considered the precursor of this sangh. It has the headquarters at New Delhi, and branches all over India.

Activities

○ Provides financial assistance to leprosy homes and clinics

○ Provides health education through publications and posters

○ Provides training to medical workers and social workers

○ Conducts research and field investigations

○ Holds periodic leprosy conferences

○ Publishes Quarterly journal "Leprosy in India"

○ Works in close collaboration with government and other agencies.

Indian Council for Child Welfare (ICCW)

Indian Council for Child Welfare established in 1952. It is affiliated with International union for child welfare. It has state and district councils all over India. It is the single largest agency, promoting development services for children. The administration includes President, Vice President, Secretary, Joint secretary, Treasurer and 15 elected members. ICCW adopts the UN Convention on the Rights of the Child (UN CRC) as a framework to guide the work. ICCW helps vulnerable and disadvantageous children by providing direct services.

Activities

○ Advocating Children's Rights

○ Establishment of crèches for children of working and sick mothers

○ Organizing training programs for child care workers

- Providing sponsorship under-privileged children to pursue school education
- Special projects for street and working children
- Scrutiny of Adoption Cases
- Rehabilitating programs for Abandoned Children
- Institutional and day care services for differently abled children
- Special focus on the girl child and support services
- Conduction of national integration and adventure camps.

Tuberculosis Association of India

Tuberculosis association of India (TAI) was established on 1939. It became a registered society in 23rd February, 1939 by incorporating the King Emperor's Anti-Tuberculosis Fund and King George Thanks-giving (Anti-Tuberculosis) Fund. It has the headquarters at New Delhi, with branches in all states.

Major Aims of TAI

- To work towards prevention, control, treatment and relief of tuberculosis
- To encourage and assist the establishments of similar objectives in whole or in part
- To perform research and investigation on matters relating to tuberculosis and allied chest diseases.

Activities

- Organizing a TB seal campaign every year to raise funds
- Training of medical, paramedical health workers and social workers in the control of TB
- Publishing of periodicals on TB and related chest disease
- Conducting annual conference
- Encouraging research on TB
- Promotion of health education.

Institutions under the Management of TAI

- The New Delhi Tuberculosis Center
- The Lady Linlithgow Sanatorium at Kasauli
- The King Edward VII Sanatorium at Dharampur
- Tuberculosis Hospital at Mehrauli.

Bharat Sevak Samaj

Bharat Sevak Samaj (BSS) is a nonofficial, nonpolitical organization started in 1952. BSS has branches in all the states and in all the districts. The basic aim of this samaj is to make people realize their potentials and help to achieve health by the own efforts and actions. The main work of BSS is to improve basic sanitation in villages.

Central Social Welfare Board (CSWB)

It was established in August 1953 by government of India. The founder Chairperson of the Board, was Dr Durgabai Deshmukh. It is an autonomous body functions under Ministry of Education.

Functions

- Surveying the needs and requirements of voluntary welfare organizations
- Promoting and setting up of social welfare organizations on voluntary basis
- Financial aid to deserving existing organizations and institutions
- Provision of family and child welfare services since 1968. This project included:
  - Craft, social education, literacy classes, educational aid for women, distribution of milk, balwadis, play centers for children
- Scheme of industrial cooperatives to supplement the income of lower middle class women in urban areas by giving them paid work.
- Short stay home program initiated in 1969 to provide temporary shelter to women and girls who are forced into prostitution and sexually assaulted.

Kasturba Memorial Fund

The Kasturba Memorial Fund was created in the name of Smt Kasturba Gandhi after her death in 1944. The principal objective was to improve women's status in rural areas through Gram-Sevikas. The fund aimed at solving various issues of women in rural India.

Family Planning Association of India

The family planning association (FPA) was formed in 1949 basing its headquarters at Mumbai. Currently FPA India functions in 17 states and in 1 Union Territory. FPA India covers about 10% of the district population and helps in fertility reduction. It has 42 branches/projects, 39 static clinics, 23 Urban Welfare Centers (funded by the Government of India), 78 outreach units and 148 adolescent's youth friendly centers/clinics.

The FPA India has been made extensive contribution in the area of family planning. Now, FPA India is devoted to promote knowledge on family planning and to advocate for sexual and reproductive health (SRH), rights and choices through its youth friendly centers.

Activities

- MCH, training and research
- Health educating students and youth workers

- Advice the couples to plan birth spacing and family
- Organizes conferences, seminars and workshop
- Educates people on STD/AIDS prevention
- FPAI had setup sex education, counseling, research, and training/therapy (SECRT) centers
- Specialized services on family life, marriage and sex counseling
- Provides sexual health program for all categories (youth, parents, educators, disabled and mentally handicapped)
- Conducts training programs for doctors, health visitors and social workers.

All India Women's Conference (AIWC)

The only women's voluntary welfare organization of India established in 1926. It has got branches all over India. This works for a society with the principles of social justice, personal integrity and equal rights and opportunities for all.

Services

- MCH clinics
- Medical centers
- Adult education center to improve female literacy
- Milk centers
- Family planning clinics.

All India Blind Relief Society

All India Blind Relief Society established in 1946. It focuses on coordinating different institutions that work with the same goal.

Main Functions

- Co-ordination with different institutions that work for the blind relief
- Eye camps for identification of preventable blindness
  - Camps for cataract screening and surgery (recently with IOL implantation)
  - Distribution of free spectacles for refractory correction

Professional Bodies

The professional bodies of India like Indian Medical Association, Indian Dental Association, and Trained Nurses Association of India are voluntary agencies who are qualified in their field and possess licenses to practice in their domain. These professional bodies conduct research, publish journals, organize scientific sessions, setup standards for professional education and works with great involvement in relief camps during disasters.

International Agencies

Rockefeller foundation, Ford foundation and CARE are examples for it and these were explained in detail in previous paragraphs.

Summary

Religion, language and culture definitely had their boundaries but diseases not. New conferences organized with great efforts to develop new organizations for the promotion of international health. These significant events are real milestones to reach to the creation of world health organization. The **First International sanitary conference** was held in 1851 to bring about uniformity in implementing quarantine measures in all the countries. **Pan American Sanitary Bureau** (PASB) was established in America in the year 1902 with the basic intention to coordinate quarantine procedures among American states.

International Agencies

Multiple international agencies and institutions extend their help and cooperation in shaping the global health. Generally, international health agencies are of three groups. They are:

(1) Multilateral organizations (2) Bilateral organizations (3) Non-governmental organizations (NGOS).

World health organization was formally established on 7th April 1947. The main objective of WHO is "The attainment by all people' of the highest level of health" which is set out in the preamble of the constitution. The two major policies that have influenced WHO are the Alma-Ata conference in 1978 on **"Primary health care"** and the **"global strategy for health for all by 2000 AD"** and **the Millennium Development goals.** The WHO includes three principal organs, they are: The World Health Assembly, the Executive Board and the Secretariat.

World health assembly: Decides on international health policy and programs. Executive board has 18 members each designated by a member state subsequently it was raised to 30. Currently it has 34 members.

Secretariat provides technical and managerial support to member states. There are 14 divisions in Secretariat and each deal with specific function.

Functions of world health organization (WHO) (1) Prevention and control of specific diseases, (2) Development of comprehensive services, (3) Family health (4) Biomedical research, (5) Health statistics, (6) Environmental health and (7) Co-operation with other organization. WHO has established its regional centers in six places.

United nations children's emergency fund (UNICEF) was one of the specialized agencies of United Nations formed in 1946 to provide relief to children of devastated countries of world war-II. In 1953, the general assembly renamed it as "United Nations Children Fund" and retained the initials UNICEF.

Services of, UNICEF includes (1) Child health, (2) Child nutrition, (3) Family and child welfare, (4) Education -**Promotion of "GOBI-FFF campaign"** to encourage four basic strategies for a "child health revolution."

United Nations Development Program (UNDP) was established in the year 1966.

The main goal of UNDP is to help poorer nations develop their human and natural resources more fully.

Food and agricultural organization (FAO): The food and agriculture organization (FAO) was formed in the year 1945 with headquarters in Rome. FAO is the lead United Nations (UN) agency for agriculture, fisheries, forestry and rural development.

The International Labor Organization (ILO) ILO was established in the year 1919 as an affiliate to league of nations to improve the living conditions of the working populations all over the world.

World Bank: The World Bank, was established in the year 1944 with the headquarters in Washington, DC. The purposes are: (1) Investments in education, (2) Health, (3) Public administration, (4) Infrastructure, (5) Financial, (6) Private sector development, (7) Agriculture, (8) Environmental and natural resource management.

UNFPA is an international development agency, created in 1968 to support the execution of projects and programs in the area of population and sexual and reproductive health.

The Colombo Plan was established on 1 July 1951 by Australia, Canada, India, Pakistan, New Zealand, Sri Lanka and the United Kingdom. This plan intended to work on a partnership concept of self-help and mutual-help in development aimed at socioeconomic progress of its member countries.

The european commission is the European Union's executive body and represents the interests of Europe as a whole (as opposed to the interests of individual countries). It is responsible for proposing legislation and implementing decisions. Members of the Commission are appointed for a renewable term of 5 years. Present commission will be in office from 2014 to 2019.

It is responsible for initiating legislation and submitting proposals for European laws.

The United Nations Educational, Scientific and Cultural Organization (UNESCO) is a specialized agency of the United Nations system based in de Fontenoy, Paris. *The main objective* of UNESCO is to contribute *peace and security* in the world by promoting international collaboration through education, science, culture and communication irrespective of race, sex, language or religion.

In 1961, President John F Kennedy created the USAID. **The United States Agency for International Development (USAID)** is the United States Government agency responsible for administering civilian foreign aid. The main aims were (1) ending extreme poverty and (2) promoting the development of resilient, democratic societies that are able to realize their potential.

Danish international development agency (DANIDA), is the brand that the Denmark uses for providing humanitarian aid and development assistance to other countries. Since 1978 India receives DANIDA's assistance for blindness control program. **Swedish international development agency (SIDA)** is a government agency works on behalf of the Swedish parliament and government.

Rockefeller foundation is a philanthropic organization started in 1913 by Mr. John D Rockefeller. Rockefeller foundation initiated its work on control of hookworm infestation in India in 1920.

Ford foundation is a private, non-profit, philanthropic organization founded in 1936.

The major goal is to strengthen democratic values and reduce poverty and injustice.

CARE is the world's largest independent, nonsectarian, nongovernmental organization founded in 1945. The mission is "To save lives, defeat poverty and achieve social justice".

Geneva Convention of 1864 established international **"Red Cross movement".**

In 1919 the League of the **Red Cross Society** was created functions at Geneva to coordinate the work of national societies. Its mission is to alleviate human suffering, protect life and health, and uphold human dignity, especially during armed conflicts and other emergencies.

Voluntary health agencies hold very important place in supporting and uplifting the health and economic status of a country. Voluntary health agencies have been involved in providing various services. **Indian Red Cross society** was established in 1920 by Jean Henry Dunant to alleviate human suffering. The **Hind Kusht Nivaran Sangh** was founded in 1950 to provide financial assistance to leprosy homes and clinics. **Indian Council for Child Welfare** established in 1952 to help vulnerable and disadvantageous children by providing direct services. **Tuberculosis association of India** was established on 1939 aimed to work toward prevention, control, treatment and relief of tuberculosis. **Bharat Sevak Samaj** is a nonofficial nonpolitical organization started in 1952. The main work of BSS is to improve basic sanitation in villages.

Central Social Welfare Board (CSWB) was established in August 1953 by government of India to promoting and setting up of social welfare organizations on voluntary basis.

The Family Planning Association was formed in 1949. FPA India has been made extensive contribution in the area of family planning. Now, FPA India is devoted to promote knowledge on family planning and to advocate for sexual and reproductive health (SRH), rights and choices through its youth friendly centers.

All India Blind Relief Society established in 1946. It focuses on coordinating different institutions that work with the same goal.

There are other professional bodies (Indian Medical Association, Trained Nurses Association of India) and international agencies (CARE) also contribute their services.

Assess Yourself

I. Multiple Choice Questions (Choose the Correct Answer)

1. Which of these is named "world health day"?
   a. 7th January
   b. 7th February
   c. 7th March
   d. 7th April

2. Which of the following *does not* fall into structure of world health organization?
   a. World health assembly
   b. The secretariat
   c. Executive board
   d. Judiciary council

3. "*GOBI-FFF*" is the campaign strategy of:
   a. WHO
   b. UNICEF
   c. USAID
   d. UNDP

4. UNDP was established in the year:
   a. 1966
   b. 1976
   c. 1986
   d. 1996

5. The organization that deals about labor issues:
   a. FAO
   b. ILO
   c. WHO
   d. USAID

6. The organization that deals about food and agriculture is:
   a. FAO
   b. ILO
   c. WHO
   d. USAID

7. Which of these *does not* belong to Colombo plan?
   a. India
   b. Pakistan
   c. Sri Lanka
   d. America

8. Which of these provides financial assistance to India in blindness control program?
   a. DANIDA
   b. USAID
   c. UNDP
   d. WHO

9. Rockefeller foundation initiated its work in India in the control of:
   a. Diabetes
   b. Blindness
   c. Hookworm
   d. Malaria

10. Indian Red Cross Society was established in the year:
    a. 1910
    b. 1920
    c. 1930
    d. 1940

11. Hind Kusht Nivaran Sangh provides financial assistance to:
    a. Malaria control program
    b. Filaria elimination program
    c. Leprosy eradication program
    d. Guinea worm eradication program

II. Short Answer Questions

1. List four functions of world health organization
2. List four functions of world health assembly
3. List four functions of UNICEF
4. State the meaning of GOBI-FFF
5. List four activities of Hind Kusht Nivaran Sangh
6. List four activities of Indian council for child welfare
7. List the aims of FAO
8. List four functions of FAO
9. List four services of ILO
10. List the services of World Bank
11. State two objectives of Colombo plan
12. List four functions of central social welfare board
13. List four functions of family planning association of India

III. Write Short Notes

1. World Health Organization (WHO), UNICEF (United Nations Children's Emergency Fund)
2. United Nations Development Program (UNDP)
3. Food and Agricultural Organization (FAO)
4. The International Labor Organization (ILO)
5. World Bank, United Nations Fund for Population Activities (UNFPA)
6. The Colombo Plan, European Commission
7. United Nations Educational
8. Scientific and Cultural Organization (UNESCO)
9. United States Agency for International Development (USAID)
10. DANIDA
11. SIDA
12. Rockefeller Foundation
13. Ford Foundation
14. Cooperative for Assistance and Relief Everywhere (CARE)
15. International Red Cross
16. Indian Red Cross Society
17. Hind Kusht Nivaran Sangh
18. Indian Council for Child Welfare (ICCW)
19. Tuberculosis Association of India (TAI)
20. Bharat Sevak Samaj (BSS), Central Social Welfare Board (CSWB)
21. Family Planning Association of India (FPA)
22. All India Women's Conference (AIWC)
23. All India Blind Relief Society

IV. Write Essays

1. State the objectives of WHO and describe its functions.
2. What is UNICEF? Describe in detail about the functions of UNICEF.
3. What are the types of health agencies? Explain the functions of voluntary health agencies.
4. List the voluntary health agencies and explain about the functions of Indian Red Cross Society.

ANSWERS

I.
1. d
2. d
3. b
4. a
5. b
6. a
7. d
8. a
9. c
10. c
11. c

INDEX

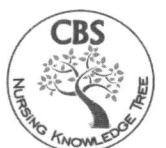

THE READING OF ALL GOOD BOOKS IS LIKE CONVERSATION WITH THE FINEST MEN OF PAST CENTURIES
– RENE DESCARTES –

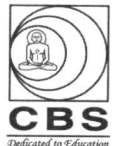

CBS Nursing Knowledge Tree (BSc Nursing Titles)

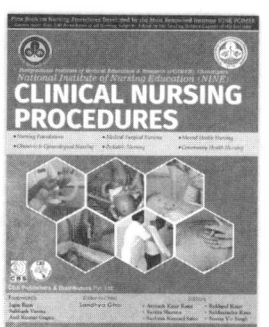
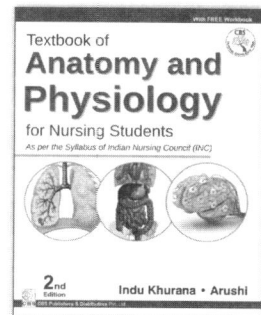
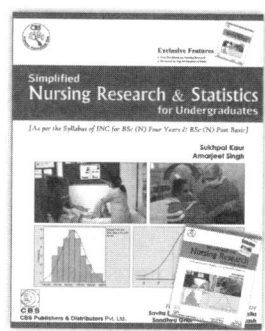

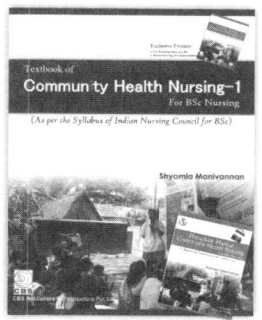
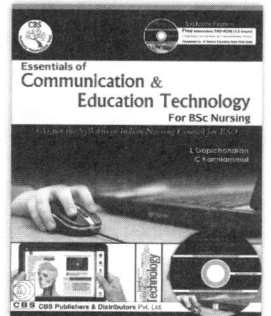
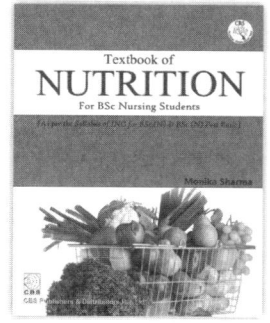
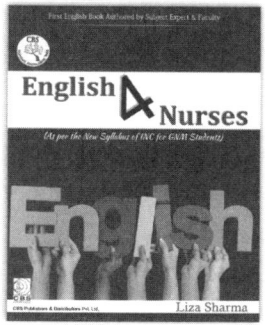

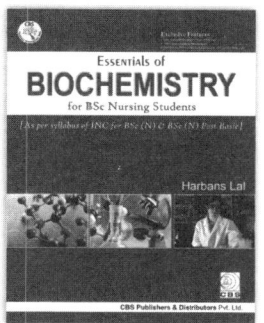
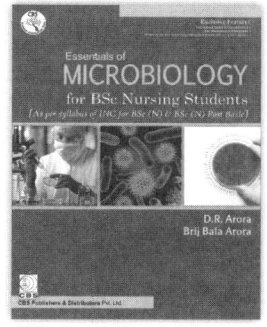
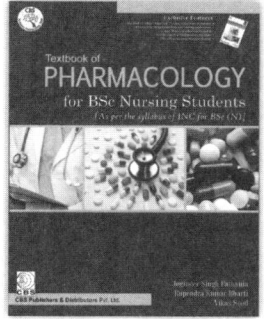
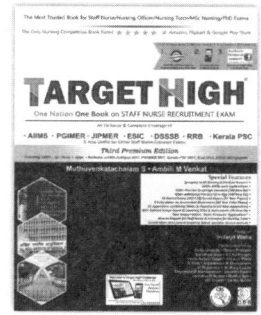

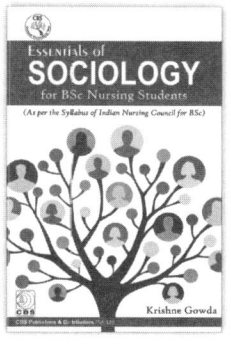
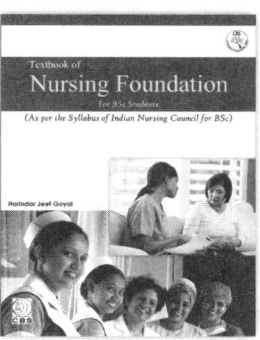
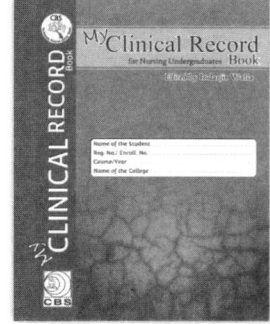
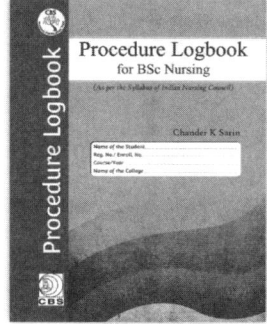

CBS Publishers & Distributors Pvt. Ltd.
• New Delhi • Bengaluru • Chennai • Kochi • Kolkata • Mumbai • Pune • Hyderabad • Nagpur • Patna • Vijayawada

Above books available at **All Medical Book Stores of India**

Buy online :

www.cbspd.co.in   amazon.in   flipkart   www.atithibooks.com   Online medical books on lowest price   prepladder.com/store   Parasredkart.com   EduLanche

For any availability issue please contact : +91-9555590180

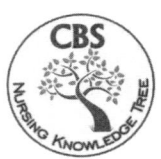
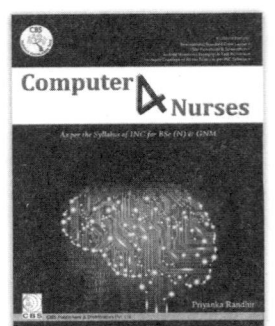
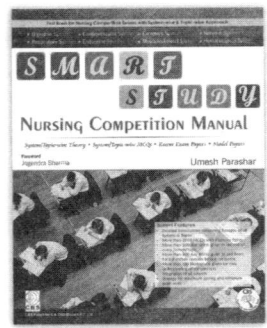
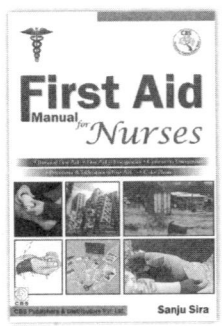
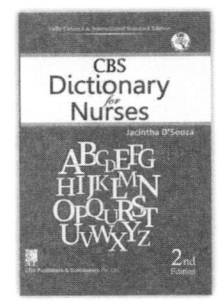
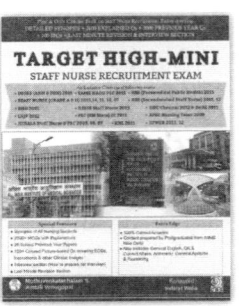
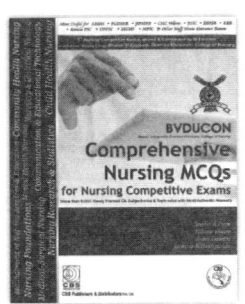
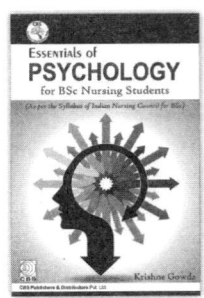
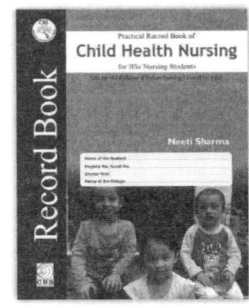
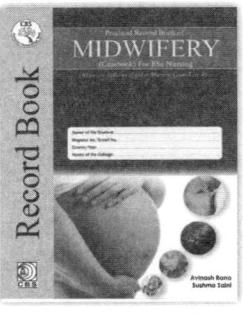
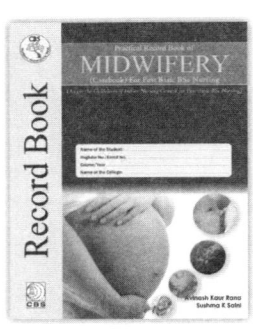
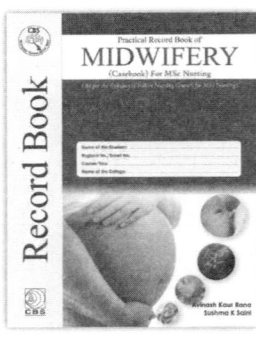
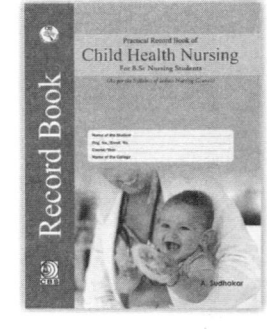
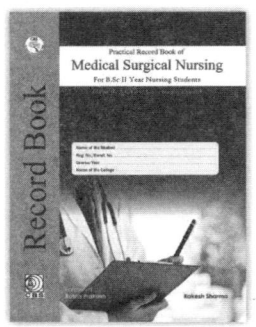
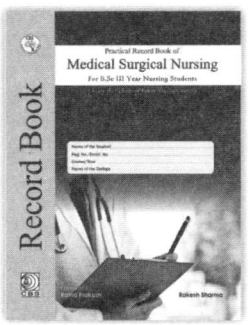
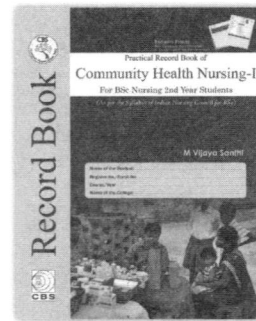
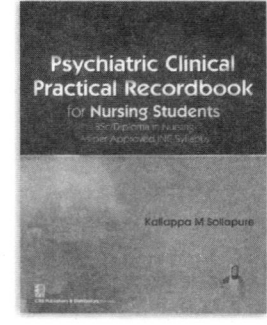
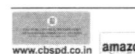
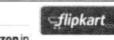
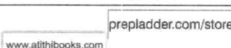